# VITAMINS AND HORMONES

VOLUME 42

# VITAMINS AND HORMONES
## ADVANCES IN RESEARCH AND APPLICATIONS

*Editor-in-Chief*

### G. D. AURBACH

*Metabolic Diseases Branch*
*National Institute of Arthritis,*
*Diabetes, and Digestive and Kidney Diseases*
*National Institutes of Health*
*Bethesda, Maryland*


*Editor*

### DONALD B. MCCORMICK

*Department of Biochemistry*
*Emory University School of Medicine*
*Atlanta, Georgia*

**Volume 42**
**1985**

**ACADEMIC PRESS, INC.** Harcourt Brace Jovanovich, Publishers

Orlando   San Diego   New York   Austin
London   Montreal   Sydney   Tokyo   Toronto

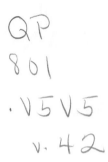

ACADEMIC PRESS, INC.
Orlando, Florida 32887


United Kingdom Edition published by
ACADEMIC PRESS INC. (LONDON) LTD.
24–28 Oval Road, London NW1 7DX


LIBRARY OF CONGRESS CATALOG CARD NUMBER: 43-10535

ISBN 0–12–709842–9

PRINTED IN THE UNITED STATES OF AMERICA

85 86 87 88      9 8 7 6 5 4 3 2 1

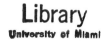

# Contents

## Ascorbic Acid in Endocrine Systems

MARK LEVINE AND KYOJI MORITA

## Vitamin K-Dependent Formation of Bone Gla Protein (Osteocalcin) and Its Function

PAUL A. PRICE

## Hormone Secretion by Exocytosis with Emphasis on Information from the Chromaffin Cell System

HARVEY B. POLLARD, RICHARD ORNBERG, MARK LEVINE, KATRINA
KELNER, KYOJI MORITA, ROBERT LEVINE, ERIK FORSBERG, KEITH W.
BROCKLEHURST, LE DUONG, PETER I. LELKES, ELI HELDMAN, AND
MOUSSA YOUDIM

## Compartmentation of Second Messenger Action: Immunocytochemical and Biochemical Evidence

JEFFREY F. HARPER, MARI K. HADDOX, ROY A. JOHANSON,
ROCHELLE M. HANLEY, AND ALTON L. STEINER

## Autoimmune Endocrine Disease

JOHN B. BUSE AND GEORGE S. EISENBARTH

# Role of Cytochromes *P*-450 in the Biosynthesis of Steroid Hormones

## PETER F. HALL

# Contributors to Volume 42

Numbers in parentheses indicate the pages on which the authors' contributions begin.

KEITH W. BROCKLEHURST, *Laboratory of Cell Biology and Genetics, National Institute of Arthritis, Diabetes, and Digestive and Kidney Diseases, National Institutes of Health, Bethesda, Maryland 20205* (109)

JOHN B. BUSE, *Duke University Medical Center, Durham, North Carolina 27710* (253)

LE DUONG, *Laboratory of Cell Biology and Genetics, National Institute of Arthritis, Diabetes, and Digestive and Kidney Diseases, National Institutes of Health, Bethesda, Maryland 20205* (109)

GEORGE S. EISENBARTH, *Joslin Diabetes Center, Brigham and Women's Hospital, New England Deaconess Hospital, Harvard Medical School, Boston, Massachusetts 02215* (253)

ERIK FORSBERG, *Laboratory of Cell Biology and Genetics, National Institute of Arthritis, Diabetes, and Digestive and Kidney Diseases, National Institutes of Health, Bethesda, Maryland 20205* (109)

MARI K. HADDOX, *Department of Pharmacology, University of Texas Medical School at Houston, Houston, Texas 77225* (197)

PETER F. HALL, *Worcester Foundation for Experimental Biology, Shrewsbury, Massachusetts 01545* (315)

ROCHELLE M. HANLEY, *Department of Internal Medicine, University of Texas Medical School at Houston, Houston, Texas 77225* (197)

JEFFREY F. HARPER, *Departments of Internal Medicine and Pharmacology, University of Texas Medical School at Houston, Houston, Texas 77225* (197)

ELI HELDMAN, *Laboratory of Cell Biology and Genetics, National Institute of Arthritis, Diabetes, and Digestive and Kidney Diseases, National Institutes of Health, Bethesda, Maryland 20205* (109)

ROY A. JOHANSON, *Department of Internal Medicine, University of Texas Medical School at Houston, Houston, Texas 77225* (197)

KATRINA KELNER, *Laboratory of Cell Biology and Genetics, National Institute of Arthritis, Diabetes, and Digestive and Kidney Diseases, National Institutes of Health, Bethesda, Maryland 20205* (109)

PETER I. LELKES, *Laboratory of Cell Biology and Genetics, National Institute of Arthritis, Diabetes, and Digestive and Kidney Diseases, National Institutes of Health, Bethesda, Maryland 20205* (109)

MARK LEVINE, *Section of Cell Biology and Biochemistry, Laboratory of Cell Biology and Genetics, National Institute of Arthritis, Diabetes, and Digestive and Kidney Diseases, National Institutes of Health, Bethesda, Maryland 20205* (1, 109)

ROBERT A. LEVINE,[1] *Laboratory of Cell Biology and Genetics, National Institute of Arthritis, Diabetes, and Digestive and Kidney Diseases, National Institutes of Health, Bethesda, Maryland 20205* (109)

KYOJI MORITA, *Laboratory of Cell Biology and Genetics, National Institute of Arthritis, Diabetes, and Digestive and Kidney Diseases, National Institutes of Health, Bethesda, Maryland 20205* (1, 109)

RICHARD ORNBERG, *Laboratory of Cell Biology and Genetics, National Institute of Arthritis, Diabetes, and Digestive and Kidney Diseases, National Institutes of Health, Bethesda, Maryland 20205* (109)

HARVEY B. POLLARD, *Laboratory of Cell Biology and Genetics, National Institute of Arthritis, Diabetes, and Digestive and Kidney Diseases, National Institutes of Health, Bethesda, Maryland 20205* (109)

PAUL A. PRICE, *Department of Biology, University of California at San Diego, La Jolla, California 92093* (65)

---

[1] Present address: Lafayette Clinic, Detroit, Michigan 48207.

ALTON L. STEINER, *Departments of Internal Medicine and Pharmacology, University of Texas Medical School at Houston, Houston, Texas 77225* (197)

MOUSSA YOUDIM,[2] *Laboratory of Cell Biology and Genetics, National Institute of Arthritis, Diabetes, and Digestive and Kidney Diseases, National Institutes of Health, Bethesda, Maryland 20205* (109)

[2]Present address: Rappaport Family Research Institute, Technion—Israel Institute of Technology, Faculty of Medicine, Department of Pharmacology, Bat Galim, Haifa, Israel.

# Preface

Volume 42 of *Vitamins and Hormones* reflects well our goal to provide informative, current, and stimulating reviews of topics important to researchers and scholars in endocrinology and nutrition. We thank the authors for their timely contributions that include a wealth of knowledge, provocative concepts, and healthy controversy.

A new look, long overdue for readers of *Vitamins and Hormones*, at ascorbic acid and its role in endocrine processes, nutrition, and enzymology is presented by M. A. Levine and K. Morita. The interactions of ascorbic acid with the endocrine system are fascinating, as is the function of the vitamin in biochemical mechanisms. The precise functions of ascorbate in endocrine systems remain elusive, but once fully understood may provide better indices than those currently used to determine nutritional figure for nutritional requirements for the vitamin.

Bone GLA protein or osteocalcin, discussed by P. A. Price, has been structurally characterized and established as a major noncollagenous protein of bone. It is known to be under the control of two vitamins, D and K, yet its actual function in bone physiology is still to be elucidated.

H. B. Pollard and coauthors have organized for us the complex array of information on secretory mechanisms in the adrenal medulla. They provide a theory on mechanisms of exocytosis, progressing from biosynthesis of catecholamines to packaging in the secretory granule, transport toward the cell periphery, fusion of the granule with the cell membrane, and lysis with release of contents to the exterior.

P. F. Hall reviews the functions of cytochrome *P*-450 in the biosynthesis of steroid hormones. This mixed function oxygenase(s) utilizes molecular oxygen in catalyzing such reactions as side-chain cleavage and hydroxylation at the 11 and 21 positions of the steroid nucleus.

J. F. Harper and colleagues discuss compartmentalization of intracellular messengers. Cyclic AMP, cyclic GMP, and calcium show distinct subcellular localizations, and such compartmentalization may constitute an important regulatory mechanism in the control of cellular function by intracellular messengers.

J. B. Buse and G. S. Eisenbarth have reviewed the fascinating clinical syndromes of autoimmune endocrine disease. In these disturbances antibodies cause disease by simulating hyper- or hypofunction of the endocrine system involved. Several of these diseases in mice and men are genetic and closely linked to the histocompatibility genes.

To the staff of Academic Press, we convey our thanks for their expert help in preparing this volume.

G. D. Aurbach
Donald B. McCormick

VITAMINS AND HORMONES, VOL. 42

# Ascorbic Acid in Endocrine Systems

## MARK LEVINE AND KYOJI MORITA

*Section of Cell Biology and Biochemistry*
*Laboratory of Cell Biology and Genetics*
*National Institute of Arthritis, Diabetes, and Digestive*
*and Kidney Diseases*
*National Institutes of Health, Bethesda, Maryland*

1

Discovery consists in seeing what everybody else has seen and thinking what nobody has thought.

ALBERT SZENT-GYORGI

## I. PROLOGUE

### A. INTRODUCTION

Ascorbic acid[1] is found in highest concentration in certain endocrine tissues of almost all mammals (Svirbely and Szent-Gyorgi, 1932; Harris and Ray, 1933; Glick and Biskind, 1935; Yavorsky et al., 1934; Hornig, 1975; Table I). Yet we have only begun to appreciate the importance of ascorbic acid physiologically, functionally, and dynamically in these tissues. In this review we emphasize emerging knowledge and the perhaps critical importance of ascorbic acid in some endocrine tissues. We will review briefly the chemistry of ascorbic acid as well as what is currently known about ascorbic acid in specific endocrine systems. We wish not to simply annotate the existing literature on ascorbate, but to pinpoint areas of controversy, propose new hypotheses, and emphasize what we believe are vital investigations for the future. Most importantly, we propose that study of ascorbic acid in endocrine systems may awaken scientists to the need to find the optimal requirements of cofactors in cells and organisms, and perhaps change medical practice accordingly.

### B. STATEMENT OF THE PROBLEM

Ascorbic acid is required by human beings (Lind, 1753; Svirbely and Szent-Gyorgi, 1932). Ingestion of ~0.9 mg/kg/day affords adequate protection against scurvy (Abt et al., 1963; Hodges et al., 1969, 1971; Baker et al., 1971; Recommended Daily Allowances, 1980). Yet ascorbic acid is synthesized by most other mammals at a rate of ~40–275 mg/kg/day (Chatterjee, 1973; Table II). These synthetic rates imply that optimal requirements for ascorbic acid in humans may exceed those required merely to prevent scurvy. Ascorbate requirements may further be affected by the milieu of the cell, tissue, or animal. Therefore, it is possible ascorbic acid requirements that afford adequate protection from scurvy are not at all equivalent to optimal require-

---

[1] Ascorbic acid and ascorbate are used interchangeably. Likewise, dehydroascorbic acid and dehydroascorbate are used interchangeably.

TABLE I

Tissue Concentrations of Ascorbic Acid

| Tissue | Ascorbic acid (mg/100 g tissue) |
|---|---|
| Rats[a] | |
| Adrenal glands | 280–400 |
| Pituitary gland | 100–130 |
| Liver | 25–40 |
| Spleen | 40–50 |
| Lungs | 20–40 |
| Kidneys | 15–20 |
| Testes | 25–30 |
| Thyroid | 22 |
| Thymus | 40 |
| Brain | 35–50 |
| Eye lens | 8–10 |
| Skeletal muscle | 5 |
| Heart muscle | 5–10 |
| Bone marrow | 12 |
| Plasma | 1.6 |
| Blood | 0.9 |
| Adult human tissues[b] | |
| Adrenal glands | 30–40 |
| Pituitary gland | 40–50 |
| Liver | 10–16 |
| Spleen | 10–15 |
| Lungs | 7 |
| Kidneys | 5–15 |
| Testes | 3 |
| Thyroid | 2 |
| Heart muscle | 5–15 |
| Skeletal muscle | 3–4 |
| Brain | 13–15 |
| Pancreas | 10–15 |
| Eye lens | 25–31 |
| Plasma | 0.4–1.0 |
| Saliva | 0.07–0.09 |

[a] Tissue concentrations of ascorbic acid in rats. Data are compiled from many investigators (modified from Hornig, 1975).

[b] Tissue concentrations of ascorbic acid in humans, from multiple autopsy studies (modified from Hornig, 1975).

ments; furthermore, optimal requirements may be dependent on homeostasis.

Until now study of optimal ascorbic acid requirements has been extremely difficult (Baker, 1967). It has not been clear what constitutes an appropriate measure of ascorbic acid need other than preven-

TABLE II

Ascorbic Acid Synthetic Rates in Mammals[a]

| Mammal | Rate (mg/kg/day) |
|--------|------------------|
| Mouse | 275 |
| Rabbit | 226 |
| Goat | 190 |
| Rat | 150 |
| Dog | 40 |
| Cat | 40 |
| Human RDA | 0.9 |

[a] Data were calculated from synthetic rates in liver homogenates. Each synthetic rate (milligram of synthesized ascorbate/gram of tissue/hour) was multiplied by the weight of the liver and then by 24 hours to obtain an estimate of daily synthetic capacity. The estimated human requirement was determined by dividing the Recommended Daily Allowance by 70 kg (modified from Chatterjee, 1973).

tion of scurvy. We believe that an ideal model system for investigation of these problems has been ascorbic acid in endocrine systems. Ascorbic acid concentration is highest in several mammalian endocrine tissues (Table I). Study of ascorbic acid function in these tissues is still in its infancy. It is first important to learn why ascorbate is present at all in these tissues, particularly adrenal medulla, cortex, and pituitary. Since the behavior of the adrenal and pituitary glands is intricately intertwined with homeostasis, further study of these tissues may provide unique models to determine optimal ascorbic acid requirements as a function of cellular milieu.

## II. Ascorbic Acid: The Substance

Overviews of the chemistry of ascorbic acid and of methods for its detection are essential for understanding ascorbic acid in biological systems. Indeed, appreciation of basic ascorbate chemistry will permit us to suggest functions for ascorbate in endocrine tissues. Knowledge of the difficulties with older ascorbate assays may help to explain why formulations for ascorbate function are just emerging now. Therefore, we will review ascorbic acid chemistry and assay techniques before considering ascorbic acid in biological systems. We will first highlight historical aspects of ascorbic acid, since these aspects are important for a basic appreciation of this field.

## A. HISTORY

The earliest physicians did not know what ascorbic acid was, but they clearly were familiar with the end results of lack of ascorbate in the diet. A disease remarkably similar to scurvy was described by the ancient Egyptians in the Papyrus Ebers (see Hodges, 1980). The ancient Greeks were likewise ravaged by a disease described in nearly identical terms (Major, 1945; Mettler, 1947). Explorers of the New World such as Jacques Cartiers were aware of a pestilence that could be cured by ingestion of the bark and leaves of the "Ameda tree" (sassafras or possibly spruce tree: see Major, 1945; Mettler, 1947). Two hundred years later, in the mid-eighteenth century, the Scottish physician James Lind described, in his "Treatise on the Scurvy" (Lind, 1753; Major, 1945, Mettler, 1947), how this disease could be prevented by consumption of citrus fruits. Physicians then were just as remarkably recalcitrant as in later ages to accept the potential value of cofactors in disease prevention. It was not for another two generations that citrus fruits were included in the rations of British sailors, or "limeys."

Although scurvy could be prevented, the substance responsible was not isolated for another 150 years. In the late 1920s Szent-Gyorgi isolated hexuronic acid (Szent-Gyorgi 1927, 1928), which was simultaneously found to be the specific antiscorbutic factor by Svirbely and Szent-Gyorgi (1932) and by Waugh and King (1932a,b). It is more than coincidence that Szent-Gyorgi used bovine adrenal glands to isolate hexuronic or ascorbic acid (Szent-Gyorgi, 1928; Svirbely and Szent-Gyorgi, 1932). We now know that the highest concentration of ascorbic acid is found in the adrenal (Table I), but we have only begun to recognize the link between ascorbate and its biological function.

## B. CHEMISTRY OF ASCORBIC ACID AND DEHYDROASCORBIC ACID

Ascorbic acid is a ketolactone, formula $C_6H_6O_8$, with a molecular weight of 176.1 (see Fig. 1). Ascorbic acid ionizes in two stages. The first p$K$ value is ~4.2 at 37°C, and the second is ~11.6. Thus, at physiological pH ascorbate is nearly totally in its anionic form. The two ionizations are thought to occur at C-2 and C-3 (Lewin, 1976; Fig. 1).

The critical function of ascorbate in biological systems may derive from its ability to donate electrons while itself undergoing reversible oxidation to dehydroascorbic acid (Bielski et al., 1975; Lewin, 1976). The oxidation pathway is shown in Fig. 2. An intermediate oxidation product is thought to exist between ascorbate and dehydroascorbic acid and has variously been called the ascorbate free radical or semidehydroascorbate (see Fig. 2).

F<sub>IG.</sub> 1. Ascorbic acid, the ascorbate anion, and dehydroascorbic acid are shown. Ionization occurs at C-2 or C-3.

Expressed in conventional terms, where oxidant + $ne^-$ = reductant, the standard oxidation–reduction potential of dehydroascorbate to ascorbate is +0.058 V (Lewin, 1976).[2] The standard redox potential of ascorbate free radical to ascorbate is +0.34 V (Everling et al., 1969). The Nernst equation expresses the relationship between the standard redox potential of a chosen conjugate pair, the observed potential, and the concentration of the oxidant and reductant as follows:

$$E_h = E'_0 + (2.303RT/nF) \log[\text{oxidant}/\text{reductant}]$$

At standard conditions, the concentrations of oxidant and reductant are equal, so that $E_h = E'_0$. Under physiological conditions the concentrations of oxidant and reductant may not at all be equal. This may be of great importance to the function of ascorbate as an electron donor in living systems.

The first chemically stable product in the oxidation of ascorbic acid is dehydroascorbate. For a basic understanding of the dehydroascorbate/ascorbate redox pair, it is easiest to conceptualize the two species as existing under some equilibruim. The conditions of the equilibrium are influenced not only by the original concentrations of the two species but by light, pH, and possibly temperature. At physiologic pH, i.e., pH 7, dehydroascorbic acid is apparently unstable with a half-life as short as a few minutes (Borsook et al., 1937; Tolbert and Ward, 1982), with subsequent hydrolysis to diketogulonic acid and loss of antiscorbutic properties. At pH of 2–3, dehydroascorbate has been reported to be stable in aqueous solutions for at least 24 hours (Tolbert and Ward, 1982), but the concentration necessary for this stability is not clear.

[2] At standard conditions, where pH 7.0 and temperature = 25°C or 298 K, all concentrations are 1.0 $M$.

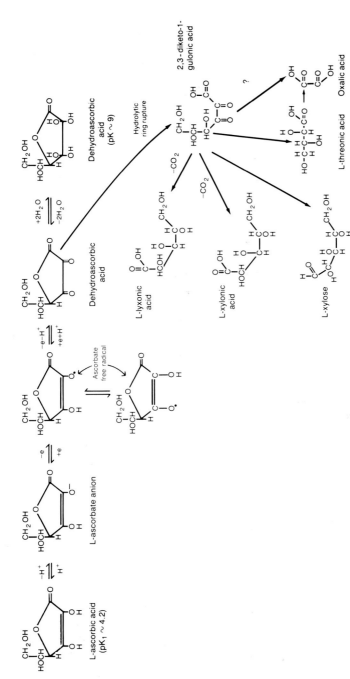

Fig. 2. Oxidation products of ascorbic acid and dehydroascorbic acid. (Modified from Lewin, 1976.)

Although dehydroascorbate is the first stable product generated by ascorbate oxidation, it is not the very first product. That place is reserved for the ascorbate free radical (Bezssonoff and Woloszyn, 1938; Yamazaki et al., 1960; Staudinger et al., 1961). In fact, it is correct to discuss equilibrium between ascorbate and ascorbate free radical and between ascorbate free radical and dehydroascorbate in a similar manner to the conceptualization of a two-step oxidation reaction involving a free radical intermediate (Bielski et al., 1975). It is the reactivity of the ascorbate free radical which may truly be responsible for ascorbate involvement in biological systems (Yamazaki, 1962), not only as a reducing agent, but as an effective free radical scavenger (Bielski et al., 1975). For example, ascorbate free radical is the intermediate in ascorbate reactions with cytochrome c (Yamasaki, 1962), ascorbic acid oxidase (Yamazaki and Piette, 1961), peroxidase (Yamazaki et al., 1960), and dopamine $\beta$-hydroxylase (Skotland and Ljones, 1980; Diliberto and Allen, 1981). Compared to other free radicals, ascorbate free radical may be a relatively nonreactive species that decays by disproportionation, thus terminating propagation of free radical reactions (Bielski et al., 1975). The involvement of the ascorbate free radical in reactions in situ is difficult to measure, however, since the free radical in tissues is still much more unstable compared to either of its progenitors. The conditions of ascorbate free radical stability are probably influenced by the same factors that affect dehydroascorbate (Lewin, 1976).

Up to this point, it has been tempting to conceptualize dehydroascorbate as simply one species. In fact, there is more than one dehydroascorbate entity (Lewin, 1976; Tolbert and Ward, 1982; see Fig. 3). An equilibrium is likely to exist between the major and minor forms of dehydroascorbate in aqueous solutions. The major forms in aqueous solutions are not clear; the two likely candidates are A and C from Fig. 3. It is unknown what is the major form found in tissues, the most active form, and the form in equilibrium with ascorbate free radical. The concentration of dehydroascorbate may be orders of magnitude less than ascorbate in biological systems because of dehydroascorbate instability relative to ascorbate (Tolbert and Ward, 1982).

The stability of ascorbate itself is influenced by several factors. Light, $O_2$, and trace metallic cations all decrease the stability markedly over minutes to hours in aqueous solutions (Lewin, 1976; Fig. 4A,B). Ascorbate stability is increased by increasing ascorbate concentration and by increasing ionic strength. Ascorbic acid can be stabilized by thiourea, perchloric acid, metaphosphoric acid, trichloroacetic acid, and dithiothreitol (Lewin, 1976; Sharma et al., 1963; Pachla and

Fɪɢ. 3. Various forms of dehydroascorbic acid in solution. Forms A and B are believed to be predominant forms. (From Tolbert and Ward, 1982 © 1982 American Chemical Society.)

Kissinger, 1979; Bradley et al., 1973; Okamura, 1980; Blank and Levine, unpublished observations).

## C. Assays

Besides stability, another problem in working with ascorbic acid is the choice of suitable assay. The assays can be divided into several classes: those based on chemical reactions of ascorbic acid, dehydroas-

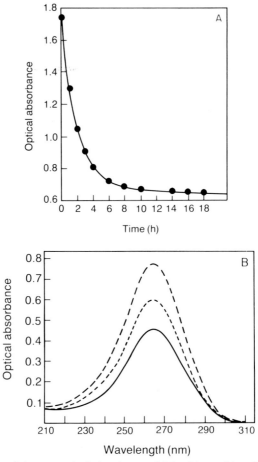

Fɪɢ. 4. (A) Effect of time on optical absorbance of 0.6 m$M$ ascorbic acid in 10% sucrose solution, pH 7.25, aerobic conditions, 25°C. Wavelength was 266 nm. (From Lewin, 1976). (B) Effect of time on the optical absorbance of 50 $\mu M$ sodium ascorbate. Conditions were pH 6.1, 25°C, anaerobic atmosphere. (– –), 9 minutes after preparation of the solution; (- - -), 70 minutes after preparation; (—), 130 minutes after preparation. (From Lewin, 1976.)

corbic acid, or diketogulonic acid, and those based on chromatography of ascorbic acid.

### 1. Chemical Assays

Most procedures for ascorbic acid analysis are based on chemical oxidation of ascorbic acid. Many agents have been used: bromine, iodine, ferric salts, and 2,6-dichlorophenol-indophenol (DCPIP). The most popular oxidant has been DCPIP, since acidic solutions of ascorbic acid can be titrated colorimetrically (Tillmans, 1930; Harris and Ray, 1933; Bessey and King, 1933). The reaction solution turns pink when excess blue DCPIP is present under acid conditions with added ascorbate. The major, and possibly insurmountable, problem with the DCPIP assay is that other reducing substances will also react with the dye, rendering analysis of biological samples difficult (Cooke and Moxon, 1981). Depending on the offending contaminant reducing substance, various controls have been suggested, but indeed these controls may simply not correct for false-positive reactions (Cooke and Moxon, 1981).

Other oxidants have used similar principles for ascorbate detection. For example, ferrozine in the presence of ascorbate forms a ferrous ferrozine chelate that can be measured at 562 nm (Butts and Mulvihill, 1975; McGown et al., 1982). The concern with this procedure is again the false-positive detection of other reducing substances also able to form the chelate.

Assays using agents that rely instead on the reactivity of dehydroascorbic acid are exemplified by the o-phenylenediamine (OPD) procedure. Dehydroascorbic acid reacts with OPD to form a quinoxalinyl lactone, which can be detected by fluorescence (Ogawa, 1953; Imhoff, 1964; Deutsch and Weeks, 1965). Ascorbic acid is first oxidized to dehydroascorbate using oxidants such as activated charcoal, DCPIP, bromine, or N-bromosuccinimide prior to reaction with OPD. As with the DCPIP assay, however, the end-point fluorescence may not be specific for ascorbate. Although blank corrections have been attempted with boric acid (Deutsch and Weeks, 1965) or DCPIP (Kirk and Ting, 1975), the specificity is uncertain (Imhoff, 1964; Bourgeois and Mainguy, 1975; Cooke and Moxon, 1981).

Another class of chemical assays for ascorbate is based on the work of Roe (Roe, 1936; Roe and Hall, 1939) and modified with Kuether (Roe and Kuether, 1942). Their assay is based on the reactivity of dehydroascorbic acid and diketogulonic acid with phenylhydrazine and its derivative 2,4-dinitrophenylhydrazine (2,4-DNP). The osazone formed is thought to be the same for dehydroascorbic acid and diketogulonic acid and may be a derivative of the latter compound (Hegenauer and Saltman, 1972). This osazone is extracted in strong acid, and the resulting red color is measured spectrophotometrically.

There are several stages of this assay, each with its drawbacks. The first step is to oxidize ascorbate to dehydroascorbate. The oxidant can potentially interfere with the subsequent measurement of the osazone, although this has been studied using only bromine or DCPIP as the oxidant (Fujita et al., 1969). The next step, reaction with 2,4-DNP, can be influenced critically by time and temperature of the incubation (Szoke-Szotyori, 1967), as well as by cations such as ferric ions (Roe and Kuether, 1943; Mills and Roe, 1947). The subsequent step, addition of strong acid, must be uniformly and carefully controlled (Zloch *et al.*, 1971; Cooke and Moxon, 1981). Finally, interfering substances in the final measurement may be the same substances expected in biological samples, such as sugars, histidine and other amino acids, and other reducing agents (Roe and Kuether, 1943; Fujita *et al.*, 1969; Bourgeios and Mainguy, 1975; Cooke and Moxon, 1981).

The 2,4-DNP assay has been used to measure ascorbate, dehydroascorbate, and diketogulonic acid. The sample may be divided into three aliquots. The first is stabilized to prevent conversion of ascorbate to dehydroascorbate, and then dehydroascorbate and diketogulonic acid are assayed. The second sample is incubated with an oxidant so as to measure all three compounds in total. The third sample is incubated with a reductant so that only diketogulonic acid is measured. Concentrations of all three substances can theoretically be calculated by subtraction. Strict precautions to minimize interference have been taken by some workers (Pelletier and Brassard, 1975,1977). Yet, as with the other chemical assays, serious concerns remain regarding interfering substances and false-positive or -negative measurements.

One recently developed chemical method depends on ascorbate oxidase to specifically oxidize ascorbic acid in biological samples, with spectrophotometric measurements made with and without L-ascorbate oxidase (Liu *et al.*, 1982). The report of this method is quite encouraging. However, the method may depend on the type of ascorbate oxidase used (Marchesini and Manitto, 1972; Marchesini *et al.*, 1974; Cooke and Moxon, 1981). It is too early to know whether the method will be affected by interfering substances and whether samples can be stored prior to analysis.

## 2. *Chromatographic Assays*

High-pressure liquid chromatography (HPLC) holds the most promise in sensitivity and specificity for measurement of ascorbic acid and dehydroascorbic acid (Sauberlich *et al.*, 1982; Erdman and Klein, 1982). A number of methods have been described utilizing electrochemical or UV detection of ascorbate (Pachla and Kissinger, 1976; Tsao and Salimi, 1981; Doner and Hicks, 1981; Lee *et al.*, 1982; Farber *et al.*, 1983; Rose and Nahrwold, 1981; Levine and Pollard, 1983; Diliberto *et al.*, 1983). The ideal method would fulfill several criteria. The method should be capable of measuring both substances in biological materials as well as artificial mixtures. An isocratic mobile phase would flow through a column which would be relatively insensitive to loss of its functional groups. To minimize confusion with other materials in biological samples, ascorbic acid should not elute close to the solvent front. The method should be suitable for processing multiple samples, perhaps with an automatic injector.

Unfortunately, there is as yet no ideal HPLC assay for both ascorbic acid and dehydroascorbic acid (Cooke and Moxon, 1981). One major difficulty seems to be the detection of dehydroascorbic acid. Several methods seem to be able to separate the two materials, but then the detection of dehydroascorbate is quite problematic. Dehydroascorbate absorbs ultraviolet (UV) light weakly at 300 nm and at 210 nm, and the signal is satisfactory only for measuring massive quantities of dehydroascorbate (Tweeten, 1979; Rose and Nahrwold, 1981). Electrochemical detection of dehydroascorbate has been unsuccessful to date (Farber *et al.*, 1983; Blank and Levine, unpublished observations). Some workers have collected fractions containing dehydroascorbate obtained during HPLC analysis of ascorbic acid, reduced the samples to ascorbate using dithithreitol, and then reinjected the samples (Farber *et al.*, 1983; Diliberto *et al.*, 1983). Such methods might be unsuitable for automated sample analysis and require intense machine operator time. Derivatization of dehydroascorbate has allowed separation from ascorbate (Keating and Haddad, 1982). Even though this analysis was not performed on biological tissue, our chief concern is that samples could be subject to interference due to the derivation. One potential method would be to separate dehydroascorbate and ascorbate without use of an HPLC column, such as with a sample preparative disposable column. If such separation were rapid and the samples not subject to instability, then dehydroascorbate could be reduced to ascorbate simply by using disposable columns with subsequent reduction of the eluates. This would allow automated analysis of the dehydroascorbate samples as measured by ascorbate HPLC.

Many reports of ascorbate HPLC analysis describe simple, artifically prepared, or food samples, as opposed to biological samples (Augustin *et al.*, 1981; Wimalasiri and Wills, 1983; Finley and Duang, 1981). Most other methods are deficient in at least one of the conditions above, particularly in the use of less stable amine columns and in the inability to satisfactorily detect dehydroascorbic acid. One advantage of the method described by Pachla and Kissinger (Pachla and Kissinger, 1976, 1979), as modified by Diliberto for use with C-18 columns (Diliberto *et al.*, 1983), is its suitability for electrochemical detection of ascorbate. In our own method we use a C-18 column with isocratic mobile phase and UV detection. Ascorbic acid elutes at 6.0 minutes and dehydroascorbic acid elutes at the solvent front. The elution time of ascorbic acid can be decreased by adding acetonitrile to the mobile phase. Our results suggest that the method is possibly suitable for electrochemical detection of ascorbate, and the assay would be ideal if dehydroascorbate were also easily detected.

## III. Ascorbic Acid in Biological Systems

### A. Biosynthesis

Ascorbic acid is synthesized in the liver in most animals (Burns *et al.*, 1956a; Grollman and Lehninger, 1957; Chatterjee *et al.*, 1961, 1975). Either glucose and glucuronic acid or galactonic acid can serve as precursors (Chatterjee *et al.*, 1961; see Fig. 5). Certain species, however, including humans, other primates, guinea pigs, Indian fruit bats, and red vested bulbuls, cannot synthesize ascorbic acid. Specifically, these species are unable to oxidize L-gulonolactone to 2-keto-L-gulono-lactone. The subsequent formation of ascorbic acid from this product is believed to occur spontaneously (Burns *et al.*, 1956; Grollman and Lehninger, 1957; Chatterjee *et al.*, 1961, 1975). The defect in ascorbate synthesis in human beings is believed due to lack of L-gulono lactone oxidase and not to endogenous inhibitors of the enzyme (Eisenberg *et al.*, 1955; Sato and Undenfriend, 1978). The available studies have not excluded the possibility that the enzyme exists, but in an inactive form.

### B. Distribution

Ascorbic acid is truly a cofactor in animals unable to synthesize it. The diet is the source of ascorbate in humans. Of what importance is this to endocrine tissues? The answer is deceptively simple. The adre-

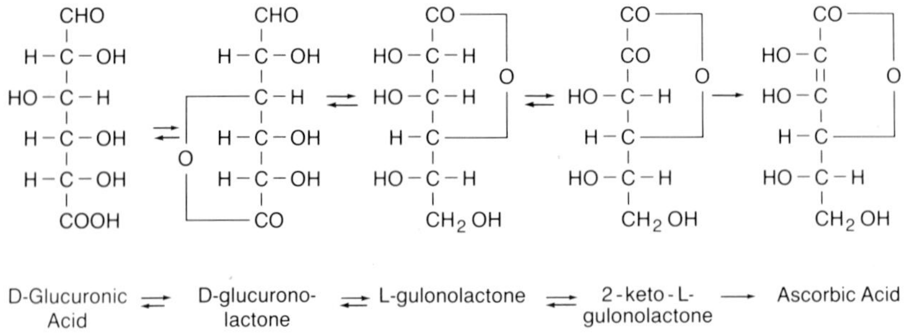

Fig. 5. Ascorbic acid biosynthetic pathway from glucuronic acid.

nal gland contains the highest concentration of ascorbate among animal tissues studied (Svirbely and Szent-Gyorgi, 1932; Bessey and King, 1933; Yavorsky et al., 1934; Glick and Biskind, 1935; Hornig, 1975). Representative data from rats, a species able to synthesize ascorbic acid, are shown in Table I. Adrenal and pituitary tissue contain as much as a 200-fold greater concentration of ascorbate than blood. Data for human beings are also shown in Table I. The ascorbate calculations for some animals, particularly humans, may be underestimates. The age of the tissue prior to analysis is often not clear, and the human material is obviously from autopsy specimens. On the other hand, some results may represent overestimates, depending on the chemical assay used. It is safe to say, however, that adrenal and pituitary tissue contain high concentrations of ascorbate, while other endocrine tissues such as testes and thyroid maintain less but still significant concentrations.

## C. MINIMUM DAILY REQUIREMENTS AND THE RECOMMENDED DAILY ALLOWANCE

What ingestion levels of ascorbic acid in humans are required for optimal tissue concentration? We can approach an answer by first addressing a minimum ascorbate requirement, that necessary to prevent scurvy in humans. Baker, Hodges, and colleagues showed clearly that clinical signs and symptoms of scurvy appeared when estimates of total body ascorbate dropped below 300 mg (Hodges et al., 1969, 1971; Baker et al., 1971; Hodges, 1980). Scurvy could be cured by administration of as little as 6–10 mg of ascorbic acid daily for 3 months (Hodges et al., 1971). The recommended requirements for humans have ranged from 30 to 70 mg/day (Baker, 1967; Recommended Dietary Allowances, 1980; Hodges, 1980). These allowances are not simply to prevent scurvy, but to provide what are thought to be satisfactory amounts for most people. The current recommended daily allowance for humans is 60 mg/day in the United States (Recommended Dietary Allowances, 1980).

But do these estimates supply optimal requirements for ascorbate? Indeed, these levels are based on ascorbate requirements to definitively prevent scurvy as determined by measurements of ascorbate body pool size and ascorbate urinary excretion. In fact, it has been very difficult to first define and then measure what is optimal (Baker, 1967; Kallner et al., 1982; Brin, 1982). Thus, we emphasize that the question of optimal tissue requirement may remain a separate issue entirely, not only from the minimum requirement, but also from the currently recommended physiologic dose.

D. COMPARISON OF THE RECOMMENDED DAILY ALLOWANCE IN
   HUMANS, MAMMALIAN SYNTHETIC RATES, AND NONHUMAN
   PRIMATE REQUIREMENTS

To learn what optimal ascorbate requirements may be, it is helpful to study synthesis rates in other animals. Chatterjee and his colleagues studied hepatic synthesis rates of ascorbic acid in many different mammals. By adjusting for hepatic weight and synthesis per 24 hours, the amount of ascorbate synthesized per kilogram was estimated in several species (Chatterjee, 1970, 1973; Table II). It is clear that over a wide range of species the ascorbate synthesis rates were 40–275 mg/kg/day, or 2.8–19.2 gm/70 kg. Such calculations may only provide rough estimates of synthetic needs in other species. These calculations assume that ascorbate synthesis rates were constant during 24 hours. Furthermore, there is inherent danger in mixing *in vitro* and *in vivo* data. In particular, it is not clear whether the rate of ascorbic acid synthesis in hepatic microsomes is directly relevant to the synthetic rate in intact cells or whole animals. It is also not know whether the rates calculated by Chatterjee reflect basal, average, ι maximal rates for whole tissue (Chatterjee, 1970, 1973). Nonetheles: these calculations stand in striking contrast to the estimates for satisfactory human requirement of 60 mg/70 kg/day.

Several other objections have been raised to comparing animal synthetic rates with estimated human requirements (Hodges, 1980), objections which we would like to address in turn. The first objection is based on early observations (Sheahan, 1947). Sheahan estimated the ascorbic acid serum levels in several barnyard animals in milligrams/deciliter as follows: cow, 0.14–0.92; bull, 0.18–0.98; sheep, 0.14–0.54; pig, 0.16–0.58. These serum levels were estimated to be reproduced by human ingestion of 40–50 mg daily. However, "It should be emphasized that neither serum, whole blood, nor buffy coat concentration of ascorbic acid can provide a valid estimate of nutritional stores" (Hodges, 1980). Furthermore, measurement of blood samples in these animals may not have been accurate due to delays of 1–2 hours between collection and assay. During such a lag time, blood ascorbate in particular may be susceptible to oxidation due to oxygen and iron, thus yielding falsely suppressed values. Sheahan in fact pointed out that other investigators found higher values. He noted that variations occurred from day to day and even from the same animal at hourly intervals.

Another criticism of making comparisons between humans and other animals is based on Srikantia's data (Srikantia *et al.*, 1970).

Srikantia found that maximal ascorbate leukocyte levels in human volunteers could be maintained by ingestion of less than 22 mg of ascorbic acid daily. However, these subjects were previously loaded with 500 mg daily doses of ascorbic acid. We are not confident that the subsequently measured leukocyte levels adequately reflect ascorbate body stores, particularly with the change in ingestion amounts from 500 to 22 mg or less. Instead, these data can be interpreted to suggest that leukocytes simply store ascorbic acid even in the face of an abrupt decline in the amount of ascorbic acid available.

Hodges has objected to the concept of tissue saturation with ascorbic acid on grounds that this concept is never applied to other cofactors (Hodges, 1980). We respond by suggesting that the concept may or may not be correct—there is not enough data at present to judge. But it is a mistake to dismiss tissue saturation simply because it has not been well studied with other cofactors. We would rephrase the issue: Our ignorance concerning one cofactor is no excuse for our ignorance regarding other cofactors.

Other factors may explain the striking discrepancy between mammalian synthesis rates of ascorbic acid as opposed to estimated human needs and therapy help clarify what may be optimal ascorbate requirements. It is possible that the functional requirements of ascorbate vary in different animals. However, an answer to this problem has not been forthcoming, since the requirements for ascorbate in animals remain unknown other than for the prevention of scurvy. In other words, it has not been clear what is an index of optimal ascorbate needs in animals (Omaye et al., 1982). It is possible that primates, including humans, may simply need less ascorbate than other animals. But indirect evidence suggests otherwise, based on the observation that so many different mammals have similar synthetic rates for ascorbate and on the discussion which now follows.

Conservation, storage, and clearance characteristics of ascorbate in different animals could affect requirements. To obtain some of these measurements, half-life and body pool size of ascorbic acid have been measured in animals and humans (Burns et al., 1951, 1956a; Curtin and King, 1955; Hellman and Burns, 1958; Von Schuching et al., 1960; Abt et al., 1963; Atkins et al., 1964; Baker et al., 1966, 1971; Hodges et al., 1971). Ascorbic acid body pools in humans have been suggested to be 15–50 mg/kg, with turnover rates of 0.19–1.4 mg/kg/day and a half-life of 13–30 days (Atkins et al., 1964). These values are quite different from data for rats and guinea pigs (Burns et al., 1951, 1956a; Curtin King, 1955; Von Schuching et al., 1960). Thus, these data have been used to suggest that ascorbic acid requirements in humans are much different than those in animals. Unfortunately, comparisons between these types of animal and human studies are flawed. Often the animals received much more ascorbate per kilogram than the human volunteers, or the animals were able to synthesize ascorbate in addition to their experimental allotment. Indeed, in guinea pigs on different ascorbate intakes, the half-life changed as the ingestion level changed (Von Schuching et al., 1960). In humans, one volunteer with a daily ascorbate dose of ~200 mg had quite different values than subjects consuming less ascorbate (Baker et al., 1966). Kallner and colleagues also found that as the ascorbate dose increased, the half-life decreased, the plasma ascorbate increased, and the total pool size tended to increase (Kallner et al., 1979, 1982). Unfortunately, these types of data are sparse, especially concerning ingestion of more than 100 mg ascorbate/day. Furthermore, it is quite difficult to compare one human study to another, given the substantial variation in these experiments. The amount of ascorbate ingested during the experiments may explain part of the variability as well as differing or uncontrolled ascorbate ingestion prior to the beginning of these experiments (Kallner et al., 1982). There are other reasons for variation in the human data. Baker has suggested that a key problem was the instability of the radiolabeled ascorbate used in these studies (Baker et al., 1963, 1966). For half-life, turnover rate, and body pool data to be meaningful, ingestion levels across a broad range with subsequent analysis may be helpful. We conclude, however, that the available data on ascorbic acid body pools, turnover rates, and half-life are not complete. These data are therefore not sufficient to explain the striking difference between animal synthetic rates of ascorbic acid versus estimated human needs.

An explanation of this difference may lie in metabolism. It is possible that ascorbate metabolism in humans differs greatly from that of other primates, guinea pigs, and animals able to synthesize ascorbic acid. Humans in fact appear to metabolize ascorbic acid without formation of $CO_2$ (Baker et al., 1966; Tolbert et al., 1967). However, these studies also did not employ a wide range in ascorbate ingestion. Other studies described generation of $CO_2$ during ascorbate metabolism in humans (Abt et al., 1963; Atkins et al., 1964; Hankes et al., 1974), but some of these results may have been attributable to degradation of radiolabeled ascorbate (Baker et al., 1963). Although there is some evidence that guinea pigs and monkeys metabolize ascorbic acid in part to $CO_2$ (Tolbert et al., 1975), this may depend on the conditioning of the animals as well as on dietary intake (Omaye et al., 1982). In addition, the dietary intakes for the animal studies may not have been comparable to the human studies. In any case, it remains to be determined whether there are consistent species differences in ascorbate metabolism, and if so, what their contribution might be toward explaining the wide variation in animal synthetic rates versus the current recommended daily allowance for humans.

Measurement of ascorbic acid requirements in humans has been attempted during stress (Henschel, 1944; Stamm *et al.*, 1944; Glickman *et al.*, 1946; Ryer *et al.*, 1954a,b; Baker, 1967). These studies have studied the effect of different ascorbic acid doses on acclimatization or resistance to cold, heat, high-altitude stress, or recovery from scurvy. The results showed generally that there was little effect of different ascorbic acid supplements under these conditions. We point out, however, that these very indirect types of assays are not specific as a measure of optimal ascorbate ingestion. Assays addressed to ascorbate function would be much more suggestive, but these simply have not been possible.

Studies with other primates could provide information regarding optimal ascorbate requirements. Data of this sort are not plentiful, although several estimates are available. DeKlerk estimated that ascorbate intake of at least 10 mg/kg/day may be necessary to maintain serum ascorbate levels in the captive baboon, similar to levels found in the wild state (De Klerk *et al.*, 1973b). Kotze reported similar findings in free-living baboons (Kotze *et al.*, 1974). Baker and colleagues were surprised to find that two rhesus monkeys required as much as 250 mg/day of ascorbic acid to maintain health (Baker *et al.*, 1975). Although no weights are given in their description of the two monkeys, we can estimate at least 20 mg/kg/day of ascorbic acid was required. Other widely varying estimates have been reported for different primate species, but in reality most requirements remain to be established. Squirrel monkeys have been suggested to require 7.5–10 mg/kg/day and rhesus monkeys anywhere from 0.5–7.5 mg/kg/day (Sahw *et al.*, 1945; Lehner *et al.*, 1968; De Klerk *et al.*, 1973a,b; Bourne, 1975; Omaye *et al.*, 1982). Other primate diets have recommended ingestion of 25 mg/kg/day of ascorbic acid (Harris, 1970; Omaye *et al.*, 1982).

Many of the above values are estimates based on ascorbate needed by primates to either prevent scurvy, to recover from scurvy, or to survive in captivity. Thus, the end points describing optimal ascorbic acid requirements were far from ideal. It is also important to note that the primates studied often were not "at rest," given the unquantifiable stress of their captivity. Clearly then, homeostasis is not comparable between primate and human volunteer studies. The difference in experimental conditions or in achievement of homeostasis could quite possibly affect ascorbate needs. Thus, the available data on nonhuman primates suggest that their ascorbate requirements are much higher than postulated human needs. Furthermore, changing conditions may indeed influence ascorbate requirements.

### E. Minimum versus Optimum and the Dynamic Requirement Hypothesis for Cofactors

Analysis of estimated ascorbate requirements in humans compared to nonhuman primate requirements and mammalian synthetic activity reveals that much work is still needed. But from what we know now, the differences have not been adequately explained and remain striking: 0.9 mg/kg/day for humans, 7.5–25 mg/kg/day for nonhuman primates, and 40–275 mg/kg/day for other mammals. We suggest that one key reason for the differences lies in what the numbers are trying to measure. For humans the estimates are to afford stringent protection against scurvy—that is one ultimate assay. The other mammalian data are quite different. These data may reflect the maximal amounts of ascorbate the animal may be able to produce, although under what conditions is not clear. The primate data are based not only on prevention of scurvy, but on survival under stress of captivity. We suggest that these three classes of data reflect three experimental paradigms that are in fact quite different. The human data are based ultimately on minimum requirements. The other mammalian data may, arguably, satisfy a potential need or optimal requirement. The primate data may be a window on the needs of ascorbate during severe and prolonged perturbation in homeostasis (i.e., "stress"). We propose that the ascorbic acid required to clearly provide a margin of safety against deficiency disease may not be at all comparable to an optimal amount. Furthermore, whatever is optimal is inextricably tied to conditions of the cell, tissue, or animal. We reiterate: Minimal is not optimal, and optimal is homeostasis dependent. More may or may not be better, but what is appropriate under resting conditions may become inappropriate as conditions change.

David Perla more than 40 years ago suggested that cofactor ingestion might influence ability of experimental animals to withstand infection (Perla and Marmorston, 1937a,b; 1941). In his visionary work, he described in detail how different amounts of cofactors in animal diets affected survival at both high and low levels of ingestion. His untimely death halted what could have been a novel approach to health and disease, i.e., the influence of diet, particularly cofactors, on prevention of disease. Other variations of this theme have appeared since Perla's time (e.g., Stone, 1972; Williams, 1971; Pauling, 1976). Many have been plagued by accusations of misrepresentation, misinterpretation, and distortion. The crux of the issue is: How do we truly know what are the right amounts of ascorbic acid, or α-tocopherol, or any other cofactor?

A large part of the problem represents deficient means to test the hypotheses. How can we really know what is optimal, insufficient, or excessively harmful? In other words, what is the assay? We propose that many questions concerning optimal requirements may be best answered by beginning on a cellular or biochemical level and not on the level of the animal. When a biochemical, cellular, or tissue function is characterized, the information can then be applied to the whole organism. Indeed, a unique and ideal system that satisfies these criteria is ascorbic acid in endocrine tissues. Ascorbic acid is present in large amounts per weight of some endocrine tissues. However, ascorbate function must be characterized in these tissues. This knowledge is necessary not only for the sake of understanding the importance of ascorbic acid, but ultimately as a key to discovery of the true optimal ascorbate requirements for cells and living systems under fixed conditions. Ascorbate requirements in endocrine tissues can then be studied as the milieu changes, for indeed the mission of endocrine tissues is the maintenance of homeostasis itself. We hope that now the purpose of the rest of our review is clear along with why we believe it is so important to review and advance our current understanding of ascorbic acid in different endocrine systems.


IV. Ascorbic Acid in Endocrine Tissues

Ascorbic acid is found in many endocrine tissues. For each, we will discuss our current understanding of ascorbic acid in four general categories: content and transport, compartmentalization and subcellular localization, function, and dynamic behavior. We begin with the tissue where our understanding is most advanced, the adrenal medulla. In this fashion perhaps we will generate new ideas for other endocrine tissues where our understanding of ascorbic acid is more primitive.


A. Adrenal Medulla

1. Content and Transport

Harris and Ray in 1933 reported that ox adrenal medulla was twice as potent as orange juice on a weight-for-weight basis in protecting guinea pigs against scurvy. Using DCPIP titrations, their measurements corresponded to ~1.1 to 1.2 mg of ascorbic acid per gram of medulla. Glick and Biskind in 1935 directly measured ascorbic acid content of beef adrenal gland slices. Instead of taking homogenates of entire layers, they measured ascorbic acid in microtome sections of tissue using DCPIP. Their results are in remarkable agreement with those of Harris and Ray. They found 1.2–1.3 mg of ascorbic acid per gram of medulla. Only in the adrenal cortex is the ascorbic acid content higher (1.5-fold) on a weight basis. The results of Harris and Ray are important because they estimated not only the amount of ascorbic acid per slice, but also the cell number per slice. Thus, ascorbic acid content per cell could be calculated as approximately $4 \times 10^{-12}$ gm of ascorbic acid per cell. These studies more than 50 years ago are truly elegant and are in fairly close agreement with experiments done years later using much more sophisticated techniques (Levine et al., 1983; Diliberto et al., 1983). The older studies suggested not just that ascorbic acid content of the cells was quite high, but that there must be some mechanism maintaining these high levels.

There are at least two explanations for the high ascorbate concentrations: Either ascorbic acid is synthesized in the tissue or it is accumulated against a concentration gradient. To address the former hypothesis, it is necessary to characterize the synthetic pathway of ascorbic acid. Isherwood and colleagues first proposed the sequence later confirmed in other laboratories (Isherwood et al., 1954, 1960; Burns et al., 1956b; Chatterjee et al., 1958, 1961; Bublitz and Lehninger, 1961; Isherwood and Mapson, 1961; Fig. 5) Several laboratories subsequently determined the capacity of tissues for synthesis of ascorbic acid. Grollman and Lehninger (1957) investigated several different tissues in nine species. In mammals the only tissue containing full activity was liver. Kidney apparently contains the enzyme systems to generate L-gulonolactone, but not 2-ketogulonolactone (see Fig. 5). Adrenal, brain, and heart do not synthesize any precursors, although in only a few species was this studied. Chatterjee has explored in detail the observation that birds and some reptiles contain the full complement of synthetic enzymes in kidney, not liver (Chatterjee, 1973). In other work, Chatterjee and co-workers (1958a,b) reported that bovine adrenal and rat brain were unable to synthesize ascorbic acid from L-gulonolactone. Based on all of these observations from the laboratories of Lehninger and Chatterjee, we feel confident that the adrenal is unable to synthesize ascorbic acid or even its precursors.

Thus, for significant accumulation of ascorbic acid in adrenal medulla, it must be concentrated there by a transport system. Such a system was recently postulated and found to exist (Levine and Pollard, 1983; Diliberto *et al.*, 1983). Cultures of free-floating bovine chromaffin cells were used as a model system to characterize ascorbic acid transport (Levine and Pollard, 1983). Transport was temperature dependent, concentration dependent, and saturable with a $K_m$ of 103 $\mu M$. Transport was blocked by omitting sodium from the medium, by the metabolic inhibitors dinitrophenol and iodoacetate, and by ouabain. There was net accumulation of ascorbic acid, with nearly $1 \times 10^{-12}$ g/cell. Diliberto and colleagues at the same time studied ascorbic acid transport into chromaffin cells in some detail (Diliberto *et al.*, 1983). Their experiments suggested that ascorbic acid uptake was concentration dependent, with a $K_m$ of 29 $\mu M$. Uptake was also temperature and sodium dependent and required calcium.

There are several explanations for the differences in the data of Levine and Diliberto. The former investigators used free-floating chromaffin cells. In this preparation many of the fibroblasts or endothelial cells attach to the sides of the culture flasts. Thus, there may be fewer contaminating cells than in standard plated cultures. The transport characteristics of these other cells have not yet been described. The differences in uniformity of the cell cultures might produce differences in $K_m$ between subgroups in the plated cells. It is also possible that free-floating cells and plated cells simply show different apparent transport properties due to differences in techniques. On the other hand, Levine and Pollard did not use the lower concentrations of ascorbic acid to calculate $K_m$, as employed by Diliberto *et al.* Although the $K_m$ in free-floating cells was more than three-fold greater than found in plated cells, the higher $K_m$ is still within the range of ascorbic acid concentrations found in adrenal venous effluents (Slusher and Roberts, 1957; Lipscomb and Nelson, 1961; Lahiri and Lloyd, 1962a,b). The transport characteristics of chromaffin cells are similar to those of adrenal cortical cells, pheochromocytoma cells, choroid plexus preparations, retina, and corpus luteum slices (Sharma *et al.*, 1963, 1964; Fiddick and Heath, 1966; Stansfield and Flint, 1967; Spector and Lorenzo, 1974; Spector and Greene, 1977; Finn and Johns, 1980).

The circulatory system of the adrenal medulla is similar to that found in only a few other tissues, notably the pituitary and the liver. The chromaffin cells receive a dual blood supply (Flint, 1900, Bennett and Kilham, 1940; Coupland, 1975; Coupland and Selby, 1976; see Fig. 6). Direct arterial perforators from outside the adrenal supply chromaffin cells with oxygen-rich blood. In addition, the chromaffin cells receive steroid- (and as we shall see, ascorbate) enriched blood from the adrenal cortex via a sinusoidal system. The system is not strictly por-

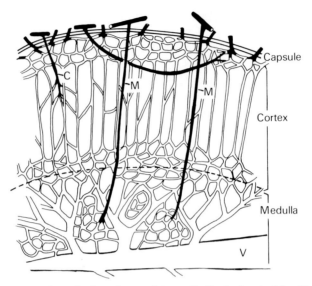

Fıg. 6. Representation of adrenal vasculature. C, Cortical arteriole; M, medullary arteriole; V, adrenal vein. (From Coupland, 1975.)

tal in that there may not be direct one-to-one correspondence between cortical and medullary sinusoids. The existence of this system may vary from animal to animal and has not been extensively described due to great experimental difficulty. There is even disagreement concerning the arrangement of the vessels directly draining the adrenal cortex in relationship to their passage through the medulla. Nonetheless, there is in most mammals studied only one great vein draining the adrenal; this vein passes through the center of the medulla (Coupland, 1975; Coupland and Selby, 1976). Thus, effluent containing steroid- (and ascorbate) enriched blood must pass through the medulla. The concentration of steroid in the effluent is extremely high. In adrenal venous samples collected at the junction with the inferior vena cava, the cortisol concentration is as much as 100-fold greater than in peripheral blood (Dunnick et al., 1979; Gill and Doppmann, unpublished observations). The steroid concentrations within the portal blood itself, before admixture with the direct arterial medullary arteries, have been estimated to be even higher, based on steroid dependence of the enzyme phenyl N-methyltransferase (PNMT) found in adrenal medulla (Wurtman, 1966; Pohorecky and Wurtman, 1971). It is likely that chromaffin cells are uniquely bathed in high concentrations of cortisol and precursors.

It has been suggested, therefore, that corticosteroid regulation of

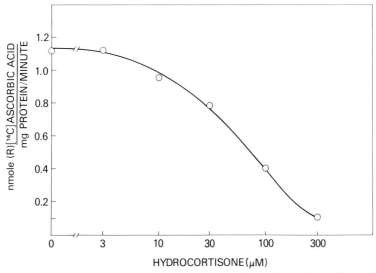

FIG. 7. Hydrocortisone inhibition of ascorbic acid uptake in chromaffin cells as a function of hydrocortisone concentration. Velocity data points, each representing eight values, were determined by measuring ascorbic acid uptake over 64 minutes at 16-minute intervals in the presence of the appropriate hydrocortisone concentration; ascorbate concentration was 132 $\mu M$. (From Levine and Pollard, 1983.)

ascorbic acid transport into chromaffin cells is unique to these cells because of their particular anatomical location (Levine and Pollard, 1983). In this study, it was shown that cortisol in concentrations found in adrenal venous effluents (Dunnick *et al.*, 1979; Gill and Doppmann, unpublished observations) regulates ascorbic acid transport. Although it might be expected that steroids would enhance transport if ascorbate were required exclusively for intracellular functions, steroids were found instead to inhibit transport. The $IC_{50}$ for inhibition of ascorbic acid uptake was ~50 $\mu M$ for cortisol (see Fig. 7). The effect was completely reversible within 30 minutes and reinducible.

The nature of this inhibition and its ultimate physiological significance remain to be determined. The actual concentration of glucocorticoid seen by chromaffin cells *in vivo* is unknown. It is conceivable that vascular barriers exist to prevent these high amounts of steroids in blood from reaching the chromaffin cells. No such barriers have yet been demonstrated. On the other hand, as already mentioned, induction of PNMT activity in experimental animals requires steroid concentrations more than 100-fold higher than are found peripherally. At high steroid concentrations, cortisol binding globulin is clearly saturated. Probably less than half of adrenal venous steroids are bound to other proteins such as albumin (Ballard, 1979); thus, steroids would be available to inhibit ascorbic acid transport. The inhibition of ascorbic acid uptake, its reversibility, and its reinducibility all suggest that ascorbic acid may have some function outside as well as inside the chromaffin cells. We will address this issue in a subsequent section.

## 2. Compartmentalization and Subcellular Localization

It was originally believed that in adrenal medullary tissue ascorbic acid was associated with subcellular particules. This concept was based on a cytological technique in which silver nitrate was reduced to metallic silver in a reaction presumed specific for ascorbic acid (Bourne, 1936). With this method, however, it was not possible to delineate whether ascorbate was outside or inside intracellular organelles. Barnett and Fisher described the pitfalls of the silver nitrate technique. Suspension of glass fragments in a geletain medium containing ascorbic acid leads to clustering of silver nitrate at the glass–medium interfaces. The staining technique suggested that ascorbic acid was within the glass fragments, even though this was not possible. Thus, the original suggestion that ascorbic acid existed within Golgi and mitochondria was questionable (Barnett and Fisher, 1943; Palade and Claude, 1949a,b).

Hagen tried to provide an answer by directly fractionating bovine adrenal medulla and measuring ascorbic acid distribution using DC-PIP (Hagen, 1954). He homogenized the tissue and centrifuged the initial homogenate at 950 $g$ for 30 minutes. The remaining supernatant was subjected to centrifugation at 22,000 $g$ and ascorbic acid measured in particulate and supernatant fractions. Hagen found 0–16% of the ascorbic acid within the crude particular fractions. Hagen himself noted that ascorbate dissociation from subcellular components was indeed possible, even though other low-molecular-weight components had been found to be retained in the crude particulate fraction. Hagen's data suggested that ascorbic acid was mainly cytosolic in chromaffin tissue.

Terland and Flatmark extended Hagen's observations by identifying ascorbic acid in chromaffin granule preparations rather than crude particulate medullary fractions (Terland and Flatmark, 1975). Chromaffin granules were isolated by sedimentation in 1.6 $M$ sucrose, providing a relatively pure granule population. A DCPIP reducing substance was found in the catecholamine free lysate. Catecholamines had to be removed because they cause reduction of DCPIP and generate false-positive results. The reducing substance was identical to ascorbic acid in UV absorption spectrum and in chromatographic behavior. The molar ratio of catecholamines to ascorbic acid was calculated to be 40:1. These data demonstrated that ascorbate was present in a preparation containing chromaffin granules, at $\sim$13 m$M$ concentration. The proposed function of ascorbic acid was to support hydroxylation of dopamine by dopamine $\beta$-monooxygenase (DBH or 3,4 dihydroxyphenylethylamine, ascorbate : oxygen oxidoreductase, EC 1.14.17.1; Friedman and Kaufman, 1965).

The relative distribution of ascorbic acid in the medulla was not addressed until several years later by workers in the same laboratory (Ingebretsen et al., 1980). Adrenal medullary tissue was subjected to homogenization, to centrifugation at 2000 $g$ for 10 minutes (postnuclear fraction) to remove debris, and to centrifugation at 26,000 $g$ for 25 minutes to generate crude particulate and supernatant fractions. Only the postnuclear and particulate fractions were analyzed for catecholamine and ascorbic acid content. It was calculated that $\sim$34% of the ascorbic acid was present in the particulate fraction compared to the total found in the postnuclear fraction, while 79% of the catecholamines were found in the same particulate fraction.

There are several possible explanations for the discrepancy between these data and that of Hagen's earlier study. The HPLC assay used by Ingebretsen et al. is presumably more definitive than the DCPIP reaction of Hagan. The DCPIP assay might be expected to yield falsely elevated ascorbate levels, although Ingebretsen et al. suggest that Hagan did not use conditions favoring ascorbate stabilization, such as acidity or cation chelation. This may be a moot point, however, since Hagan's values for ascorbate content were slightly higher than Ingebretsen's: 0.72 mg/g tissue (Ingebretsen et al., 1980) and 0.85 mg/g tissue (Hagen, 1954). It was not possible to compare the results of the two studies without knowing percentage recovery from the original homogenates.

One explanation of the difference in the ascorbate measurements in the particulate fractions in these experiments may be related to sample preparation. Ascorbic acid appears to be more stable at higher concentrations (Lewin, 1976). Ingebretsen et al. might have unknowingly created a difference in ascorbate concentrations between particulate and postnuclear tissue fractions during sample deproteinization. The volumes of the two fractions may have varied greatly, depending on the resuspension volume of the particulate fraction. If the resuspension volume of the particulate fraction were small, the ascorbate concentration in the particulate fraction may have been higher than in the postnuclear fraction, even though there was more total ascorbate in the postnuclear fraction. The different concentrations of ascorbate could then have resulted in differing stabilities for the two fractions during the 1- to 2-hour deproteinization of the samples. There might have been greater ascorbate oxidation in the postnuclear fraction leading to an artificially high proportion of ascorbate in the particulate fraction. An answer to this problem would have been a determination of ascorbate in each of the three fractions: low-speed centrifugation (postnuclear), high-speed pellet (particulate fraction), and high-speed supernatant. This would provide an index of percentage recovery. Hagen showed these data, with good agreement among all three fractions. It is possible that the lower total values of ascorbate content measured by Ingebretsen *et al.* might reflect an oxidation problem in their experiments. Thus, we believe that the distribution of ascorbic acid in acutely isolated adrenal medullary tissue is not yet accurately known.

These results do show that ascorbic acid is found in particulate fractions of adrenal medulla, presumably contained at least partially in chromaffin granules. An important issue, therefore, is the mechanism of ascorbate entry into the granules themselves (Tirrell and Westhead, 1979a). The data obtained by Tirrell and Westhead are very important. These investigators incubated crude chromaffin granules in radiolabeled ascorbate with or without excess cytochrome *c* to form dehydroascorbate. Autoradiograms of incubation mixtures spotted on thin-layer chromatography plates demonstrated that radiolabeled ascorbate was indeed oxidized. Only the oxidized product of radiolabeled ascorbate, presumed to be dehydroascorbate, was found in the granules. Dehydroascorbate uptake was ATP independent but temperature dependent and probably represented diffusion. Ascorbic acid itself appeared not to be transported.

In future experiments, it will be important to ascertain that the oxidized radiolabel is in fact dehydroascorbate. Dehydroascorbate is extremely unstable at approximately pH 7 (Borsook *et al.*, 1937; Tolbert and Ward, 1982), the pH range used by many investigators who study chromaffin granules. In future studies, it may be necessary to prove the reversibility of the oxidation of radiolabeled material to show clearly that the product is dehydroascorbate and not diketogulonic acid. Perhaps application of direct assays for ascorbate and dehydroascorbate will be needed. Such assays will also be able to characterize the effects on uptake of endogenous granule ascorbate or dehydroascorbate. Pursuit of the findings of Tirrell and Westhead should provide further characterization of other granule functions during exposure to ascorbate or dehydroascorbate.

Despite the cited limitations, the data of Tirrell and Westhead provide a strong case for diffusion-mediated uptake of only dehydroascorbate into crude chromaffin granules. These data are important and raise critical questions. Since ascorbic acid is present in crude granules, do granules reduce dehydroascorbate, and if so, how? Is dehydroascorbate found in isolated chromaffin granules? Are granules from intact cells able to accumulate ascorbic acid? Do granules from intact cells contain dehydroascorbate? Will findings from purified chromaffin granule preparations confirm these first studies?

Most of these issues remain incompletely answered, but we can consider the available evidence. To answer the first question, the existence of an NADH:dehydroascorbate oxidoreductase was investigated in isolated chromaffin granule membranes by Tirrell and Westhead (1979b). No such activity was detected. Future investigations might characterize possible oxidoreductase activity over a wide pH range, since intragranular and extragranular pH are quite different. Possibly such activity may be present in intact granules and is lost during membrane preparation. Thus, how and whether dehydroascorbate is reduced to ascorbate by chromaffin granules continues to be an unsolved aspect of chromaffin granule biology (see next section).

The possible existence of such reduction in chromaffin cells was suggested by several investigators. Levine et al. (1983) found that 3-day-old chromaffin cells rapidly accumulated ascorbic acid from ~95 to 850 ng per $10^6$ cells. The particulate fraction obtained from these cells by Dounce homogenization and centrifugation accumulated ascorbate from 30 to 155 ng in the same experiment. Diliberto and colleagues (1983) found nearly identical data in 2- or 3-day-old chromaffin cells. Neither of these groups, however, reported direct determination of dehydroascorbate in granules during the ascorbate accumulation. Most importantly, there was no further characterization of the crude particulate fraction that accumulated ascorbate and contained chromaffin granules. Thus, it is not certain that the chromaffin granules themselves contained in these fractions had actually accumulated ascorbic acid.

Tirrell and Westhead (1979a) prepared chromaffin granules directly, incubated them with radiolabeled dehydroascorbate, and subjected them to sucrose density gradient centrifugation to purify the granules. These investigators stated that the distribution of radiolabeled material paralleled the distributions of epinephrine and DBH. Given the possible uncertainty in using only radiolabeled dehydroascorbate, further characterizations are necessary of crude and purified granules isolated from tissue and from chromaffin cells.

If the ascorbate accumulation in the crude particulate cell fractions did indeed reflect ascorbate accumulation in chromaffin granules, the mechanism of this accumulation remains unknown. On the one hand, granules in cells may simple accumulate dehydroascorbate by diffusion, which then is reduced back to ascorbic acid, as previously suggested (Tirrell and Westhead, 1979a). On the other hand, it is also possible that granules in intact cells may be able to transport ascorbate as ascorbate, with loss of such function during granule isolation. It is even possible that little ascorbate is present in purified granules and that ascorbate measurements in crude particulate fractions reflect contamination from other subcellular organelles. We will discuss the possibilities further in the next section. Certainly, the subcellular localization and distribution of ascorbate is an area of study where exciting discoveries are still to be made.

## 3. Function

We now return to one of our original questions: Why is the concentration of ascorbic acid in the adrenal medulla so high? The function of ascorbic acid in the adrenal medulla is still incompletely understood. Perhaps we can best conceptualize ascorbate function in three general areas: as a cofactor for DBH, as a cofactor for an amidation enzyme, and as a secreted neuromodulator. We will consider each potential function in turn.

*a. Dopamine β-Hydroxylase. i. The enzyme reaction, its requirements, and its stoichiometry.* Blaschko (1939) postulated that one rate-limiting step in the synthesis of norepinephrine might be the hydroxylation of 3,4-dihydroxyphenylethylamine (dopamine). Goodall and Kirshner (1957) showed that the pathway proposed by Blashko was correct. The hydroxylating enzyme, DBH, was solubilized from adrenal medullary homogenates in 1960 and purified in the next decade (Levin et al., 1960; Levin and Kaufman, 1961; Friedman and Kaufman, 1965; Goldstein et al., 1965; Foldes et al., 1972). Reducing agents, it was postulated, function as cofactors for some hydroxylation enzymes; thus, requirements for such a cofactor were investigated with DBH. Ascorbic acid was found to enhance the activity of the solubilized and partially purified enzyme. More purified preparations showed almost complete dependence on ascorbic acid (Levin et al., 1960; Levin and Kaufman, 1961; Friedman and Kaufman, 1965), but other reducing agents, such as reduced 2,6-DCPIP, were also satisfactory cofactors for DBH. These results were frankly discussed by the investigators who noted the original requirement for ascorbic acid (Friedman and Kaufman, 1965). Dopamine itself was a possible cofactor for DBH in the absence of another reducing agent (Levin and Kaufman, 1961; Friedman and Kaufman, 1965).

Kaufman and co-workers in their studies with almost completely purified enzyme determined that 1 mol of enzyme could oxidize between one and two equivalents of ascorbic acid to dehydroascorbate. At the same time, the enzyme appeared to be reduced. The reduced enzyme, even without an electron donor, could subsequently interact with dopamine and oxygen to form the hydroxylated product, norepinephrine (Friedman and Kaufman, 1965). A possible reaction sequence was proposed as follows:

$$E + \text{ascorbate} \rightarrow E^{2-} + \text{dehydroascorbate} + 2H^+$$
$$E^{2-} + O_2 + RH + 2H^+ \rightarrow E + ROH + H_2O$$

The amounts of dehydroascorbate and hydroxylated product generated appeared to be equivalent. The enzyme was found by these investigators to contain copper, with $\sim 2$ $\mu$mol of $Cu^{2+}$ per $\mu$mol of enzyme. Copper had originally been proposed to undergo cyclic reduction and oxidation (Fig. 8A), with formation of dehydroascorbate (Friedman and Kaufman, 1965).

The copper content of DBH was subsequently found to vary, which seemed to depend on the purity of the enzyme (see Rosenberg and Lovenberg, 1980, for review). Preparations of DBH with high specific activities were reported to contain four copper atoms per tetramer of DBH. Recent reports have suggested that DBH requires 8 copper atoms per tetramer for full activity (Ash *et al.*, 1984; Klinman *et al.*, 1984). Since DBH contains more copper content than originally envisioned, the scheme in Fig. 8A can be amended to reflect one-electron transfers. Indeed, Skotland and Ljones (1980) and Diliberto and Allen (1981) proposed modified schemes with semidehydroascorbate, or ascorbate free radical, as the immediate product of the hydroxylation instead of dehydroascorbate. Thus, instead of a two-electron transfer, one example of a proposed reaction sequence incorporated two one-electron transfers in series, with an unidentified reduced intermediary moiety (Fig. 8B). The fate of semidehydroascorbate in this scheme is open to interpretation. Diliberto and Allen (1981) suggested that the free radical is not terribly unstable, but other investigators have disagreed (Lewin, 1976). Of course, it is quite possible that stability is a function of pH and the tissue itself. Adrenal medullary tissue contains semidehydroascorbate reductase, localized to mitochondrial membranes (Diliberto *et al.*, 1982) and not to chromaffin granules, which contain virtually all of the DBH (Kirshner, 1957, 1962; Belpaire and Laduron, 1968; Laduron, 1975). Diffusion of the semidehydroascorbate to mitochondria has been postulated (Diliberto *et al.*, 1981). Another possibility is that ascorbate and dehydroascorbate are formed from two

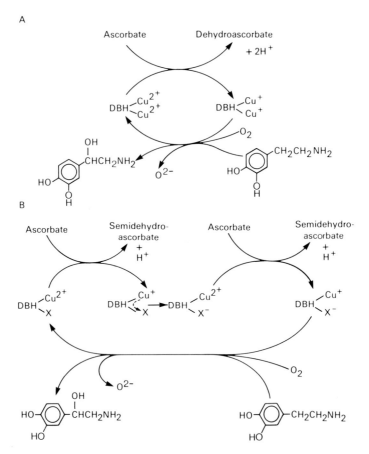

Fig. 8. Schemes for the mechanism of DBH action. (A) Mechanism proposed by Fried-man and Kaufman (1965), with transfer of two electrons to DBH in one step. (B) Mechanism suggested by Diliberto *et al.* (1981), with reduction of DBH occurring by successive single electron transfers. (From Diliberto *et al.*, 1981.)

molecules of semidehydroascorbate. Not only the identity of the intermediates in cells, but also their location and fate remain to be characterized.

*ii. Localization.* The location of DBH is unique compared to other biosynthetic enzymes for catecholamines. Kirshner (1962) discovered that dopamine transport into chromaffin granules was necessary for hydroxylation to occur. One implication of Kirshners's important investigations (1957, 1962) was that the enzyme must be within or associated with chromaffin granules. His predictions were subsequently confirmed (Belpaire and Laduron, 1968; Laduron, 1975). Approximately one-half of DBH activity is recoverable as a soluble component of the chromaffin granule matrix (Hortnagl *et al.*, 1972) and is released from stimulated chromaffin cells (Viveros *et al.*, 1971; Ledbetter and Kirshner, 1981; Pollard *et al.*, 1984). Whether both membrane-bound and soluble DBH are physiologically active is unknown. The resolution of this issue may be of critical importance in understanding the catalytic behavior of the enzyme.

*iii. Function of DBH in cells.* The reaction, requirements, and characteristics of isolated DBH were elegantly described 25 years ago (Levin *et al.*, 1960; Levin and Kaufman, 1961; Friedman and Kaufman, 1965). Yet, the original observations regarding the high ascorbic acid concentration in adrenal medulla were made more than 50 years ago, and seemed to languish. *In vitro* and *in vivo* discoveries did not converge again until 1975 when Terland and Flatmark rediscovered high concentrations of ascorbic acid in the adrenal medulla, and specifically in chromaffin granules. The cast was assembled: the enzyme, substrate, product, and cofactor in fact appeared to be in the chromaffin granules, as required for the *in vitro* system to work. But the drama is still to be played out.

One critical player to be cast is ascorbic acid. Even though ascorbic acid and DBH are found in granules, most of the cellular ascorbate is not in granules (Levine *et al.*, 1983; Diliberto *et al.*, 1983), and crude granules cannot transport ascorbate (Tirrell and Westhead, 1979a; Levine *et al.*, 1985a). The isolated enzyme, in turn, requires reducing equivalents. Thus, if ascorbate cannot enter chromaffin granules, how does DBH acquire and replenish reducing equivalents? Does our understanding of the isolated enzyme reflect its true behavior in the cell?

These key issues are as yet unresolved. But there are several possible answers.

1. Ascorbic acid is not needed at all as a cofactor by DBH in chromaffin cells.

2. Ascorbic acid is a cofactor for DBH, but ascorbic acid enters chromaffin granules only in intact cells.

3. The amount or concentration of ascorbic acid within granules is sufficient for DBH, and the transport of more ascorbic acid is unnecessary.

4. Ascorbic acid increases DBH activity. Ascorbic acid's reducing equivalents are transferred across the chromaffin granule membrane without actual transport of ascorbic acid.

There are several reasons why we favor variations of the last hypothesis (Levine *et al.*, 1985a,b). We believe that ascorbic acid is present in such high concentration in chromaffin cells for a purpose. It is possible, although unlikely, that ascorbate function is vestigial and

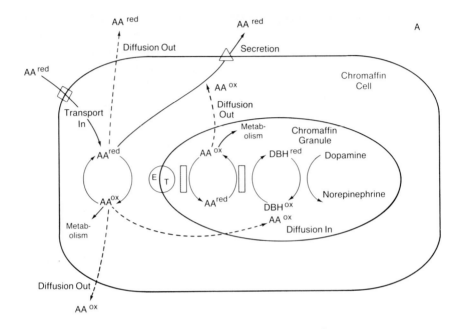

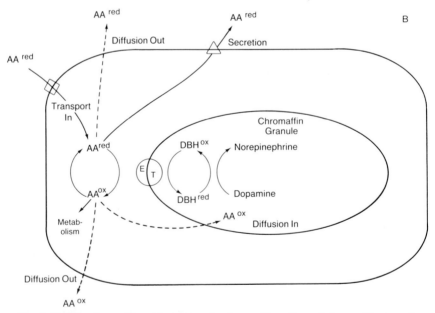

FIG. 9. Models of ascorbic acid economy in chromaffin cells and chromaffin granules. (A) Ascorbic acid (AA$^{red}$ for reduced ascorbic acid) is actively transported into chromaffin cells. Ascorbate electrons are transferred across the chromaffin granule membrane by an electron transporter (E/T). The electron transporter may be cytochrome $b_{561}$, but there

DBH requirement for reducing equivalents is met by another mechanism. It may be correct to conclude that ascorbic acid can enter chromaffin granule fractions in intact cells despite ascorbate's inability to be transported into isolated crude granules. In addition to the pitfalls we have already raised in interpreting these data, however, it is clear that most of newly transported ascorbic acid in chromaffin cells is cytosolic and not in chromaffin granules (Levine *et al.*, 1983; Diliberto *et al.*, 1983). Quite simply, we believe that since most ascorbic acid is cytosolic, its location may be indicative of its function (Levine *et al.*, 1983).

We believe that ascorbic acid enhances DBH activity, but that cytosolic ascorbic acid need not enter chromaffin granules. Ascorbic acid's reducing equivalents are transferred across the chromaffin granule membrane by a carrier system. There may still be ascorbate present within granules, however. The electron transport system may reduce semidehydroascorbate or dehydroascorbic acid formed from the intragranular ascorbate interaction with DBH (Njus *et al.*, 1983). Thus, ascorbate within the granules may be regenerated from extragranular ascorbate via the electron transport system (Fig. 9A). Alternatively, it is conceivable that the final electron donor to DBH is not ascorbic acid and is in fact either a component of the electron transport system or another electron carrier which accepts electrons from intragranular regenerated ascorbate (Fig. 9A). It is even possible that electrons are transferred from cytosolic ascorbate across the chromaffin granule membrane to DBH with no subsequent involvement of intragranular ascorbic acid (Fig 9B). In this model, ascorbate would not have to be present in purified chromaffin granules. We favor the alternatives that account for intragranular ascorbate, since its possible presence suggests (but does not prove) a purpose. Some similar suggestions have been advanced by Njus and co-workers (1983) based on the chromaffin granule ghost.

To support the hypothesis that ascorbic acid is necessary for dopamine hydroxylation in chromaffin cells and granules it must be es-

---

may be other intermediary electron carriers. Electrons may reduce intragranular oxidized ascorbate ($AA^{ox}$) directly or reduce $AA^{ox}$ via other intermediates. Shaded bars indicate that electron transfers may either be direct or require unknown intermediates. It is not certain whether $AA^{ox}$ represents ascorbate free radical or dehydroascorbic acid. This model requires that ascorbic acid is localized to purified chromaffin granules. (B) In this alternative proposal, ascorbic acid transfers electrons by the electron transporter (E/T) to DBH with no subsequent steps involving intragranular reduction of $AA^{ox}$. The shaded bar indicates that electron transfers may either be direct or require unknown intermediates. This model does not require ascorbate to be localized within purified chromaffin granules. See text for other details.

tablished that (1) ascorbic acid enhances DBH activity in chromaffin cells and/or modified chromaffin cell preparations; (2) ascorbic acid is not transported into isolated crude or purified chromaffin granule preparations; and (3) ascorbic acid enhances norepinephrine synthesis in isolated chromaffin granules under conditions in which ascorbic acid does not enter granules and in a manner which is specific for ascorbic acid and DBH.

In addition, crude chromaffin granules must be purified and the content of ascorbic acid and dehydroascorbic acid determined in the different fractions. Granules prepared directly and granules prepared from cells should be analyzed. If ascorbic acid is found in purified granule fractions, then some ascorbic acid must enter chromaffin granules in intact cells to be available for DBH utilization and subsequent extragranular reduction.

Chromaffin granule ghosts (Phillips, 1974) and biochemical preparations will also provide key pieces of evidence for proof of the hypothesis.

1. An electron carrier must exist on the chromaffin granule membrane.

2. The carrier system specifically transports reducing equivalents from ascorbic acid in the extragranular space to an electron acceptor in the intragranular space.

3. The carrier system reduces intragranular component (semidehydroascorbate or dehydroascorbate?) which is then available to DBH directly or indirectly.

There is some support for the proposal that ascorbic acid increases DBH activity. Data from our laboratory suggest that ascorbic acid is necessary as a cofactor for norepinephrine biosynthesis in chromaffin cells and isolated chromaffin granules, without concurrent transport of ascorbic acid into isolated granules (Levine et al., 1985a,b). Additional data are available in chromaffin granule ghosts. Njus and colleagues measured electron transfer across the chromaffin granule membrane (Njus et al., 1983). These investigators used ghosts loaded with ascorbic acid and assayed the change in membrane potential associated with transfer of electrons from inside to outside the membrane vesicles. Ferricyanide added to ascorbate-loaded ghosts causes an increase in membrane potential (inside positive), an increase reversible with the proton ionophore carbonyl cyanide p-trifluoromethoxyphenylhydrazone (FCCP). These experiments indeed suggest the existence of a transmembrane electron shuttle. The direction of transfer, however, is opposite to that required for ascorbate action. Njus suggested that the electron carrier was cytochrome $b_{561}$, the second most abundant protein in the chromaffin granule membrane, as recently characterized (Duong and Fleming, 1982; Duong et al., 1984). Investigators in Fleming's laboratory have extended these experiments elegantly. Purified cytochrome $b_{561}$ was reconstituted into phosphatidylcholine vesicles (Srivastava et al., 1984). In vesicles preloaded with ascorbic acid, external cytochrome $c$ was reduced. Specifically, the reduction of cytochrome $c$ was dependent on cytochrome $b_{561}$ in the membrane and was not due to leakage of ascorbate from the vesicles. Conclusively, cytochrome $b_{561}$ can catalyze transmembrane electron transfer. Although in this case it may not matter, the direction of electron transfer was inside to outside the vesicle, again opposite to the direction necessary for ascorbate action in the chromaffin cell.

Grouselle and Phillips (1982) tested directly whether chromaffin granule ghosts could increase their DBH activity. These investigators incubated granules with external ascorbate and used ascorbate-loaded ghosts. In these ghosts, however, there was no utilization of external or internal ascorbate to increase DBH activity. DBH activity, however, was stimulated in these ghosts by potassium ferricyanide externally, but not internally. Since ascorbate did not successfully increase DBH activity and cytochrome $b_{561}$ cannot be reduced by ferrocyanide, the investigators concluded that DBH can accept electrons across the granule membrane, but that neither ascorbate nor cytochrome $b_{561}$ is involved. It is possible, however, that soluble DBH in the milieu of the intact granule displays entirely different behavior. In the chromaffin granule ghost, soluble DBH is missing as well as much of the rest of the intact granule interior (Phillips, 1974; Njus et al., 1981). We can conclude that electron transfer across the chromaffin granule membrane is an attractive hypothesis for norepinephrine synthesis, but is as yet unsubstantiated.

In the context of the ascorbate–electron transfer hypothesis, it is important to reemphasize that ascorbic acid is likely to be found in granules, as first noted by Terland and Flatmark (1975). We have already discussed the possibility that ascorbate may enter chromaffin granules in intact cells. If indeed ascorbate exists in chromaffin granules, potential mechanisms that could explain its uptake have already been alluded to. Unfortunately, each mechanism can be criticized. Ascorbate in the cytosol may simply be incorporated into newly formed chromaffin granules. This is a questionable explanation, given the rapid appearance of ascorbate in particulate fractions of intact cells as compared to relatively slow turnover rates for granules. There may be a transport system in intact cells that is lost in preparation of granules; perhaps it is a cytosolic factor or loosely associated membrane moiety. This idea is hard to reconcile with subcellular distribution data of ascorbate, which indicate that most ascorbate is cytosolic. Alternatively, there may be diffusion of dehydroascorbate into granules with subsequent reduction, as proposed by Tirrell and Westhead (1979a). It might be problematic to account for diffusion of dehydroascorbate because of its presumed instability at intracellular pH. Dehydroascorbate, however, is believed to be transported in leukocytes (Bigley and Stankova, 1974). The measurement and role of dehydroascorbate will be critical to the understanding of ascorbate in chromaffin granules. The existence of semihydroascorbate, or ascorbate free radical, and its transient nature complicate further an already difficult area. Nonetheless, the solutions to these problems are important to our understanding of ascorbate function with DBH and ascorbate function in the chromaffin cell.

b. *Amidation.* The primary function of ascorbic acid as an electron donor may be to provide electrons to DBH, but it is also reasonable to propose that ascorbic acid may donate electrons for synthesis of other hormones, proteins, or peptides in chromaffin cells. One such candidate may be adrenorphin, a newly discovered carboxy-terminal amidated peptide found in human pheochromocytoma, human and bovine adrenal medulla, and in brain (Matsuo *et al.,* 1983). Adrenorphin is an amidated octapeptide with potent opioid activity, but unknown biological function. Ascorbic acid is an ideal cofactor for amidation activity in pituitary tissue (Bradbury *et al.,* 1982; Eipper *et al.,* 1983a,b; and see below). Thus, another function of ascorbic acid may be as a reducing agent for amidation enzymes involved in the synthesis of medullary opioid peptides.

## 4. *Dynamic Behavior*

It had been assumed that the amount of ascorbic acid in the adrenal medulla remains relatively constant in animals, unless scurvy intervenes. However, recent evidence suggests that the amount of ascorbate in the chromaffin cell may change. Specifically, dynamic behavior has been proposed when chromaffin cells are stimulated to secrete: Ascorbic acid secretion has been postulated and demonstrated from cultured chromaffin cells (Daniels *et al.,* 1982, 1983; Levine *et al.,* 1983).

Secretion of ascorbic acid was postulated for several reasons. Chromaffin granules were estimated (perhaps incorrectly) to have ascorbate concentrations as high as 22 m$M$ (Ingebretsen *et al.,* 1980). Since DBH as well as catecholamines are secreted from chromaffin granules, ascorbate secretion seemed plausible if ascorbate were in soluble form in the granule interior. Another suggestion that ascorbate might be secreted derived from ascorbate transport experiments. Glucocorticoids were found to inhibit ascorbate uptake into chromaffin cells (Levine and Pollard, 1983). Glucocorticoids and ascorbate released from the adrenal cortex would be expected to bathe chromaffin cells in high concentration (Wurtman, 1966; Pohorecky and Wurtman, 1971; Coupland, 1975, 1976; Dunnick et al., 1979; Levine and Pollard, 1983; see transport sections, adrenal medulla, and adrenal cortex). Since glucocorticoids block ascorbate uptake into chromaffin cells under conditions where the whole adrenal was stimulated, it was possible that there was an extracellular as well as intracellular function for ascorbate. We therefore predicted that some ascorbic acid already present in chromaffin cells might be secreted, possibly as a neuromodulator in a paracrine fashion (Levine et al., 1983).

Ascorbic acid secretion was indeed found with cultured chromaffin cells. Since chromaffin cells in culture lose nearly 90% of their ascorbate, cultured cells were preloaded with ascorbate prior to induction of secretion. These experiments therefore measured secretion of newly transported ascorbic acid. Ascorbic acid was secreted along with catecholamines, but the time course of release differed. Ascorbate secretion was induced with nicotine, acetylcholine, KCl, and veratridine, and was calcium dependent (see Fig. 10).

Although there is no doubt that ascorbic acid secretion occurs, the origin of the secreted material and the mechanism of secretion are controversial. Daniels and his co-workers suggested that ascorbic acid is secreted from a vesicular compartment by exocytosis (Daniels et al., 1982). Part of this hypothesis is based on the behavior of aminoisobutyric acid. Cells were preloaded with aminoisobutyric acid, an amino acid which is transported but not metabolized and has been shown to be in cytosolic fractions of brain tissue homogenates. Nicotine induced secretion of ascorbic acid and catecholamines, but did not induce release of aminoisobutyric acid. We believe that these data simply show aminoisobutyric acid is not secreted and does not distinguish between cytosolic or particulate release of ascorbic acid. The data do show that aminoisobutyric acid does not leak out of the cell during stimulation.

We have proposed that ascorbic acid secretion occurs predominantly from a nonchromaffin granule cytosolic compartment, which may be the cytosol itself (Levine et al., 1983; Morita et al., 1985). Comparison of percentage release of ascorbic acid and catecholamines supports this contention. More ascorbic acid is secreted from chromaffin cells than is found in particulate fractions of chromaffin cells. Ascorbate might yet be released from another vesicular compartment, but we have been unable to identify it. It is possible, as pointed out by Daniels, that such a vesicular compartment is fragile and disrupted during cellular fractionation (Daniels et al., 1983). Recent experiments using the digitonin-treated chromaffin cell model further support the concept of nonexocytotic ascorbic acid release (Morita et al., 1985).

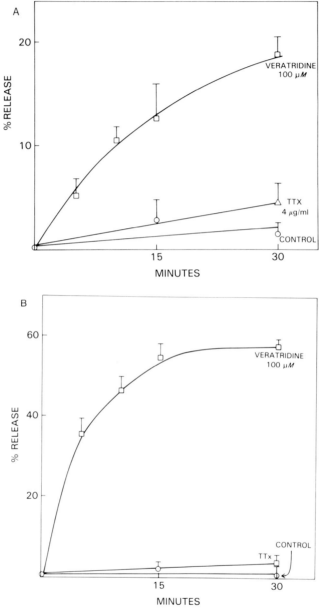

FIG. 10. Ascorbic acid and catecholamine secretion from cultured chromaffin cells. Veratridine-induced release of ascorbic acid (A) and catecholamines (B) over time from chromaffin cells; data are displayed as percentage material released. TTX, tetrodotoxin (From Levine *et al.*, 1983.)

Identification of the source of the secreted ascorbic acid is necessary for suggesting a mechanism of secretion. Daniels and co-workers propose that secretion of ascorbate is exocytotic and that the ascorbate originates from a fragile vesicular compartment such as the endoplasmic reticulum (Daniels *et al.*, 1983). We suggest that while some ascorbate is secreted from chromaffin granules, most ascorbate is secreted directly from the cell cytosol. Secretion is then mediated by an "ascorbate pump" on the plasma membrane which may or may not be identical to the ascorbate uptake site. Further experiments are necessary to resolve the issue, as this field is in its infancy.

Of greater importance will be to determine why ascorbate is secreted from the chromaffin cell. Although many possibilities exist, none have been addressed. Perhaps ascorbic acid is a neuromodulator, regulating secretion of catecholamines, neuropeptides, or other secreted materials. Ascorbic acid may have a local stabilizing role for secreted substances from the medulla or even cortex. The local or paracrine nature of ascorbate function seems correct, since high ascorbate concentrations measured in adrenal venous effluents are reduced when the adrenal vein joins the inferior vena cava (Slusher and Roberts, 1957; Lipscomb and Nelson, 1961; Lahiri and Lloyd, 1962a,b). It is also possible that ascorbate is necessary for maintaining the vascular integrity, structure, or function of the sinusoidal portal system. Whether as a local modulator of adrenal neurohormone release, as an antioxidant, or as an integral part of the response to stress, ascorbic acid secretion may be an important aspect of adrenal medullary function.

## B. ADRENAL CORTEX

### 1. *Content and Transport*

Ascorbic acid was originally isolated from bovine adrenal cortex (Szent-Gyorgi, 1928; Svirbely and Szent-Gyorgi, 1932), and its concentration in adrenal cortex is the highest of any tissue in mammals (Table I). Analyses, however, have ignored potential differences between glomerulosa, fasciculata, and reticularis. These measurements may be important in determining the function of ascorbate in adrenal cortex.

Sharma and others found ascorbic acid uptake in guinea pig adrenal cortical slices (Sharma *et al.*, 1963, 1964; De Nicola *et al.*, 1968; Clayman *et al.*, 1970). Transport appeared to proceed against a concentration gradient, since the tissue:medium ratio exceeded unity. Uptake of the radiolabeled material was inhibited by 1 m$M$ dinitrophenol or lack of sodium or calcium in the incubation medium. This work unfortunately did not provide detailed kinetics of ascorbate transport and was more concerned with regulation of ascorbate uptake by corticosteroids, as described in the next section.

Despite long-standing knowledge of high cortical ascorbate content, ascorbate transport in cortical tissue has only recently been more extensively characterized (Finn and Johns, 1980). Ascorbic acid transport was concentration dependent and saturable, with an apparent $K_m$ of 16.6 $\mu M$. Ascorbate transport was calcium dependent. Radiolabeled ascorbic acid was used to assay transport, and total ascorbic acid was measured using 2,4-dinitrophenylhydrazine. Dehydroascorbate was not analyzed extensively. Since these studies used cells acutely isolated, newly transported ascorbate accounted for 16–50% of total cellular ascorbate, depending upon the incubation time. Characteristics of ascorbate transport were similar to those reported for other cell types (Fiddick and Heath, 1966; Spector and Lorenzo, 1974; Spector and Greene, 1977; Levine and Pollard, 1983; Diliberto et al., 1983).

## 2. Compartmentalization and Subcellular Localization

Limited information is available about subcellular distribution of cortical ascorbic acid. Hagen (1954) found 96% of ascorbic acid in soluble fractions of cortical homogenates. His analysis did not take into account possible differences in ascorbate content and distribution between the three layers of the adrenal cortex. De Nicola et al. (1968) and Finn and Johns (1980) also analyzed whole cortical ascorbate content and found results in agreement with Hagen. Other studies were vague about the localization of particulate ascorbate (Fiddick and Heath, 1966). We shall see in the next section why subcellular localization of ascorbate may be very important.

## 3. Function and Dynamic Behavior

The function of ascorbic acid in adrenal cortex is not known. Since ascorbate function may be intimately linked to its dynamic behavior, we will discuss these two aspects together. Just 2 years after the isolation of ascorbic acid, Harde discovered that the ascorbate content of guinea pig adrenal was reduced in animals that died from diphtherial intoxication (Harde, 1934). These reports were confirmed by others (see Torrance, 1940), but their significance remained uncertain. In 1944, Clark and Rossiter found that ascorbic acid content of the rabbit adrenal was depleted by a severe, nonfatal burn to the animal. Sayers and colleagues then conducted a truly remarkable series of investigations during the next several years (Sayers et al., 1944a,b, 1945, 1946,

1948; Sayers and Sayers, 1947). They showed that hemorrhage induced ascorbic acid depletion from rat and guinea pig adrenal glands (Sayers *et al.*, 1945) and realized that theirs as well as earlier studies pointed toward stress as the cause of ascorbate depletion. They further realized that "following stress of a diverse character, the functional activity of the adrenal cortex is increased" (Sayers *et al.*, 1945). Thus, ascorbate depletion from adrenal glands was associated with increased adrenal metabolic activity, since this is linked to increased corticosteroid secretion. Indeed, Sayers and co-workers demonstrated specifically that ACTH preparations induced adrenal ascorbate depletion (Sayers *et al.*, 1946). They devised a bioassay for ACTH, still used today, based on ascorbate depletion of rat adrenal glands (Sayers *et al.*, 1948).

The classical experiments of Sayers and Sayers showing ascorbate depletion from adrenal have been confirmed repeatedly and in several species (Vogt, 1948; Fortier *et al.*, 1950; Pirani, 1952; Slusher and Roberts, 1957; Briggs and Toepel, 1958; Munson and Toepel, 1958; Brodish and Long, 1960; Lipscomb and Nelson, 1960; Lahiri and Llyod, 1962a,b; Harding and Nelson, 1963; Bhattacharyya *et al.*, 1966; Honjo and Imaizumi, 1967; Greenman *et al.*, 1967; Freeman, 1970; Llorens *et al.*, 1973). In all likelihood, most of the ascorbate secreted in response to ACTH originates from the cortex, although this issue was not explored in much detail by Sayers *et al.*, nor by most subsequent investigators. Sayers *et al.*, in fact, noted only that the effect on the whole gland reflected changes in the cortex (Sayers *et al.*, 1946), but were not necessarily specific for the cortex. This may be important, given the recent finding of ascorbic acid secretion from chromaffin cells (Daniels *et al.*, 1982; Levine *et al.*, 1983). Moreover, it remains to be determined which cortical layers are responsive to ACTH.

The Sayers' experiments raise several important questions worth exploring in detail. One concerns the secreted ascorbic acid. What happens to it? Is it oxidized or found in the adrenal vein? Vogt (1948) first addressed this issue, but was unable to obtain consistent results. Slusher and Roberts (1957) found that ascorbic acid lost from adrenal glands upon administration of ACTH was quantitatively recovered in the adrenal vein. The release of ascorbic acid preceded release of corticosteroids by as much as 15 minutes. The assay used by Slusher and Roberts was for total ascorbate and did not distinguish between ascorbate, dehydroascorbate, and diketogulonic acid. Neither their results nor those of Briggs and Toepel (1958) or Munson and Toepel (1958) answered the question definitively. Lahiri and Lloyd specifically measured each compound in adrenal venous effluents of rats (Lahiri and

Lloyd, 1962 a,b). They found 30–60 minutes after ACTH that nearly all of the depleted adrenal ascorbate appeared in the adrenal vein, and that almost all of the secreted material was ascorbate. The DCPIP assay used by Lahiri and Lloyd, however, did not discriminate among other reducing substances in adrenal venous blood. Harding and Nelson (1963) assayed adrenal venous blood using an ascorbate oxidase assay and a DCPIP assay. They found a fairly large discrepancy. The DCPIP assay detected a higher concentration than the ascorbate oxidase assay; thus, some of the secreted material may have been dehydroascorbate. A concurrent analysis of depletion from adrenal tissue was not performed, however, and the ascorbate oxidase assay may not have been totally reliable (Marchesini and Mannito, 1972; Marchesini et al., 1974; Cooke and Moxon, 1981). Harding and Nelson (1963) postulated that the "extra" reducing substance measured by DCPIP might have been glutathione, found in high concentrations in adrenal cortex. Yet, in their experiments, there was no depletion of glutathione induced by ACTH. Thus, ascorbic acid depletion induced by ACTH may still reflect ascorbic acid secretion into adrenal venous blood. While some of the ascorbic acid may be utilized, it seems that most is in fact elaborated into the blood. Ascorbate itself may indeed be the primary species in adrenal venous blood, but the issue is not completely resolved.

In the Sayers' experiments, more than 30% of ascorbic acid was depleted from rat adrenals in 20 minutes, and more than 55% at 60 minutes. In the guinea pig, however, only a 15% depletion was evident at 1 hour, with the 50% depletion maximum occurring finally at 3 hours. These species differences may reflect the guinea pig dietary requirement for ascorbate, or the higher ascorbate concentrations found in rat tissue. Slusher and Roberts (1957) measured ascorbate in rat adrenal venous effluents within 15 minutes, as did Lahiri and Lloyd (1962a,b). Lipscomb and Nelson (1960) measured significant increases in ascorbic acid in adrenal venous effluents as early as 1–2 minutes after ACTH challenge in cannulated rats. Whether this ascorbate was of cortical or medullary origin is not clear, especially at the earliest time points. For example, impurities in ACTH or the stress of the injection technique may have induced medullary ascorbate secretion. The rapid falloff in ascorbate secretion in the adrenal vein as measured by Lipscomb and Nelson is puzzling, since Sayers et al. (1946) found continuing ascorbate secretion for 1 hour. Possibly variation in dosage of ACTH accounts for these differences. It is likely that the experiments measuring ascorbate secretion at 15 or 30 minutes do indeed reflect ascorbate secretion from the cortex, since the cortex makes up most of the rat adrenal and the concentration of ascorbate is probably similar in the rat cortex and medulla.

The mechanism of cortical ascorbic acid secretion or depletion is unknown. Implicit in many of the earlier studies was the hypothesis that ascorbic acid was actively secreted. In contrast, Sharma *et al.* (1963, 1964) proposed that ascorbate depletion could reflect inhibition of ascorbic acid uptake mediated through a response of the cortex to ACTH. ACTH added to rat adrenal cortical slices inhibited ascorbic acid uptake by 50% (Sharma *et al.*, 1963, 1964; De Nicola *et al.*, 1968; Clayman *et al.*, 1970). Although it was claimed that ACTH did not affect radiolabeled ascorbate efflux from adrenal slices for at least 1 hour, ACTH inhibited ascorbate influx within 15 minutes of incubation (De Nicola *et al.*, 1968). This critical observation unfortunately was not elaborated upon. The transport inhibitor induced by ACTH was initially believed to be a steroid. However, corticosteroids incubated with cortical slices did not generally inhibit ascorbate transport unless the steroid concentration was greater than 50–100 $\mu M$. These investigators thought these concentrations too high for endogenous cortical steroids. It was postulated that an unknown substance, still possibly a steroid, was released in response to ACTH to inhibit ascorbate transport (De Nicola *et al.*, 1968; Clayman *et al.*, 1970).

The steroid concentrations may in fact not be too high to reflect adrenal cortical origin, given the results obtained for the adrenal vein and for regulation of phenylethanolamine-$N$-methyl transferase (Wurtman, 1966; Pohorecky and Wurtman, 1972; Dunnick *et al.*, 1979). The main problem in these experiments, however, is that much of the inhibition data were taken from 2- to 3-hour incubations with ACTH or corticosteroids. Although inhibition of ascorbate uptake was noted within 15 minutes of adding ACTH, no time course was given for ACTH-induced inhibition of ascorbic acid transport (De Nicola *et al.*, 1968). Such a time course with concurrent steroid analyses would help to characterize the mechanism of ascorbate depletion or secretion in the adrenal cortex. It is also not possible from the literature to distinguish between a steroid-induced effector versus the steroids themselves as inhibitors of ascorbate uptake. It may have been technically difficult to determine both ascorbate uptake and secretion using a single radiolabeled tracer. Despite the unanswered issues, the observations raised in these studies are quite important and unresolved.

Finn and Johns (1980) tried to discern how ACTH induced ascorbic acid secretion. They characterized ascorbic acid uptake by acutely isolated bovine cortical cells and then studied the effect of ACTH on ascorbic acid transport. They found that while ACTH induced a maximal steroid response in 40 minutes, there was only a small inhibition of ascorbic acid uptake by that time. ACTH-induced ascorbic acid depletion from cells amounted to only 6% at 1 hour.

There are several potential explanations for the lack of ascorbic acid depletion in these experiments. Positive effects might have been noted at longer times of incubation for either ascorbate uptake or depletion. It is thus important to recall the differences in the time course of ascorbic acid depletion observed by Sayers *et al.* (1946) between guinea pigs and rats. Perhaps acutely isolated bovine cells were impaired by the digestion procedure. Finn and Johns (1980) suggested that possibly the cells contained two reservoirs of ascorbate and that the ACTH-sensitive pool had been lost during isolation (Salomon, 1958). We believe that this explanation is not correct, since no change in total ascorbate content was noted after a 1-hour incubation in 100 $\mu M$ exogenous ascorbate. The suggestion could have been tested by preincubating the cells in ascorbate for longer periods of time prior to the experiments.

Other groups have studied ascorbic acid depletion induced by ACTH (Kitabchi and West, 1975; Leonard *et al.*, 1983). Both groups were able to demonstrate that ACTH could inhibit ascorbic acid transport into isolated or cultured cells. These investigations, however, did not lead to an understanding of how ACTH induces ascorbic acid depletion. Again, a detailed comparison between the kinetics of ascorbate depletion and steroid biosynthesis would be revealing. We conclude that the mechanism of ascorbic acid depletion or secretion from adrenal cortex remains to be determined.

There are two further intertwined issues of great importance: Why is ascorbic acid present in adrenal cortex, and why is it depleted after ACTH stimulation? Ascorbic acid may be necessary in several steps in cortisol biosynthesis and is reported to accelerate 11-hydroxylation *in vitro* (Jenkins, 1962). Ascorbate increased the induction of 11$\beta$-hydroxylase activity in cultured adrenal cells under some conditions, although in most experiments the effect was reproducible with other antioxidants (Hornsby, 1980). Ascorbic acid has also augmented the action of $\Delta^5$-3$\beta$-hydroxysteroid dehydrogenase. The animals used in the latter experiments, however, were also deficient in vitamin A (Gruber *et al.*, 1976). Hornsby has proposed from comprehensive experiments that ascorbate might maintain reducing conditions in the cortex to protect cytochrome *P*-450s against steroid-induced destruction (Hornsby, 1980). However, under conditions of ascorbate depletion in cells, steroidogenesis has been reported to be inducible by ACTH stimulation without ascorbate addition, as noted by Hornsby himself

(Hornsby *et al.*, 1979; Hornsby and Crivello, 1983). In scorbutic guinea pigs with definitive adrenal ascorbate depletion, steroid biosynthesis was still clearly responsive to ACTH (Hodges and Hotston, 1970). These conflicting points of view are in need of resolution.

Another role for ascorbate has been promoted by Kitabchi, who suggested that ascorbate acted as an inhibitor of steroid biosynthesis and that ascorbate secretion would permit steroid synthesis to proceed unimpaired (Kitabchi, 1967a). Some evidence for this hypothesis in fact suggested that ascorbate enhanced lipid peroxidation, which then inhibited 21-hydroxylase activity (Kitabchi, 1967b; Greenfield *et al.*, 1980). Effects of ascorbate on lipid peroxidation and subsequent inhibition of enzymatic activity may be quite nonspecific, however (Milewich *et al.*, 1980). For example, catalase was not included in some of these experiments. Without catalase, DBH activity in the medulla is inhibited by ascorbic acid. During the reaction, ascorbic acid generates hydrogen peroxide, which greatly diminishes DBH activity. Indeed, the same false-positive inhibition could be induced by ascorbate in adrenal cortical homogenates.

Ascorbic acid is also secreted or depleted from ovarian tissue (Parlow, 1958; Stansfield and Flint, 1967). This similarity between adrenal cortex and corpus luteum may be a clue to one function of ascorbate. Perhaps ascorbate secretion bears some relationship to steroid synthesis or secretion. While conclusive data for ascorbic acid enhancement of steroid biosynthesis are lacking, there may yet be a role for ascorbate in steroid synthesis. Ascorbate might also be important for steroid secretion, although again there is little information at present. Ascorbate may act as a stabilizer, protector, enhancer, or inhibitor in relationship to the high local concentrations of steroids in the adrenal or ovary.

Perhaps cortical ascorbate is secreted for use by the chromaffin cells in the adrenal medulla. Indeed, ascorbic acid enhancement of DBH activity has recently been demonstrated in isolated chromaffin cells (Levine *et al.*, 1985a). Yet ascorbate also is secreted from the chromaffin cells. Medullary secretion would occur concurrently with ACTH-induced ascorbate cortical depletion under most circumstances *in vivo*. Although ascorbate may indeed be important for function in the medulla, cortical ascorbate probably has other functions as well.

In general terms, we believe that the initial function of the secreted cortical and medullary ascorbate may be local, since high ascorbate concentrations in adrenal venous blood are diluted in the inferior vena cava. Possibly ascorbate secreted from both cortex and medulla acts as a paracrine effector or neuromodulator. The secreted ascorbate may be used by other cortical or medullary cells in an as yet unknown way. Perhaps structural cells of the adrenal sinusoidal system require ascorbate, or the high local concentrations are utilized by the constituents of the blood. A stablizing role of ascorbate for other secreted materials from cortex or medulla is, as mentioned, another possibility. The facts remain that ACTH induces ascorbate depletion in many species, presumably from the adrenal cortex, and that ascorbate is secreted from the adrenal medulla. The role of ascorbic acid in the functions of both cortical and medullary tissue requires intensive investigation. The implications may be profound for species such as the human, which are unable to synthesize ascorbic acid. When functions for adrenal ascorbate are ascertained, ascorbate requirements in terms of these specific functions can then be addressed.

## C. Pituitary

The amount of ascorbic acid in pituitary tissue is similar to that found in adrenal tissue (Table I). However, little information is available concerning transport, subcellular localization, and compartmentalization of ascorbic acid in pituitary tissue (Phillips and Stare, 1934; Salhanick et al., 1949; Pirani, 1952; Lahiri and Lloyd, 1962b). Kabrt (1983) reported that ~75% of pituitary ascorbic acid was unbound. Unfortunately, reports did not often distinguish between anterior, intermediate, and posterior pituitary, although Kabrt did make the distinction clear. Salhanick et al. (1949) studied the effects of external stresses or pharmacologic agents on pituitary ascorbic acid content. In rats, pituitary ascorbate remained remarkably constant, between 112 and 157 mg/100 g of pituitary tissue, even with stress to the animal. These results are somewhat less than for adrenal tissue in rats, yet the pituitary ascorbate content is quite high. Kabrt reported similar findings using the 2,4-DNP assay (1983).

The function of ascorbic acid in pituitary tissue is only of recent interest, and it is an exciting story. Bradbury and colleagues presented evidence that porcine pituitary granules contain an enzyme that amidates terminal glycine residues on pituitary peptides (Bradbury and Smyth, 1982; Bradbury et al. 1982). Such peptides with terminal glycine–amide groups include oxytocin and vasopressin, both found in posterior pituitary. In fact, other bioactive peptides isolated from endocrine tissues contain an amide moiety at the carboxyl terminus. Concurrently, Eipper and colleagues demonstrated an enzymatic activity in pituitary tissue which was capable of $\alpha$-amidation and required oxygen, copper, and ascorbic acid (Eipper et al., 1983a). Ascorbic acid was noted to be the most potent stimulator of $\alpha$-amidation. Although the comparison between ascorbic acid and other reducing substances in cells remains to be completed, Eipper *et al.* (1983b) had previously reported that primary cultures of rat intermediate pituitary cells lost the ability to amidate the carboxyl terminus of α-melanocyte-stimulating hormone (MSH). This observation is consistent with loss of ascorbic acid from cultured pituicytes, in much the same way chromaffin cells in culture lose ascorbic acid rapidly. Indeed, ascorbic acid supplementation of intermediate pituitary cells resulted in a dramatic increase of the cells to form α-amidated peptide (Glembotski, 1984). It is very exciting that the amidating enzyme contains copper and requires both oxygen and reducing equivalents. These are in fact the same requirements of the monooxygenase in adrenal medulla, DBH! Furthermore, the recent isolation of cytochrome $b_{561}$ in posterior pituitary suggests that this cytochrome may mediate electron transport from ascorbate to the enzymes not only in adrenal medulla, but in posterior pituitary (Duong *et al.*, 1984). Indeed, our most recent experiments with isolated posterior pituitary granules suggest that there is electron transfer across pituitary granules (Russell *et al.*, 1985), analogous to electron transfer across chromaffin granule ghosts (Njus *et al.*, 1983). Thus, these studies suggest that the ability of ascorbic acid to act as a specific electron donor may be present in more than one endocrine tissue. Perhaps one general function of ascorbic acid in endocrine systems is to donate electrons for transfer across membranes, perhaps for utilization in amidation or hydroxylation reactions. The next few years should see profound advances in our understanding of the function of ascorbic acid in pituitary tissues.

## D. PANCREAS AND GLUCOSE HOMEOSTASIS

Very little is known about pancreatic ascorbic acid except that it is found in human tissues (Table I). Ascorbate distribution among the pancreatic cell types and within the cells themselves is unknown.

Incomplete and indirect evidence exists concerning the role of ascorbic acid in glucose homeostasis. Patterson (1950) noted that dehydroascorbate acid is structurally similar to alloxan, a compound that produces experimental diabetes (Dunn *et al.*, 1943). Patterson found in rats that a dose of ~1 g/kg of dehydroascorbic acid induced hyperglycemia and 1.5 g/kg induced permanent diabetes (Patterson, 1950; Patterson and Lazarow, 1950). These extremely large doses led to degranulation of β cells as well as hyperglycemia (Merlini and Caramia, 1965). The significance of these findings to ascorbic acid ingestion and glucose homeostasis was not at all clear (Meglasson and Hazelwood, 1982).

Nandi *et al.* found that ascorbic acid at 600 mg/kg was toxic to guinea pigs fed very high carbohydrate diets (Nandi *et al.*, 1973). De-hydroascorbic acid content of blood, urine, and liver of the guinea pigs increased markedly (Chatterjee *et al.*, 1975) and in proportion to the ascorbate dose. Concomitant increases in blood glucose were found with doses of ascorbic acid beginning at 200 mg/kg. The rise in blood glucose was reversible upon discontinuation of ascorbic acid adminis-tration. Animals fed diets without high carbohydrate content dis-played normal blood glucose and dehydroascorbate levels, using ascor-bate doses as high as 1 g/kg body weight.

Similar experiments were conducted in normal human volunteers in India (Chatterjee *et al.*, 1975). They were fed diets of 80–85% cereal, 8–10% legumes, and 4–5% fish with average calorie intake of 1700. As-corbic acid supplements were 4 g daily for 15 days. There were 5- to 50-fold or greater increases in blood dehydroascorbate, but no abnormal responses in glucose tolerance tests. Upon discontinuation only of the ascorbic acid, the dehydroascorbate levels returned to the preexperi-mental values.

Chatterjee and colleagues (1975) and Banerjee (1982) then studied dehydroascorbic acid content of blood in patients with frank diabetes. They found that dehydroascorbate concentrations in blood were ~20- to 50-fold higher in diabetic patients than in controls. Increases were recorded in both type I and type II diabetics (Banerjee, 1982). The concentrations remained persistently abnormal over 18 months. Pa-tients with acute illness or severe physical trauma also showed higher dehydroascorbate than normal controls, but these levels returned to normal or near normal during convalescence. Interestingly, some first-degree relatives of patients with unspecified types of diabetes showed elevated dehydroascorbate concentrations (Banerjee, 1982). Two of them developed frank diabetes within 6 months (Chatterjee *et al.*, 1975). The increased dehydroascorbate was located in plasma and pri-marily in erythrocytes, although for which diabetic patients was not clear. Other investigators studied ascorbate content in mononuclear leukocytes in patients with type II diabetes and found decreased ascor-bate in these cells as compared to controls (Chen *et al.*, 1983). Stankova *et al.* (1984) found that granulocytes from diabetics had impaired dehy-droascorbate uptake. In striking contrast to the Indian patients, this last group of diabetic patients did not show elevated plasma dehy-droascorbate.

The findings of increased dehydroascorbic acid in some diabetic pa-tients and some first-degree relatives are provocative. Of concern is the experimental assay for dehydroascorbate, especially use of the older DCPIP and 2,4-DNP assays. In this regard it is worrisome that the findings reported in the Indian patients (Chatterjee *et al.*, 1975; Banerjee, 1982) could not be repeated in patients in Portland, Oregon (Stankova *et al.*, 1984). Indeed, the Indian patient samples were measured using the DCPIP technique and the Oregon patient samples were measured using the 2,4-DNP technique. Also, the possibility of generally lower ascorbate intake in the Calcutta patients needs to be considered as well as other dietary variations (Stankova *et al.*, 1984). These experiments need to be repeated using newer more specific techniques. Nevertheless, the results are suggestive of aberrant ascorbate metabolism in diabetics, as reflected either by possibly elevated red blood cell dehydroascorbate or by possibly impaired ascorbate or dehydroascorbate uptake in leukocytes. Perhaps imparied insulin action is coupled to the inability to transport or reduce dehydroascorbate in these patients. Furthermore, as Banerjee suggested, erythrocyte ascorbate might someday serve as a marker for some prediabetic patients. Further work is necessary to clarify these findings and their relationship to glucose homeostasis in blood cells.

## E. GONADS

Ascorbic acid has been found in gonadal tissue (Table I). Further characterization is sparse. Ovarian slices appear to concentrate radiolabeled ascorbate, although kinetic studies are not available (Stansfield and Flint, 1967). Depletion of ascorbate from luteal tissue has been reported as a bioassay for luteinizing hormone, similar to the ACTH ascorbate depletion assay (Parlow, 1958). Luteinizing hormone was found to deplete ascorbic acid from ovarian slices within 3–4 hours (Stansfield and Flint, 1967). This suggested that the ascorbate depletion was mediated indirectly by luteinizing hormone. High concentrations of progesterone inhibited ascorbic acid uptake in ovarian tissue slices, similar to observations of ascorbate transport inhibition in adrenal cortex. It is interesting that both steroid-synthesizing tissues display ascorbate depletion mediated by pituitary hormones. Indeed, ascorbate depletion in ovary and adrenal suggests a similar role for ascorbate in both tissues, and perhaps in testes as well. Unfortunately, the common thread of steroid biosynthesis and ascorbate depletion has not helped decipher the function of ascorbate in any of these steroid-synthesizing tissues. Although there are reports that ascorbic acid inhibited ovarian steroidogenesis (Sanyal and Datta, 1979), these findings may represent ascorbate-mediated lipid peroxidation, as previously discussed.

F. Other Endocrine Tissues

Ascorbic acid has been found in the thyroid gland and hypothalamus, but has not been measured in parathyroid glands (Table I) (Mefford *et al.*, 1981). Recent evidence suggests that ascorbic acid may be necessary for $\alpha$-amidation of the hypothalamic peptide thyrotropin releasing hormone (Glembotski *et al.*, 1985). In the next few years it is likely that the role of ascorbic acid in the biosynthesis of hypothalamic hormones will be elucidated.

## V. Conclusions

Ascorbic acid is required for survival in mammals. To meet this need, most animals synthesize ascorbic acid by a multistep process in hepatic tissue. Human beings, other primates, and guinea pigs are representative of animals that lack the terminal enzyme in the ascorbic acid synthetic pathway and that must obtain ascorbic acid in the diet. Requirements for ascorbic acid in humans and guinea pigs have been estimated from measurements of ascorbate pool size and from doses of ascorbate required to prevent scurvy. The latter estimates, however, may not represent optimal requirements for ascorbate. Many species that synthesize ascorbate make far more ascorbic acid per kilogram than the estimated human requirements. It is estimated that even primates, unable to synthesize ascorbate, need far more ascorbate per kilogram than is currently recommended for us.

There have been several difficulties in determining optimal ascorbate requirements for human beings. Of great importance has been the lack of suitable assays to determine ascorbate requirements in biological systems. Indeed, the basic functions of ascorbate in many biological systems have been poorly understood. Our conception of optimal requirements also may be in need of revision. What is satisfactory for a resting state may not be adequate for different metabolically active states. Thus, optimal requirements for ascorbate may be homeostasis dependent. If these issues could be addressed, ascorbate requirements for humans might be reexamined in a scientific manner. Potential to begin to answer these problems now exists through study of ascorbic acid in endocrine systems. Endocrine tissues in mammals show the highest concentrations of ascorbic acid per weight of tissue. The functions of ascorbic acid as a neuromodulator and specific electron donor in some endocrine tissues are beginning to be characterized. A greater understanding of ascorbic acid in endocrine cellular and subcellular systems may eventually permit estimation of optimal ascorbic acid concentrations first in tissues, and then in animals.

One critical purpose of endocrine systems is maintenance of homeostasis. Since ascorbic acid is found in its highest concentration in endocrine tissues, ascorbic acid may therefore be important for endocrine function and maintenance of homeostasis. Optimal ascorbic acid needs in a given endocrine system may differ depending on maintenance of homeostasis, deviation from homeostasis, and ability of the organism to reestablish homeostasis. Thus, optimal requirements for ascorbic acid in endocrine systems may change, depending upon the vicissitudes of endocrine function in maintaining a constant internal milieu.

Further investigation of ascorbic acid function in endocrine systems is of critical importance. Only with new knowledge will we be able to determine optimal tissue concentration and organism requirements. We believe that working toward these goals may have profound and unique implications for maintenance of human health.

## ACKNOWLEDGMENTS

We would like to thank Pat Fleming and David Blank for their editorial assistance and Shelley Sturman and Harvey Pollard for their wholehearted support of this work.

## REFERENCES

Abt, A. F., Von Schuching, S., and Enns T. (1963). Vitamin C requirements of man reexamined. *Am. J. Clin. Nutr.* **12**, 21–29.

Ash, D. E., Papadopoulos, N. J., Colombo, G., and Villafranca, J. S. (1984). Kinetic and spectroscopic studies of the interaction of copper with dopamine $\beta$-hydroxylase. *J. Biol. Chem.* **259**, 3395–3398.

Atkins, G. L., Dean, B. M., Griffin, W. J., and Watts R. W. E. (1964). Quantitative aspects of ascorbic acid metabolism in man. *J. Biol. Chem.* **239**, 2975–2980.

Augustin, J., Beck, C., and Marousek, G. J. (1981). A quantitative determination of ascorbic acid in potatoes and potato products by high pressure liquid chromatography. *J. Food Sci.* **46**, 316–318.

Baker, E. M. (1967). Vitamin C requirements in stress. *Am. J. Clin. Nutr.* **20**, 583–590.

Baker, E. M., Levandoski, N. G., and Sauberlick, H. E. (1963). Respiratory catabolism in man of the degradative intermediates of L-ascorbic 1-[14]C-acid. *Proc. Soc. Exp. Biol. Med.* **113**, 379.

Baker, E. M., Saari, J. C., and Tolbert B. M. (1966). Ascorbic acid metabolism in man. *Am. J. Clin. Nutr.* **19**, 371–378.

Baker, E. M., Hodges, R. E., Hood, J., Sauberlich, H. E., March, S., and Canham, J. E. (1971). Metabolism of [14]C- and [3]H-labelled L-ascorbic acid in human scurvy. *Am. J. Clin. Nutr.* **24**, 444–454.

Baker, E. M., Halver, J. E., Johnsen, D., Joyce, B. E., Knight, M. K., and Tolbert, B. M. (1975). Metabolism of ascorbic acid and ascorbic 2-sulfate in man and the subhuman primate. *Ann. N.Y. Acad. Sci.* **258**, 72–80.

Ballard, P. L. (1979). Delivery and transport of glucocorticoids to target cells. *In* "Glucocorticoid Hormone Action" (J. D. Baxter and G. G. Rousseau, eds.), pp 25–48. Springer-Verlag, Berlin and New York.

Banerjee, A. (1982). Blood dehydroascorbic acid and diabetes mellitus in human beings. *Ann. Clin. Biochem.* **19,** 65–70.

Barnett, S. A., and Fisher, R. B. (1943). Experiments on the silver nitrate method for the histological demonstration of ascorbic acid. *J. Exp. Biol.* **20,** 14–15.

Belpaire, F., and Laduron, P. L. (1968). Tissue fractionation and catecholamines. *Biochem. Pharmacol.* **17,** 411–421.

Bennett, H. W., and Kilham, L. (1940). The blood vessels of the adrenal gland of the adult cat. *Anat. Rec.* **77,** 447–471.

Bessey, O. A., and King, C. G. (1933). The distribution of vitamin C in plant and animal tissues and its determination. *J. Biol. Chem.* **103,** 687–698.

Bezssonoff, M., and Woloszyn, M. (1938). Surl'existence d'une forme oxyd'ee, interm'ediaire entre la vitamine C et l'acide d'ehyudroascorbique. *Bull. Soc. Chim. Biol.* **20,** 93–122.

Bhattacharyya, T. K., Sarkar, A. K., Ghosh, A., and Ganguli, A. (1966). A comparative study on avian adrenocortical response to exogenous and endogenous corticotropin. *J. Exp. Zool.* **165,** 301–308.

Bielski, B. H. J., Richter, H. W., and Chan, P. C. (1975). Some properties of the ascorbate free radical. *Ann. N.Y. Acad. Sci.* **258,** 231–238.

Bigley, R. H., and Stankova, L. (1974). Uptake and reduction of oxidized and reduced ascorbate by human leukocytes. *J. Exp. Med.* **139,** 1084–1092.

Blaschko, H. (1939). The specific action of L-dopa decarboxylase. *J. Physiol. (London)* **96,** 50p–51p.

Borsook, H., Davenport, H. W., Jeffreys, C. E. P. and Warner, R. C. (1937). The oxidation of ascorbic acid and its reduction *in vitro* and *in vivo. J. Biol. Chem.* **117,** 237–249.

Bourgeois, C. F., and Mainguy, P. R. (1975). Determination of vitamin C. *Int. J. Vitam. Nutr. Res.* **45,** 70–84.

Bourne, G. (1936). The vitamin C technique as a contribution to cytology. *Anat. Rec.* **66,** 369–385.

Bourne, G. H. (1975). "The Rhesus Monkey," Vol. II, pp. 111–113. Academic Press, New York.

Bradbury, A. F., and Smyth, D. G. (1982). Amidation of synthetic peptides by a pituitary enzyme: Specificity and mechanism of the reaction. *In* "Peptides" (K. Blaha and P. Malon, eds.), pp. 381–386. Walter de Gruyter and Co., Berlin and New York.

Bradbury, A. F., Finnie, M. D. A., and Smyth, D. G. (1982). Mechanism of C-terminal amide formation by pituitary enzymes. *Nature (London)* **298,** 686–688.

Bradley, D. W., Emery, G., and Maynard, J. E. (1973). Vitamin C in plasma: A comparative study of the vitamin stabilized with trichloroacetic acid or metaphosphoric acid. *Clin. Chim. Acta* **44,** 47–52.

Briggs, F. N., and Toepel, W. (1958). The effect of adrenocorticotrophic hormone on the ascorbic acid concentration of adrenal venous plasma of the rat. *Endocrinology* **62,** 24–29.

Brin, M. (1982). Nutritional and health aspects of ascorbic acid. *In* "Ascorbic Acid: Chemistry, Metabolism, Uses" (P. A. Seib and B. M. Tolbert, eds.), pp. 369–380. American Chemical Society, Washington, D.C.

Brodish, A., and Long, C. N. H. (1960). Characteristics of the adrenal ascorbic acid response to adrenocorticotrophic hormone in the rat. *Endocrinology* **66,** 149–159.

Bublitz, C., and Lehninger, A. L. (1961). The role of aldonolactonase in the biosynthesis of L-ascorbic acid. *Ann. N.Y. Acad. Sci.* **92,** 87–90.

Burns, J. J., Burch, H. B., and King, C. G. (1951). The metabolism of L-$^{14}$C ascorbic acid in guinea pigs. *J. Biol. Chem.* **191**, 501–514.

Burns, J. J., Dayton, P. G., and Schulenberg, S. (1956a). Further observations on the metabolism of L-ascorbic acid in guinea pigs. *J. Biol. Chem.* **218**, 15–21.

Burns, J. J., Peyser, P., and Moltz, A. (1956b). Missing step in guinea pigs required for the biosynthesis of L-ascorbic acid. *Science* **124**, 1148–1149.

Butts, W. C., and Mulvihill, H. J. (1975). Centrifugal analyzer determination of ascorbate in serum or urine with $Fe^{3+}$/ferrozine. *Clin. Chem.* **21**, 1493–97.

Chatterjee, I. B. (1970). Biosynthesis of ascorbic acid in animals. *In* "Methods in Enzymology" (D. B. McCormick and L. D. Wright, eds.), Vol. 18, Pt. A, pp. 28–34. Academic Press, New York.

Chatterjee, I. B. (1973). Evolution and the biosynthesis of ascorbic acid. *Science* **182**, 1271–1272.

Chatterjee, I. B., Ghosh, J. J., Ghosh, N. C., and Guha, B. C. (1958a). Effect of cyanide on the biosynthesis of ascorbic acid by an enzyme preparation from goat liver microsomes. *Biochem. J.* **70**, 509.

Chatterjee, I. B., Ghosh, N. C., Ghosh, J. J., and Guha, B. C. (1958b). Site of the enzyme system involved in the biosynthesis of ascorbic acid. *Sci. Cult.* **23**, 382.

Chatterjee, I. B., Kar, N. C., Ghosh, N. C., and Guha, B. C. (1961). Aspects of ascorbic acid biosynthesis in animals. *Ann. N.Y. Acad. Sci.* **92**, 36–56.

Chatterjee, I. B., Majumder, A. K., Nandi, B. M., and Subramanian, N. (1975). Synthesis and some major functions of vitamin C in animals. *Ann. N.Y. Acad. Sci.* **258**, 24–47.

Chen, M. S., Hutchinson, M. L., Pecoraro, R. E., Lee, W., and Labbe, R. (1983). Hyperglycemia induced intracellular depletion of ascorbic acid in human mononuclear leukocytes. *Diabetes* **32**, 1078–1082.

Clark, E. J., and Rossiter, R. J. (1944). Carbohydrate metabolism after burning. *Q. J. Exp. Physiol.* **32**, 279–300.

Clayman, M., Tsang, A., DeNicola, A. F., and Johnstone, R. M. (1970). Specificity of action of ACTH *in vitro* on ascorbate transport in rat adrenal glands. *Biochem. J.* **118**, 283–289.

Cooke, J. R., and Moxon, R. E. D. (1981). Detection and measurement of vitamin C. *In* "Vitamin C: Ascorbic Acid" (J. N. Counsell and D. H. Hornig, eds.), pp. 167–198. Applied Science Publ., London.

Coupland, R. E. (1975). Blood supply of the adrenal gland. *In* "Handbook of Physiology, Section 7, Endocrinology" (H. Blaschko, G. Sayers, and A. D. Smith, eds.), pp. 283–294. American Physiological Society, Washington, D.C.

Coupland, R. E., and Selby, J. E. (1976). The blood supply of the mammalian adrenal medulla: A comparative study. *J. Anat.* **122**, 539–551.

Curtin, C. O., and King, C. G. (1955). The metabolism of ascorbic acid L-$^{14}$C and oxalic acid $^{14}$C in the rat. *J. Biol. Chem.* **216**, 539–548.

Daniels, A. J., Dean, G., Viveros, O. H., and Diliberto, E. J., Jr. (1982). Secretion of newly taken up ascorbic acid by adrenomedullary chromaffin cells. *Science* **216**, 737–739.

Daniels, A. J., Dean, G. Viveros, O. H., and Diliberto, E. J., Jr. (1983). Secretion of newly taken up ascorbic acid by adrenomedullary chromaffin cells originates from a compartment different from the catecholamine storage vesicle. *Mol. Pharmacol.* **23**, 437–444.

DeKlerk W. A., Duplessis, D. P., Van Der Watt, J. J., De Jager, A., and Laubscher, N. F. (1973a). Vitamin C requirements of the vervet monkey. *S. Afr. Med. J.* **47**, 705–708.

DeKlerk, W. A., Kotze, J. P., Weight, M. J., Menne, I. U., Matthews, A., and McDonald,

T. (1973b). The influence of various dietary ascorbic acid levels on serum ascorbic acid and serum cholesterol values of the baboon (*Papio ursinus*) during captivity. *S. Afr. Med. J.* **47**, 1503.

DeNicola, A. F., Clayman, M., and Johnstone, R. M. (1968). Hormonal control of ascorbic acid transport in rat adrenal glands. *Endocrinology* **82**, 436–446.

Deutsch, M. J., and Weeks, C. E. (1965). Microfluorometric assay for vitamin C. *J. Assoc. Off. Anal. Chem.* **48**, 1248–1256.

Diliberto, E. J., Jr., and Allen P. L. (1981). Mechanism of dopamine β-hydroxylation. *J. Biol Chem.* **256**, 3385–3393.

Diliberto, E. J., Jr., Dean G., Carter, C., and Allen, P. L. (1982). Tissue, subcellular and submitochondrial distributions of semidehydroascorbate reductase. *J. Neurochem.* **39**, 563–568.

Diliberto, E. J., Jr., Heckman, G. D., and Daniels A. J. (1983). Characterization of ascorbic acid transport by adrenomedullary chromaffin cells. *J. Biol. Chem.* **258**, 12886–12994.

Doner, L., and Hicks, K. B. (1981). High performance liquid chromatographic separation of ascorbic acid, erythorbic acid, dehydroascorbic acid, dehydroerythorbic acid, diketogulonic acid, and diketogluconic acid. *Anal. Biochem.* **115**, 225–230.

Dunn, J. S., Sheehan, H. L., and McLetchie, N. G. B. (1943). Necrosis of islets of Langerhans produced experimentally. *Lancet* **1**, 484.

Dunnick, N. R., Doppman, J., Mills, S. R., and Gill, J. R., Jr. (1979). Pre-operative, diagnosis and localization of aldosteronomas by measurement of corticosteroids in adrenal venous blood. *Radiology* **133**, 331–333.

Duong, L., and Fleming, P. (1982). Isolation and properties of cytochrome $b_{561}$ from bovine adrenal chromaffin granules. *J. Biol. Chem.* **257**, 8561–8564.

Duong, L., Fleming, P., and Russel, J. (1984). An identical cytochrome $b_{561}$ is present in bovine adrenal chromaffin vesicles and posterior pituitary neurosecretory vesicles. *J. Biol. Chem.* **259**, 4885–4889.

Eipper, B. A., Glembotski, C. A., and Mains, R. E. (1983a). Selective loss of α-melanotropin amidating activity in primary cultures of rat intermediate pituitary cells. *J. Biol. Chem.* **258**, 7292–7298.

Eipper, B. A., Mains, R. E., and Glembotski, C. (1983b). Identification in pituitary tissue of a peptide α-amidation activity that acts on glycine extended peptides and requires molecular oxygen, copper, and ascorbic acid. *Proc. Natl. Acad. Sci. U.S.A.* **80**, 5144–5148.

Eisenberg, F., Field, J. B., and Stetten, D. (1955). Studies on glucuronide conjugation in man. *Arch. Biochem. Biophys.* **59**, 297–299.

Erdman, J. W., and Klein, B. P. (1982). Harvesting, processing, and cooking influences on vitamin C in foods. In "Ascorbic Acid: Chemistry, Metabolism, and Uses" (P. A. Seib and B. M. Tolbert, eds.), pp. 499–532. American Chemical Society, Washington, D.C.

Everling, F. B., Weis, W., and Staudinger, H. (1969). Bestimmung des Standard Redoxypotentials (pH 7.0) von L-(+)-ascorbat/semidehydro-L(+)—Ascorbinsäure durch nichtenzymatische Reaktion von L(+)-ascorbat/semidehydro-L(+)-Ascorbinsäure mit cytochrom $b_5(Fe^2)$/cytochrom $b_5(Fe^3)$. *Hoppe-seyler's Z. Physiol. Chem.* **350**, 886–888.

Farber, C. M., Kanengiser, S., Stahl, R., Liebes, L., and Silber, R. (1983). A specific HPLC assay for dehydroascorbic acid shows an increased content in CLL lymphocytes. *Anal. Biochem.* **134**, 355–360.

Fiddick, R., and Heath, H. (1966). The in vivo uptake of L-1-$^{14}$C ascorbic acid by the rat retina and adrenal gland. *Exp. Eye* Res. **5**, 329–334.

Finley J. W., and Duang, E. (1981). Resolution of ascorbic, dehydroascorbic, and diketo-gulonic acids by paired ion reversed-phase chromatography. *J. Chromatogt.* **207**, 449–453.

Finn, F. M., and Johns, P. A. (1980). Ascorbic acid transport by isolated bovine adrenal cortical cells. *Endocrinology* **106**, 811–817.

Flint, J. M. (1900). The blood vessels, angiogenesis, organogenesis, reticulum, and histology of the adrenal. *Johns Hopkins Hosp. Rep.* 153–229.

Foldes, A., Jeffrey, P. L., Preston, B. N., and Austin, L. (1972). Dopamine $\beta$-hydroxylase of bovine adrenal medulla. *Biochem. J.* **126**, 1209–1217.

Fortier, C., Skelton, F. R., Constantinides, P., Timiras, P. S., Herland, M., and Selye, H. (1950). A comparative study of some of the chemical and morphological changes elicited in the adrenals by stress and adrenocorticotropic hormone. *Endocrinology* **46**, 21–29.

Freeman, B. M. (1970). The effects of ACTH on adrenal weight and adrenal ascorbic acid in the normal and bursectomized fowl. *Comp. Biochem. Physiol.* **32**, 755–761.

Friedman, S., and Kaufman, S. (1965). 3,4-Dihydroxyphenylethylamine $\beta$-hydroxylase. *J. Biol. Chem.* **240**, 4763–4773.

Fujita, A., Hirose, F., and Uchiyama, Y. (1969). Studies on the determination of vitamin C by the hydrazine method and the determination of true vitamin C by thin layer chromatography. *Vitamins* **40**, 17–26.

Glembotski, C. (1984). The $\alpha$ amidation of $\alpha$-melanocyte stimulating hormone in intermediate pituitary requires ascorbic acid. *J. Biol. Chem.* **259**, 13041–13048.

Glembotski, C. C., Maneker, S., Winokur, V., and Gibson, T. R. (1985). Ascorbic acid increases the thyrotropin releasing hormone immunoactivity of hypothalamic cell cultures. *Endocrinology* **116** (Supp), 130.

Glick, D., and Biskind, G. R. (1935). The histochemistry of the adrenal gland. 1. The quantitative distribution of vitamin C. *J. Biol. Chem.* **110**, 1–7.

Glickman, N. R., Keeton, R. W., Mitchell, H. H., and Fahnestock, M. K. (1946). The tolerance of man to cold as affected by dietary modifications: High versus low intake of certain water-soluble vitamins. *Am. J. Physiol.* **146**, 538–558.

Goldstein, M., Lauber, E., and McKereghen, M. R. (1965). Studies on the purification and characterization of 3,4-dihydroxyphenylethylamine-$\beta$-hydroxylase. *J. Biol. Chem.* **240**, 2066–2072.

Goodall, McC., and Kirshner, N. (1957). Biosynthesis of adrenaline and noradrenaline *in vitro*. *J. Biol. Chem.* **226**, 213–221.

Greenfield, N., Ponticorvo, F., Chasalow, F., and Lieberman, S. (1980). Activation and inhibition of the adrenal steroid 21-hydroxylation system by cytosolic constituents: Influence of glutathione, glutathione reductase, and ascorbate. *Arch. Biochem. Biphys.* **200**, 232–244.

Greenman, D. L., Whitley L. S., and Zarrow, M. X. (1967). Ascorbic acid depletion and corticosterone production in the avian adrenal gland. *Gen. Comp. Endocrinol.* **9**, 422–427.

Grollman, A. P., and Lehninger A. L. (1957). Enzymatic synthesis of L-ascorbic acid in different animal species. *Arch. Biochem. Biophys.* **69**, 458–467.

Grouselle, M., and Phillips, J. H. (1982). Reduction of membrane-bound dopamine $\beta$-hydroxylase from the cytoplasmic surface of the chromaffin granule membrane. *Biochem. J.* **202**, 759–770.

Gruber, K., O'Brian, L., and Gerstner, R. (1976). Vitamin A: Not required for adrenal steroidogenesis in rats. *Science* **191**, 472–474.

Hagen, P. (1954). The distribution of ascorbic acid between the particulate and non-particulate components of adrenal and liver cells. *Biochem. J.* **56**, 44–46.

Hankes, L. V., Janson, C. R., and Schmaeler, M. (1974). Ascorbic acid catabolism in Bantu with hemosiderosis (scurvy). *Biochem. Med.* **9**, 244.

Harde, E. (1934). Acide ascorbique (vitamine C) et intoxications. *C. R. Acad.* **199**, 618–620.

Harding, B. W., and Nelson, D. H. (1963). Changes in rat adrenal ascorbic acid and glutathione following hypophysectomy and ACTH stimulation. *Endocrinology* **73**, 97–102.

Harris, L. J., and Ray, S. N. (1933). Vitamin C in the suprarenal medulla. *Biochem J.* **27**, 2006–2010.

Harris, R. S. (1970). "Feeding and Nutrition of Non-Human Primates," page 97. Academic Press, New York.

Hassan, M., and Lehninger, A. L. (1956). Enzymatic formation of ascorbic acid in rat liver extracts. *J. Biol. Chem.* **223**, 123–138.

Hegenauer, J., and Saltman, P. (1972). Resolution of ascorbic, dehydroascorbic, and diketogulonic acids by anion exchange column chromatography. *J. Chromatogr.* **74**, 133–137.

Hellman, L., and Burns, J. J. (1958). Metabolism of L-ascorbic acid 1-$^{14}$C in man. *J. Biol. Chem.* **230**, 923–928.

Henschel, A. H. (1944). Vitamin C and ability to work in hot environments. *Am. J. Trop. Med.* **24**, 259–265.

Hodges, R. E. (1980). Ascorbic acid. *In* "Modern Nutrition in Health and Disease" (R. S. Goodhart and M. E. Shils, eds.), pp. 259–273. Lea & Febiger, Philadelphia.

Hodges, J. R., and Hotston, R. T. (1970). Ascorbic acid deficiency and pituitary adrenocortical activity in the guinea pig. *Br. J. Pharmacol.* **40**, 740–746.

Hodges, R. E., Baker, E. M., Hood, J., Sauberlich, H. E., and March, H. C. (1969). Experimental scurvy in man. *Am. J. Clin. Nutr.* **22**, 535–543.

Hodges, R. E., Hood, J., Canham, J. E., Sauberlich, H. E., and Baker, E. M. (1971). Clinical manifestations of ascorbic acid deficiency in man. *Am. J. Clin. Nutr.* **24**, 432–443.

Honjo, S., and Imaizumi, K. (1967). Ascorbic acid content of adrenal and liver in cynomolgus monkeys suffering from bacillary dysentery. *Jpn. J. Med. Sci. Biol.* **20**, 97–102.

Hornig, D. (1975). Distribution of ascorbic acid, metabolites and analogues in man and animals. *Ann. N.Y. Acad. Sci.* **258**, 103–118.

Hornsby, P. (1980). Regulation of cytochrome *P*-450 supported 11-hydroxylation of deoxycortisol by steroids, oxygen, and antioxidants in adrenocortical cell cultures. *J. Biol. Chem.* **255**, 4020–4027.

Hornsby, P. J., and Crivello, J. F. (1983). The role of lipid peroxidation and biological antioxidants in the function of the adrenal cortex. *Mol. Cell. Endocrinol.* **30**, 123–147.

Hornsby, P. J., Simonian, M. H., and Gill, G. N. (1979). Aging of adrenocortical cells in culture. *Int. Rev. Cytol. Suppl.* **10**, 131–162.

Hortnagl, H., Winkler, H., and Lochs H. (1972). Membrane proteins of chromaffin granules. *Biochem. J.* **129**, 187–195.

Imhoff, U. (1964). Eine fluorometrische bestimmung nes vitamin C in Hahrungsmitteln. *Z. Ernähr.* **5**, 135–141.

Ingrebretsen, O. C., Terland O., and Flatmark, T. (1980). Subcellular distribution of ascorbate in bovine adrenal medulla. *Biochim. Biophys. Acta* **628**, 182–189.

Isherwood, F. A., and Mapson, L. W. (1961). Biosynthesis of L-ascorbic acid in animals and plants. *Ann. N.Y. Acad. Sci.* **92**, 6–20.

Isherwood, F. A., Chen, Y. T., and Mapson, L. W. (1954). Synthesis of ascorbic acid in plants and animals. *Biochem. J.* **56**, 1–15.

Isherwood, F. A., Mapson, L. W., and Chen, Y. T. (1960). Synthesis of L-ascorbic acid in rat liver homogenates. *Biochem. J.* **76**, 157–171.

Jenkins, J. S. (1962). The effect of ascorbic acid on adrenal steroid synthesis *in vitro*. *Endocrinology* **70**, 267–272.

Kabrt, J. (1983). Ascorbic acid in the pituitary gland. *Acta Univ. Carol. Med.* **28**, 267–366.

Kallner, A., Hartmann, D., and Hornig, D. (1979). Steady-state turnover and body pool of ascorbic acid in man. *Am. J. Clin. Nutr.* **32**, 530–539.

Kallner, A., Hartmann, D., and Hornig, D. (1982). Kinetics of ascorbic acid in humans. *In* "Ascorbic Acid: Chemistry, Metabolism, Uses" (P. A. Seib and B. M. Tolbert, eds.), pp. 335–348. American Chemical Society, Washington, D.C.

Keating, R. W., and Haddad, P. R. (1982). Simultaneous determination of ascorbic acid and dehydroascorbic acid by reversed-phase ion-pair HPLC with pre-column derivatization. *J. Chromatogr.* **245**, 249–255.

Kirk, J. R., and Ting, N. (1975). Fluorometric assay for total vitamin C using continuous flow analysis. *J. Food. Sci.* **40**, 463–466.

Kirshner, N. (1957). Pathway of noradrenaline formation from dopa. *J. Biol. Chem.* **226**, 821–825.

Kirshner, N. (1962). Uptake of catecholamines by a particulate fraction of the adrenal medulla. *J. Biol. Chem.* **237**, 2311–2317.

Kitabchi, A. E. (1967a). Ascorbic acid in steroidogenesis. *Nature (London)* **215**, 1385–1386.

Kitabchi, A. E. (1967b). Inhibition of steroid C-21 hydroxylase by ascorbate: Alteration of microsomal lipids in beef adrenal cortex. *Steroids* **10**, 567–577.

Kitabchi, A., and West, W. H. (1975). Effect of steroidogenesis on ascorbic acid content and uptake in isolated adrenal cells. *Ann. N.Y. Acad. Sci.* **258**, 422–431.

Klinman, J. P., Krueger, M., Brenner, M., and Edmondson, D. E. (1984). Evidence for two copper atoms/subunit in dopamine $\beta$-monooxygenase catalysis. *J. Biol. Chem.* **259**, 3399–3402.

Kotze, J. P., DeKlerk, W. A., Weight, M. J., Menne, I. V., Horn L. P., and Laubscher, N. F. (1974). Seasonal variation in serum ascorbic acid and serum lipid composition of free living baboons (*Papio ursinus*). *S. Afr. Med. J.* **48**, 1700.

Laduron, P. (1975). Evidence for a localization of dopamine $\beta$-hydroxylase within the chromaffin granules. *FEBS Lett.* **52**, 132–134.

Lahiri, S., and Lloyd, B. B. (1962a). The form of vitamin C released by the rat adrenal. *Biochem. J.* **84**, 474–478.

Lahiri, S., and Lloyd, B. B. (1962b). The effect of stress and corticotropin on the concentrations of vitamin C in blood and tissues of the rat. *Biochem. J.* **84**, 478–483.

Ledbetter, F. H., and Kirshner, N. (1981). Quantitative correlation between secretion and cellular content of catecholamines and dopamine $\beta$-hydroxylase in cultures of adrenal medulla cells. *Biochem. Pharmacol.* **30**, 3246–3249.

Lee, W., Hamernyik, P., Hutchinson, M., Raisys, V., and Labbe, R. (1982). Ascorbic acid in lymphocytes: Cell preparation and liquid chromatographic assay. *Clin. Chem.* **28**, 2165–2169.

Lehner, N., Bullock, B. C., and Clarkson, T. B. (1968). Ascorbic acid deficiency in the squirrel monkey. *Proc. Soc. Exp. Biol. Med.* **128**, 512–514.

Leonard, R. K., Auersperg, N., and Parkes, C. O. (1983). Ascorbic acid accumulation by cultured rat adrenocortical cells. *In Vitro* **19**, 46–52.

Levin, E. Y., and Kaufman, S. (1961). Studies on the enzyme catalyzing conversion of 3,4-dihydroxyphenylethylamine to norepinephrine. *J. Biol. Chem.* **236**, 2043–2049.

Levine, E. Y., Levenberg, B., and Kaufman, S. (1960). The enzymatic conversion of 3,4-dihydroxyphenylethylamine to norepinephrine. *J. Biol. Chem.* **235,** 2080–2086.

Levine, M., and Pollard, H. B. (1983). Hydrocortisone inhibition of ascorbic transport by chromaffin cells. *FEBS Lett.* **158,** 134–38.

Levine, M., Morita, K., and Pollard, H. B. (1985a). Enhancement of norepinephrine biosynthesis by ascorbic acid in cultured bovine chromaffin cells. *J. Biol. Chem.,* in press.

Levine, M., Morita, K., and Pollard, H. B. (1985b). Ascorbic acid regulation of norepinephrine biosynthesis in cultured bovine chromaffin cells and isolated chromaffin granules. *Endocrinology* **116** (Suppl.), 116.

Levine, M., Asher, A., Pollard, H. B., and Zinder, O. (1983). Ascorbic acid and catecholamine secretion in cultured chromaffin cells. *J. Biol. Chem.* **258,** 13111–13115.

Lewin, S. (1976). "Vitamin C: Its Molecular Biology and Medical Potential," pp. 1–125. Academic Press, New York.

Lind, J. (1753). "A Treatise on the Scurvy." Millar, London (republished Edinburgh Univ. Press, Edinburgh, 1953).

Lipscomb, H. S., and Nelson, D. H. (1961). Dynamic changes in ascorbic acid and corticosteroids in adrenal vein blood after ACTH. *Endocrinology* **66,** 144–146.

Liu, T. Z., Chin, N., Kiser, M. D., and Bigler, W. (1982). Specific spectrophotometry of ascorbic acid in serum or plasma by use of ascorbate oxidase.

Llorens, I., Borrell, J., and Borrell, S. (1973). Effects of insulin, glucagon, and ACTH on the levels of corticosteroids, noradrenaline, adrenaline and ascorbic acid in the adrenal glands of cats. *Horm. Res.* **4,** 321–330.

McGown, E. L., Rusnak, M. G., Lewis, C. M., and Tillotson, J. A. (1982). Tissue ascorbic acid analysis using ferrozine compared with the dinitrophenylhydrazine method. *Anal. Biochem.* **119,** 55–61.

Major, R. H. (1945). "Classic Descriptions of Disease," pp. 585–594. Thomas, Baltimore.

Marchesini, A. M., and Manitto, P. (1972). Un noivo metodo enzimatuo per dosare l'acido ascorbica, deidroascorbica riduttoni nei vegetali freschi e conservati. *Agrochimica* **4–5,** 351.

Marchesini, A. M., Montuori, F., Muffat, O. D., and Maestri, D. (1974). Application and advantages of the enzymatic method for assay of ascorbic acid, dehydroascorbic acid, and reductones. *J. Food Sci.* **39,** 568–571.

Matsuo, H., Miyata, A., and Mizuno, K. (1983). Novel C-terminally amidated opioid peptide in human phaeochromocytoma tumour. *Nature (London)* **305,** 721–723.

Mefford, I. N., Oke, A. F., and Adams, R. N. (1981). Regional distribution of ascorbate in human brain. *Brain Res.* **212,** 223–226.

Meglasson, M. D., and Hazelwood, R. L. (1982). Ascorbic acid diabetogenesis in the domestic fowl. *Gen Comp. Endocrinol.* **47,** 205–212.

Merlini, D., and Caramia, F. (1965). The effects of dehydroascorbic acid on the islets of Langerhans of the rat pancreas. *J. Cell Biol.* **26,** 245–257.

Mettler, C. C. (1947). "History of Medicine," pp. 323, 368–369. McGraw-Hill (Blakiston), New York.

Milewich, L., Chien, G. T., MacDonald, P. C., and Peterson, J. A. (1981). Ascorbic acid inhibition of aromatase activity in human placental tissue. *J. Steroid Biochem.* **14,** 185–193.

Mills, M. B., and Roe, J. H. (1947). A critical study of proposed modifications of the Roe and Kuether method for the determination of ascorbic acid with further contributions to the chemistry of the procedure. *J. Biol. Chem.* **170,** 159–164.

Morita, K., Levine, M., Heldman, E., and Pollard, H. B. (1985). Ascorbic acid and catecholamine secretion from digitonin-treated chromaffin cells. *J. Biol. Chem.,* submitted.

Munson, P. L., and Toepel, W. (1958). Detection of minute amounts of ACTH by the effect on adrenal venous ascorbic acid. *Endocrinology* **63**, 785–793.

Nandi, B. K., Majumder, A. K., Subramanian, N., and Chatterjee, I. B. (1973). Effects of large doses of vitamin C in guinea pigs and rats. *J. Nutr.* **103**, 1688–1695.

Njus, D., Knoth, J., and Zallakian, M. (1981). Proton-linked transport in chromaffin granules. *Curr. Top. Bioenerg.* **11**, 107–147.

Njus, D., Knoth, J., Cook, C., and Kelley, P. M. (1983). Electron transfer across the chromaffin granule membrane. *J. Biol. Chem.* **258**, 27–30.

Ogawa, S. (1953). Fluorescent reaction of vitamin C: Mechanism of the reaction. *J. Pharm. Soc. Jpn.* **73**, 309–316.

Okamura, M. (1980). An improved method for determination of L-ascorbic acid and L-dehydroascorbic acid in blood plasma. *Clin. Chim. Acta* **103**, 259–268.

Omaye, S. T., Tillotson, J. A., and Sauberlich, H. E. (1982). Metabolism of L-ascorbic acid in the monkey. *In* "Ascorbic Acid: Chemistry, Metabolism, Uses" (P. A. Seib and B. M. Tolbert, eds.), pp. 317–334. American Chemical Society, Washington, D.C.

Pachla, L. A., and Kissinger, P. T. (1976). Determination of ascorbic acid in foodstuffs, pharmaceuticals, and body fluids by liquid chromatography with electrochemical detection. *Anal. Chem.* **48**, 364–367.

Pachla, L. A., and Kissinger, P. T. (1979). Analysis of ascorbic acid by liquid chromatography with amperometric detection. *In* "Methods in Enzymology" (D. B. McCormick and L. D. Wright, eds.), Vol. 62, pp. 15–24. Academic Press, New York.

Palade, G. E., and Claude, A. (1949a). The nature of the Golgi apparatus I. *J. Morphol.* **85**, 35–70.

Palade, G. E., and Claude, A. (1949b). The nature of the Golgi apparatus II. *J. Morphol.* **85**, 71–112.

Parlow, A. F. (1958). A rapid bioassay method for LH and factors affecting LH secretion. *Fed. Proc., Fed. Am. Soc. Exp. Biol.* **17**, 402.

Patterson, J. W. (1950). The diabetogenic effect of dehydroascorbic acid and dehydroisoascorbic acids. *J. Biol. Chem.* **183**, 81–88.

Patterson, J. W., and Lazarow, A. (1950). Sulfhydryl protection against dehydroascorbic acid diabetes. *J. Biol. Chem.* **186**, 141–144.

Pauling, L. (1976). "Vitamin C, The Common Cold, and the Flu." Freeman, San Francisco.

Pelletier, O., and Brassard, R. (1975). Automated analysis of vitamin C in food products. *J. Assoc. Off. Anal. Chem.* **58**, 104–109.

Pelletier, O., and Brassard, R. (1977). Determination of vitamin C in food by manual and automated photometric methods. *J. Food Sci.* **42**, 1471–1477.

Perla D., and Mormorston J. (1937a). The role of vitamin C in resistance. *Arch. Pathol.* **23**, 543.

Perla, D., and Marmorston J. (1937b). The role of vitamin C in resistance. *Arch. Pathol.* **23**, 683.

Perla, D., and Marmorston, J. (1941). "Natural Resistance and Clinical Medicine," Chs. 35, 36. Little, Brown, Boston.

Phillips, J. (1974). Steady-state kinetics of catecholamine transport by chromaffin granule "ghosts." *Biochem. J.* **144**, 319–325.

Phillips, P. H., and Stare, F. J. (1934). The distribution of a reducing substance (vitamin C) in the tissues of fluorine fed cows. *J. Biol. Chem.* **104**, 301.

Pirani, C. (1952). Review: Relation of vitamin C to adrenocortical function and stress phenomena. *Metabolism* **1**, 197–222.

Pohorecky, L. A., and Wurtman, R. J. (1971). Adrenocortical control of epinephrine synthesis. *Pharm. Rev.* **23**, 1–30.

Pollard, H. B., Pazoles, C. J., Cruetz, C. C., Scott, J. H., Zinder, O., and Hotchkiss, A.

(1984). An osmotic mechanism for exocytosis from dissociated chromaffin cells. *J. Biol. Chem.* **259**, 1114–1121.

Recommended Daily Allowances (1980). 9th Ed., p. 76. Food and Nutrition Board, National Academy of Sciences, National Research Council, Washington D.C.

Roe, J. H. (1936). The determination of ascorbic acid as furfural and a comparison of results obtained by this method and by indophenol titration. *J. Biol. Chem.* **116**, 609–619.

Roe, J. H., and Hall, J. M. (1939). The vitamin C content of human urine and its determination through the 2,4-dinitrophenylhydrazine derivative of dehydroascorbic acid. *J. Biol. Chem.* **128**, 329–337.

Roe, J. H., and Kuether, C. A. (1942). A color reaction of dehydroascorbic acid useful in the determination of vitamin C. *Science* **95**, 77.

Roe, J. H., and Kuether, C. A. (1943). The determination of ascorbic acid in whole blood and urine through the 2,4-dinitrophenylhydrazine derivative of dehydroascorbic acid. *J. Biol. Chem.* **147**, 399–407.

Rose, R. C., and Nahrwold, D. L. (1982). Quantitative analysis of ascorbic acid and dehydroascorbic acid by high performance liquid chromatography. *Anal. Biochem.* **114**, 140–145.

Rosenberg, R. C., and Lovenberg W. (1980). Dopamine β-hydroxylase. *Essays Neurochem. Neuropharmacol.* **4**, 163–209.

Russell, J., Levine, M., and Njus, D. (1985). Electron transfer across posterior pituitary neurosecretory vesicles. *J. Biol. Chem.,* **260**, 226–231.

Ryer, R., Grossman, M. J., Friedemann, T. E., Best, W. R., Consolazio, C. F., Kuhl, W. J., Fusull, W., and Hatch, F. T. (1954a). The effect of vitamin C supplementation of soldiers residing in a cold environment: Part I. *Am. J. Clin. Nutr.* **2**, 97–132.

Ryer, R., Grossman, M. J., Friedemann, T. E., Best, W. R., Consolazio, C. F., Kuhl, W. J., Fusull, W., and Hatch, T. T. (1954b). The effect of vitamin C supplementation on soldiers residing in a cold environment: Part II. *Am. J. Clin. Nutr.* **2**, 179–194.

Salhanick, H. H., Zarrow, I. G., and Zarrow, M. X. (1949). Ascorbic acid in the pituitary of the rat. *Endocrinology* **45**, 314–316.

Salomon, K. K. (1958). Studies on adrenal ascorbic acid: III; exchangeability with extracellular ascorbic acid. *Tx. Rep. Biol. Med.* **16**, 153.

Sanyal, S., and Datta, S. (1979). Effect of ascorbic acid on *in vitro* rat adrenal and ovarian steroidogenesis. *Indian J. Exp. Biol.* **17**, 86–88.

Sato, P., and Vden Friend, S. (1978). Studies on ascorbic acid related to the genetic basis of scurvy. *Vits. and Horms.* **36**, 33–52.

Sauberlich, H. E., Green, M. D., and Omaye, S. T. (1982). Determination of ascorbic acid and dehydroascorbic acid. *In* "Ascorbic Acid: Chemistry, Metabolism, Uses" (P. A. Seib and B. M. Tolbert, eds.), pp. 199–221. American Chemical Society, Washington, D.C.

Sayers, G., and Sayers, M. A. (1947). Regulation of pituitary adrenocorticotrophic activity during the response of the rat to acute stress. *Endocrinology* **40**, 265–273.

Sayers, G., Sayers, M. A., Fry, E. G., White, A., and Long, C. N. H. (1944a). The effect of the adrenotrophic hormone of the anterior pituitary on the cholesterol content of the adrenals. *Yale J. Biol. Med.* **16**, 361.

Sayers, G., Sayers, M. A., Lewis, H. L., Long, C. N. H. (1944b). Effect of adrenotrophic hormone on ascorbic acid and cholesterol content of the adrenal. *Proc. Soc. Exp. Biol. Med.* **55**, 238–239.

Sayers, G., Sayers, M. A., Liang, T., and Long, C. N. H. (1945). The cholesterol and ascorbic acid content of adrenal, liver, brain, and plasma following hemorrhage. *Endocrinology* **37**, 96–110.

Sayers, G., Sayers, M. A., Liang T., and Long, C. N. H. (1946). The effect of the pituitary adrenotrophic hormone on the cholesterol and ascorbic content of the adrenal of the rat and the guinea pig. *Endocrinology* **38**, 1–9.

Sayers, M. A., Sayers, G., and Woodbury, L. A. (1948). The assay of adrenocorticotrophic hormone by the adrenal ascorbic acid depletion method. *Endocrinology* **42**, 379–393.

Sharma, S. K., Johnstone, R. M., and Quastel, J. H. (1963). Active transport of ascorbic acid in adrenal cortex and brain cortex *in vitro* and the effects of ACTH and steroids. *Can. J. Biochem.* **41**, 597–604.

Sharma, S. K., Johnstone, R. M., and Quastel, J. H. (1964). Corticosteroids and ascorbic acid transport in adrenal cortex *in vitro. Biochem. J.* **92**, 564–573.

Shaw, J. H., Phillips, P. H., and Elvehjem, C. A. (1945). Acute and chronic ascorbic acid deficiency in the squirrel monkey. *J. Nutr.* **29**, 365–372.

Sheahan, M. M. (1947). The ascorbic acid content of the blood serum of farm animals. *J. Comp. Pathol.* **57**, 28–35.

Skotland, T., and Ljones, T. (1980). Direct spectrophotometric detection of ascorbate free radical formed by dopamine β-monooxygenase and by ascorbate oxidase. *Biochim. Biophys. Acta* **630**, 30–35.

Slusher, M. A., and Roberts, S. (1957). Fate of adrenal ascorbic acid: Relationship to corticosteroid secretion. *Endocrinology* **64**, 98–105.

Spector, R., and Greene, L. A. (1977). Ascorbic acid transport by a clonal line of pheochromocytoma cells. *Brain Res.* **136**, 131–140.

Spector, R., and Lorenzo, A. V. (1974). Specificity of ascorbic acid transport system of the central nervous system. *Am J. Physiol.* **226**, 1468–1473.

Srikantia, S. G., Mohanram, M., and Krishnaswamy, K. (1970). Human requirements of ascorbic acid. *Am. J. Clin. Nutr.* **23**, 59–62.

Srivastava, M., Duong, L., and Fleming, P. (1984). Cytochrome $b_{561}$ catalyzes transmembrane electron transfer. *J. Biol. Chem.,* 259, 8072–8075.

Stamm, W. P., McCrae, T. F., and Yudkin, S. (1944). Incidence of bleeding gums among R.A.F. personnel and the value of ascorbic acid treatment. *Br. Med. J.* **2**, 239–241.

Stankova, L., Riddle, M., Larned, J., Burry, K., Menaske, D., Hart, J., and Bigley R. (1984). Plasma ascorbate concentrations and blood cell dehydroascorbic acid transport in patients with diabetes mellitus. *Metabolism* **33**, 347–353.

Stansfield, D. A., and Flint, A. P. (1967). The entry of ascorbic acid into the corpus luteum *in vivo* and *in vitro* and the effect of luteinizing hormone. *J. Endocrinol.* **39**, 27–35.

Staudinger, H., Krisch, K., and Leonhauser, S. (1961). Role of ascorbic acid in microsomal electron transport and the possible relationship to hydroxylation reactions. *Ann. N.Y. Acad. Sci.* **91**, 195–207.

Stone, I. (1972). "The Healing Factor." Grosset & Dunlap, New York.

Svirbely, I., and Szent-Gyorgi, A. (1932). The chemical nature of vitamin C. *Biochem. J.* **26**, 865–870.

Szent-Gyorgi, A. (1927). The chemistry of the adrenal cortex. *Nature (London)* **119**, 782–783.

Szent-Gyorgi, A. (1928). Observations on the function of peroxidase systems and the chemistry of the adrenal cortex. *Biochem. J.* **22**, 1387–1409.

Szoke-Szotyori, K. (1967). Eine Methode zur Bestim mung der ascorbinsäure mittels Papier chromatographischer Trennung ihres Osazone. *Nahrung* **11**, 129–138.

Terland, O., and Flatmark, T. (1975). Ascorbate as a natural constituent of chromaffin granules from bovine adrenal medulla. *FEBS Lett.* **59**, 52–56.

Tillmans, J. (1930). *Z. Lebensmitteluntersuch.* **60**, 34.

Tirrell, J. G., and Westhead, E. W. (1979a). The uptake of ascorbic acid and dehydroascorbic acid by chromaffin granules of the adrenal medulla. *Neuroscience* **4**, 181–186.

Tirrell, J. G., and Westhead, E. W. (1977b). Ascorbate uptake and metabolism by adrenal medullary chromaffin granules. *Int. Catecholamine Symp., 4th*, pp. 316–319.

Tolbert, B. M., and Ward, J. B. (1982). Dehydroascorbic acid. *In* "Ascorbic Acid: Chemistry, Metabolism, Uses" (P. A. Seib and B. M. Tolbert, eds.), pp. 101–123. American Chemical Society, Washington, D.C.

Tolbert, B. M., Chen, A. W., Bell, E., and Baker, E. M. (1967). Metabolism of L-ascorbic 4-$^3$H-acid in man. *Am. J. Clin. Nutr.* **20**, 250.

Tolbert, B. M., Downing, M., Carlson, R. W., Knight, M., and Baker, E. M. (1975). Chemistry and metabolism of ascorbic acid and ascorbate sulfate. *Ann. N.Y. Acad. Sci.* **258**, 48–69.

Torrance, C. C. (1940). Diphtherial intoxication and vitamin C content of the suprarenals of guinea pigs. *J. Biol. Chem.* **132**, 575.

Tsao, C. S., and Salimi, S. L. (1981). Ultramicromethod for the measurement of ascorbic acid in plasma and white blood cells by high performance liquid chromatography with electrochemical detection. *J. Chromatogr.* **224**, 477–480.

Tweeten, T. (1979). Simultaneous analysis for ascorbic acid and dehydroascorbic acid. *Hewlett-Packard Appl. Brief:* 1.3.4.100.

Viveros, O. H., Arqueros, L., and Kirshner, N. (1971). Mechanism of secretion from the adrenal medulla. *Mol. Pharmacol.* **7**, 444–454.

Vogt, M. (1948). Ascorbic acid in adrenal blood. *J. Physiol. (London)* **107**, 239–243.

Von Schuching, S., Enns, T., and Abt, A. F. (1960). Connective tissue studies: IV. L-ascorbic 1-$^{14}$C acid excretion in intact and wounded guinea pigs on varying vitamin C intakes. *Am J. Physiol.* **199**, 423–428.

Waugh, W. A., and King, C. G. (1932a). Isolation and identification of vitamin C. *J. Biol. Chem.* **97**, 325–331.

Waugh, W. A., and King, C. G. (1932b). The chemical nature of vitamin C. *Science* **75**, 357–358.

Williams, R. (1971). "Nutrition Against Disease." Putnam, New York.

Wimalasiri, P., and Wills, R. B. H. (1983). Simultaneous analysis of ascorbic acid and dehydroascorbic acid in fruit and vegetables by high performance liquid chromatography. *J. Chromatogr.* **256**, 368–371.

Wurtman, R. J. (1966). Control of epinephrine synthesis in the adrenal medulla by the adrenal cortex: Hormonal specificity and dose–response characteristics. *Endocrinology* **79**, 608–614.

Yamazaki, I. (1962). The reduction of cytochrome *c* by enzyme-generated ascorbate free radical. *J. Biol. Chem.* **237**, 224–229.

Yamazaki, I., and Piette, L. H. (1961). Mechanism of free radical formation and disappearance during the ascorbic acid oxidase and peroxidase reactions. *Biochim. Biophys. Acta* **50**, 62–69.

Yamazaki, I., Mason, H. S., and Piette, L. (1960). Identification by electron paramagnetic resonance spectroscopy of free radicals generated from substrates by peroxidase. *J. Biol. Chem.* **235**, 2444–2449.

Yavorsky, M., Almaden, P., and King, C. G. (1934). The vitamin C content of human tissues. *J. Biol. Chem.* **106**, 525–529.

Zloch, Z., Cerven, J., and Ginter, E. (1971). Radiochemical evaluation of the 2,4-dinitrophenylhydrazine method for determination of vitamin C. *Anal. Biochem.* **43**, 99–106.

VITAMINS AND HORMONES, VOL. 42

# Vitamin K-Dependent Formation of Bone Gla Protein (Osteocalcin) and Its Function

## PAUL A. PRICE

*Department of Biology*
*University of California at San Diego*
*La Jolla, California*

## I. INTRODUCTION

The bone Gla protein (BGP, osteocalcin) is presently the best characterized noncollagenous bone protein. Characteristic chemical features are small size, typically 49 or 50 residues, and existence within the molecule of three residues of the vitamin K-dependent amino acid, $\gamma$-carboxyglutamic acid (Gla). BGP is among the most abundant noncollagenous bone proteins and appears to be a universal constituent of the skeleton and tooth dentine of all vertebrates. Since its synthesis is regulated by 1,25-dihydroxyvitamin $D_3$, it is likely that BGP plays a role in the action of this hormone on bone.

In spite of the concerted efforts of an increasing number of scientists, the precise function of BGP in the formation and metabolism of bone remains uncertain. Considerable progress has, however, been made in identifying bone abnormalities associated with BGP depletion in vitamin K-deficient animals. The first objective of this review will be to examine our current knowledge of BGP as it bears on the possible functions of the protein.

Since the last review of BGP was written (1), there has been an explosion of interest in the use of serum BGP measurements in the clinical evaluation of bone disease. While a detailed analysis of this area will not be undertaken, a second aim of the present review is to evaluate the general relationships between serum BGP levels and bone metabolism.


II. Occurrence


BGP has been detected in the calcified tissues of all vertebrates examined to date. In most species, it is one of the most abundant noncollagenous bone proteins. For example, the BGP content of rat, bovine, chicken, and swordfish bone is typically 1–3 mg per gram of dry undemineralized tissue (2,3). The number of BGP molecules in the skeleton of such vertebrates ranks the protein as numerically one of the 10 most abundant proteins in the entire animal. There are, in fact, approximately as many BGP molecules in bone as there are molecules of tropocollagen or crystals of hydroxyapatite (3). Tooth dentine contains BGP in amounts comparable to those found in bone (4), an observation which is consistent with the fact that dentine has a calcified collagenous matrix generally similar to that of bone (5). BGP cannot, however, be detected in tooth enamel (3), a mineralized tissue which differs from dentine and bone in that the average size of its hydroxyapatite crystals is far larger and that it lacks a collagenous matrix. The presence of $\gamma$-carboxyglutamic acid in renal calculi (6), calcified atherosclerotic plaques (3,7), and ectopic calcifications (8) indicates that pathological calcifications contain vitamin K-dependent proteins, and so possibly contain BGP.

In addition to calcified tissues, BGP has been detected in the plasma of all vertebrates examined (9–11). The amount of BGP in rat plasma is typically only 100–300 ng/ml and plasma BGP is cleared by kidney filtration with a $t_{1/2}$ of 5 minutes (12). A significant amount of daily

BGP synthesized by bone cells appears in plasma instead of bone. For example, a 100 g rat will replace half of its 300 ng/ml concentration of plasma BGP ~300 times per day. This requires the secretion into plasma of 0.5 mg BGP per day. For comparison, a rat of this size will deposit between 2 and 4 mg of BGP per day into the extracellular bone matrix.

Tissue content of BGP is unusually low in humans. For example, BGP levels in human bone are 0.05–0.1 mg per gram (13), about 5% of that in the bones of most other vertebrates. BGP levels are also unusually low in human plasma, 5–10 ng/ml (9,14) compared to 100–300 ng/ml for rat and calf plasma (9,10). The dramatically lower BGP levels in humans suggests that the protein plays a less crucial role in the metabolism of the human skeleton and could therefore provide an important clue to its function.

## III. ISOLATION

We have used two general procedures for the isolation of BGP from bone (3,15). Both entail first removing the adhering connective tissue and then freeze-drying the bone. If the bone is particularly oily, it is useful to extract it with acetone before freeze-drying. Dry bone samples are then ground to the consistency of coarse sand in a blender or, for large-scale preparations, a mill. Ground bone is washed extensively with cold water to remove blood proteins and then dried with acetone. In one extraction method, ground bone is placed within dialysis tubing with two parts by volume of 0.5 $M$ EDTA, pH 7.4, and dialyzed against the same buffer in the cold (3). BGP emerges from bone in parallel with demineralization and is retained within the dialysis tubing. Purification of BGP from the extract is then achieved by a combination of gel filtration over Sephadex G-100 and gradient elution from DEAE-Sephadex (3).

One drawback to this procedure has been the occasional appearance of proteolytic cleavage products. While this has never been a consistent problem in the isolation of BGP from calf bone, it is a problem in the extraction of BGP from rat or human bone. The second procedure was developed to enable the isolation of BGP when endogenous proteases are present (3). BGP is first extracted by demineralization of bone with 10 parts by weight of 10% formic acid. Purification of BGP from the extract can then be accomplished by gel filtration over a Sephacryl S-200 column equilibrated with 6 $M$ guanidine-HCl (3) and gradient elution from DEAE-Sephadex. While it should be noted that this procedure probably disrupts the tertiary structure of BGP more than EDTA extraction does, in our experience BGP purified by the formic acid procedure retains such indices of normal function as hydroxyapatite and $Ca^{2+}$ binding, the ability to retard hydroxyapatite formation, and antigenicity.

## IV. Structure

### A. Primary Structure of BGP

The molecular weights of calf and chicken BGP have been determined by sedimentation equilibrium centrifugation and are 5800 and 6500, respectively (16,17). Both molecular weight values agree well with those computed from the corresponding covalent structures. In contrast, the apparent molecular weight of BGP determined by gel filtration and by SDS–gel electrophoresis is about 12,000 (2,3,18). Since sedimentation equilibrium centrifugation studies carried out under the same conditions used in the gel filtration study do not reveal BGP dimerization (3), it seems probable that the anomalously high apparent molecular weights are due to the shape or charge density of the molecule.

The primary structure has been determined for BGP isolated from calf, swordfish, human, chicken, and monkey bone (15–17, 19–21), and the N-terminal sequence has been reported for BGP isolated from rat bone (22) and dentine (4). A comparison of these structures reveals a remarkable degree of conservation over evolutionary time. This is well illustrated by the comparison of calf and human BGP with swordfish BGP (Fig. 1). The structural features common to these three proteins, which must be sufficiently important to BGP function to have survived the 400 million years since swordfish diverged from terrestrial vertebrates, include the sequence positions of the three Gla residues and the associated disulfide bond. Indeed, in the region from residues 16–31, which contains the three Gla residues, only four amino acids have changed. While considerable sequence homology is found between the Gla-containing N-terminal regions of the different vitamin K-dependent coagulation factors, there is no homology between the Gla-containing region of these proteins and BGP. In addition, the adjacent pairs of Gla residues which are found in all Gla-containing blood coagulation factors are absent in BGP. The Gla-containing regions of BGP and of the blood coagulation factors must therefore have arisen independently in evolution to serve specialized functions in bone and in blood coagulation.

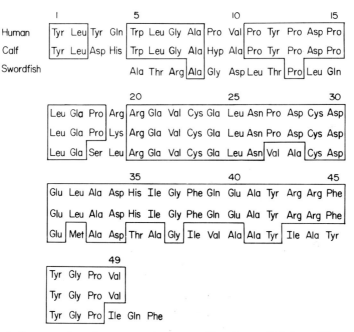

Fɪɢ. 1. Sequence homology among human, calf, and swordfish bone Gla proteins. From Poser *et al.* (15), used with permission.

A new Gla-containing protein has recently been discovered in urea extracts of demineralized bovine bone (23). This protein, termed matrix Gla protein (MGP) because of its affinity for the organic matrix of bone, contains five Gla residues and has an apparent $M_r$ of 15,000. Preliminary sequence analysis of the Gla-containing region of matrix Gla protein has revealed a striking homology with BGP (24). Indeed, three of the five Gla residues in MGP are in exactly the same sequence positions relative to the single disulfide bond, as are the three Gla residues in BGP relative to its disulfide bond. This sequence homology indicates that the Gla-containing regions of MGP and BGP may have common specialized functions, probably in the binding to hydroxyapatite in bone (see later).

In both the vitamin K-dependent coagulation factors and BGP, γ-carboxyglutamic acid residues are restricted to the N-terminal region of the protein. In this region, all glutamic acid residues have been γ-carboxylated. There is no structural feature common to BGP and the coagulation factors to explain targeting of these particular proteins for γ-carboxylation, but all of these proteins are secreted and might have a leader peptide with the appropriate recognition site for the γ-carboxylase.

## B. Structure of the BGP Message

A significant portion of the rat BGP message structure has recently been established (25). A cDNA clone for rat BGP was first isolated from a λgtll cDNA library for the 17/2 rat osteosarcoma cell line. This 314 base-pair partial BGP cDNA contains the entire coding region for the 50-residue protein found in bone, the 3′-untranslated region, and a short segment of the leader peptide (25). Two basic amino acid residues separate the leader peptide from BGP, suggesting that the secreted form of BGP is produced by proteolytic cleavage of an intracellular precursor in a manner analogous to the processing of several prohormones and other serum proteins (26). Preliminary results from Northern blot analysis of ROS 17/2 RNA further showed that the BGP cDNA hybridized strongly to a single RNA band of ~600 nucleotides. This putative BGP messenger RNA is large enough to encode the 9000-Da immunoreactive intracellular precursor previously identified in ROS 17/2 cells (see below) as well as a postulated signal peptide of 18–33 residues, which is cotranslationally cleaved from most secreted proteins after insertion of the nascent polypeptide chain into the endoplasmic reticulum (27). Given the limited coding capacity of this small messenger RNA, it seems unlikely that the 35- and 85-kDa components of developing chicken bone identified by a chicken BGP radioimmunoassay (28) could be precursors to the 5.7-kDa protein.

The complete 50 amino acid sequence of secreted rat BGP can be predicted from its cDNA. The nucleotide sequence codes for asparagines at positions 4 and 28, which were previously reported to be aspartic acids in the partial sequence of rat cortical bone BGP (22). Comparison of rat and calf BGPs reveals only two nonidentical residues between postions 6 and 42 inclusive, and these are the relatively conservative substitutions of histidine for lysine at position 19 and asparagine for aspartic acid at position 28. In contrast, the amino and carboxy-terminal regions of these two proteins are significantly different. In particular, nonhomologies within the carboxy-terminal peptides may account for the lack of cross-reactivity between rat and calf BGP antibodies. Human BGP, which does cross-react with antibody to bovine BGP, is identical to the calf protein in the carboxy-terminal region (15).

## V. Properties

BGP is a very acidic protein, with an isoelectric point of 4.0 and a net negative charge at pH 8 of 9 (18,29). Because of its high negative charge density and its small size, BGP has a mobility at pH 8.9 of $R_f$ 0.57 in 20% polyacrylamide gels and $R_f$ 1.0 in 10% polyacrylamide gels (30). In our experience, no other protein in demineralization extracts of bone has a mobility in 20% polyacrylamide gels which is as great as that of BGP.

## A. SPECIFIC CHEMICAL MODIFICATION OF GLA RESIDUES IN BGP

To explore the role of $\gamma$-carboxyglutamic acid residues in the interaction of BGP with $Ca^{2+}$ and with hydroxyapatite, we have developed two procedures for the specific decarboxylation of $\gamma$-carboxyglutamate to glutamate (29) (Fig. 2). These decarboxylation reactions yield a modified BGP which appears to be identical to that found in a vitamin K-deficient animal (12). Both procedures are based on the fact that the protonated side chain of Gla decarboxylates readily in the absence of water. Thus, by drying a sample of BGP from 50 m$M$ HCl or 50 m$M$ NH$_4$HCO$_3$ and then heating, decarboxylation can be achieved in the complete absence of hydrolytic side reactions which would otherwise occur.

We have also developed a specific and nondegradative method to

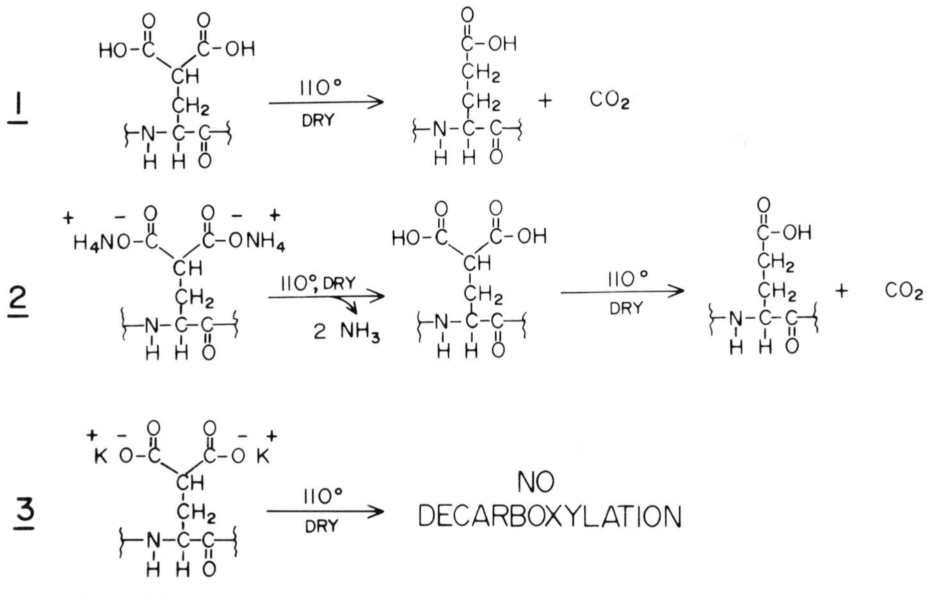

FIG. 2. Models for the thermal decarboxylation of $\gamma$-carboxyglutamic acid to yield glutamic acid in dry salts of Gla-containing proteins.

tritium label proteins that contain Gla residues (31). This procedure is
based on our discovery that the $\gamma$-proton of Gla exchanges readily with
tritium-labeled water below pH 5, but is resistant to exchange at
higher values of pH. Since no proton found in the 20 common amino
acids has this pH dependence for exchange with water, it is possible to
introduce $^3$H label by equilibration with $^3$H$_2$O at pH 5 and then remove
$^3$H from all acid-exchangeable sites other than Gla by desalting into
base. Recent reviews are available which discuss the methods for
chemical modification of Gla residues in proteins (32–34) and for the
quantitative determination of Gla by the analysis of alkaline hydroly-
zates of proteins (35).

## B. Interaction of BGP with Ca$^{2+}$ and Hydroxyapatite

Bone Gla protein binds Ca$^{2+}$, although the strength of this association is relatively weak. Scatchard plot analysis of Ca$^{2+}$ binding to
bovine BGP revealed the presence of three Ca$^{2+}$ binding sites with an
average dissociation constant of 2–3 m$M$ (19,30,37). The corresponding
analyses of Ca$^{2+}$ binding to chicken BGP revealed two Ca$^{2+}$ binding
sites with an average dissociation constant of 0.8 m$M$ (17). Since there
are three Gla residues in bovine BGP, it seems reasonable to postulate
that the three Ca$^{2+}$ binding sites are provided by the side chain of Gla.
This interpretation is supported by the observation that decarboxylation of Gla to Glu abolishes Ca$^{2+}$ binding to BGP (29). Such coordination of Ca$^{2+}$ by Gla residues in BGP would leave two Ca$^{2+}$ coordination
sites unoccupied by protein ligands and therefore free to function in
binding interactions with bone mineral.

Ca$^{2+}$ binding to fully carboxylated BGP alters the circular dichroism
spectrum and the immunochemical properties of the protein (36,37).
The apparent $\alpha$-helical content of BGP, which can be estimated from
the circular dichroism spectrum, increases from 1% in the absence of
Ca$^{2+}$ to 14% in the presence of Ca$^{2+}$ for bovine BGP (36), and from 8%
in the absence of Ca$^{2+}$ to 35% in the presence of Ca$^{2+}$ for chicken BGP
(37). Since the apparent $\alpha$-helical content of decarboxylated BGP is
closer to that of native BGP in the presence of Ca$^{2+}$ (36), it appears
likely that Ca$^{2+}$ binding to the Gla residues in the native protein
enables it to adopt a conformation similar to that of the decarboxylated
BGP molecule. This inference is supported strongly by the discovery
that an antibody which reacts only with native bovine BGP in the
presence of Ca$^{2+}$ reacts equally well with decarboxylated BGP whether
or not Ca$^{2+}$ is present (36). One interpretation of these observations
(36) is that the Gla-containing region of BGP, a region previously

predicted to be $\alpha$-helical on the assumption that Gla stabilizes an $\alpha$-helix to an extent similar to Glu (37), can in fact only exist as an $\alpha$-helix when the Gla residues bind $Ca^{2+}$. In the absence of $Ca^{2+}$, Gla residues would destablize the $\alpha$-helix, perhaps because of the extra negative charge on the Gla side chains.

The affinity of BGP for hydroxyapatite is far greater than for $Ca^{2+}$. At high concentrations of BGP (over $10^{-6}$ $M$), the addition of hydroxyapatite simply titrates the protein from solution (29). This titration is a measure of the binding capacity of a particular hydroxyapatite preparation for BGP. One preparation used extensively in our own studies gives, for example, a binding capacity of 1 mg of BGP per 17 mg of hydroxyapatite (29). In general, the best binding data for any type of interaction are those collected when the participants are studied at concentrations near the dissociation constant for the interaction. To satisfy this condition for BGP, given the high affinity of BGP for hydroxyapatite, it is necessary to use quantities of protein below the limits of UV detection. Two procedures have been employed in our laboratory, $^{125}I$ labeling of BGP and specific radioimmunoassay; both procedures yield the same estimate of BGP binding affinity for hydroxyapatite. As can be seen in Fig. 3, the binding of native BGP to hydroxyapatite exhibits a simple logarithmic binding isotherm. At pH 7.4 in 0.15 $M$ NaCl at 25°C, the dissociation constant for BGP binding

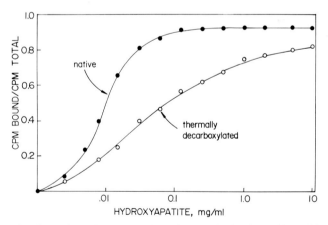

FIG. 3. Role of $\gamma$-carboxyglutamic acid residues in the binding of bone Gla protein to synthetic hydroxyapatite. After 1 hour of incubation at pH 7.4, 25°C, in 0.15 $M$ NaCl, the extent of binding was assayed by measuring the extent of $^{125}I$-labeled BGP in the supernatant after sedimentation of hydroxyapatite. From Price et al. (38), used with permission.

to hydroxyapatite is $\sim 10^{-7}$ $M$ in apatite binding sites, or 0.021 mg/ml in weight of apatite (38).

The binding of BGP to hydroxyapatite probably involves the bidentate chelation of $Ca^{2+}$ atoms on the crystal surface by the malonate side chain of Gla. This is supported by the fact that binding to hydroxyapatite completely prevents the thermal decarboxylation of Gla residues to Glu residues. As expected, decarboxylation of Gla residues in BGP markedly reduces the affinity of the protein for hydroxyapatite in buffered saline (Fig. 3) or in serum (12). In addition, the non-γ-carboxylated BGP synthesized in an animal treated with the vitamin K antagonist warfarin neither binds strongly to hydroxyapatite nor accumulates significantly in bone (39).

## C. Regulation of Hydroxyapatite Formation

BGP is a potent inhibitor of hydroxyapatite formation *in vitro* (3,29), a property which may be important to its biological function (40). In supersaturated solutions of calcium phosphate at pH 7.4, inhibition of crystallization by BGP requires the presence of Gla residues and an intact disulfide bond (Fig. 4). The degree to which BGP retards crystallization in this system depends critically on the concentration of BGP, with a doubling of the time required for half-maximal crystal formation at a BGP concentration of 6 $\mu M$ (29). Since the final amount of hydroxyapatite formed is not affected by BGP, the effect of BGP is exclusively on the kinetics of mineral formation rather than on the thermodynamic end point (solubility product) of the mineral phase.

The effect of BGP on mineralization has also been tested in supersaturated solutions of calcium phosphate seeded with a small amount of hydroxyapatite (41). The results of these investigations are in agreement with the earlier investigations outlined above: BGP is a potent inhibitor of mineralization only if it contains Gla residues and an intact disulfide bond, and the effect of BGP is kinetic rather than thermodynamic. All the above studies demonstrate that BGP has the *in vitro* ability to regulate the rate of mineralization, and so could function as a regulator of the mineralization rate in bone.

## VI. Biosynthesis

The most direct evidence that BGP is synthesized in bone has been obtained by the analysis of proteins labeled with [³H]proline in the primary culture of 1 mm thick cross-sectional wafers of calf trabecular

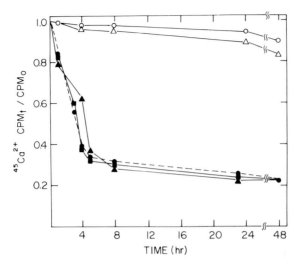

Fɪɢ. 4. Inhibition of hydroxyapatite crystallization by native, decarboxylated, and reduced and S-carboxyamidomethylated bone Gla protein. Hydroxyapatite formation was monitored by the precipitation of $^{45}Ca^{2+}$ from a solution which contained 15 m$M$ PIPES, pH 7.4, 0.15 $M$ KCl, and an initial Ca x P product of 25 m$M^2$. (○), 35 $\mu M$ native BGP; (△), 35 $\mu M$ BGP after heating as potassium salt (no decarboxylation); (▲), 35 $\mu M$ BGP after reduction and S-carboxyamidomethylation; (■), 140 $\mu M$ BGP after heating as NH$_4^+$ salt (complete decarboxylation of Gla to Glu); (●), no protein. From Poser and Price (29), used with permission.

and cortical bone (30). These studies showed that [³H]proline label is incorporated into a protein identical to BGP in molecular weight, electrophoretic mobility, isoelectric focusing position, and tryptic peptide mapping. Additional evidence that BGP is synthesized in bone has been provided by the demonstration that ¹⁴C is incorporated into protein-bound γ-carboxyglutamate during incubation of chick bone microsomes with ¹⁴CO₂ in the presence of vitamin K (42). One of the proteins labeled in such experiments has an apparent molecular weight on SDS–gel electrophoresis which is the same as that of BGP (43).

Several lines of evidence point to osteoblasts as the cells in bone which synthesize BGP. BGP has a residue of 4-hydroxyproline in its structure (16), an observation which indicates that the cells that synthesize BGP have proline 4-monooxygenase. This enzyme has been used as a marker for osteoblasts in culture. BGP is synthesized by those clonal rat osteosarcoma cells which display features of the osteoblastic phenotype such as high PTH responsiveness and high alkaline phosphatase activity (44,45). BGP is also synthesized by primary cultures of osteoblastic cells derived from human trabecular bone (46).

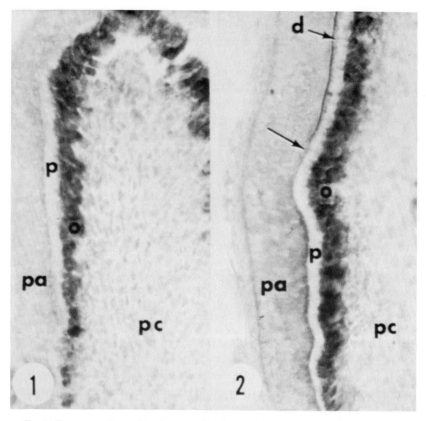

F₁ɢ. 5. Frozen sections of undemineralized rat tooth germs treated with antisera to BGP. pa, Preameloblasts; d, dentine; p, predentine; o, odontoblasts; pc, pulp cells. The unlabeled arrow in (2) denotes the approximate onset of dentine formation. Note the intense immunoperoxidase staining of odontoblasts.

Finally, recent immunohistologic studies indicate that osteoblasts in the proximal tibia and calvaria of 3-day-old rats stain intensely with antibody raised against rat BGP (47). Osteoclasts, distinguished from osteoblasts in the bone sections by staining for acid phosphatase, did not react with the anti-BGP antibody (47).

BGP is also synthesized by the odontoblasts in teeth (48,49). Studies with cultured rat tooth germs have shown that labeled amino acids are incorporated into a protein identical in size and immunoreactivity with rat BGP (48). As shown in Fig. 5, the only cells in the developing tooth which react with antibody raised against rat BGP are the odontoblasts (49). Ameloblasts, which synthesize enamel, and the pulpal cells in the tooth core do not react with the antibody.

The developing tooth germ shown in Fig. 5 encompasses several stages of dentine formation. The upper part of the figure shows that odontoblasts synthesize the unmineralized collagenous matrix of predentine and, further from the cell at the interface with enamel, mineralize predentine to dentine. In the lower part of this figure, odontoblasts synthesize predentine, but will not begin to mineralize predentine to dentine for at least 1 day. It is intriguing to note that the odontoblasts engaged in synthesizing predentine but not yet in mineralizing predentine to form dentine already stain intensely with the antibody raised against BGP. This observation reveals a temporal dissociation between BGP synthesis and mineralization and suggests that the protein could act to delay the mineralization of predentine.

The clonal rat osteosarcoma cell line which produces BGP, ROS 17/2, has provided a useful system to explore molecular aspects of BGP synthesis and secretion (44). The ROS 17/2 cells secrete into culture medium a protein which is identical to BGP isolated from bone in molecular weight and electrophoretic mobility. BGP can also be detected within ROS 17/2 cells at a level sufficient to sustain 2–3 hours of secretion. The intracellular antigen, however, is a mixture of a component identical to the 5800-MW BGP isolated from bone (20%) and a 9000-MW component (80%). It seems likely that the higher molecular weight immunoreactive protein inside ROS 17/2 cells is a BGP precursor analogous to proinsulin or procalcitonin. The presence of both putative precursor and BGP itself inside cells indicates that precursor is fully processed to product BGP prior to secretion, a result expected from the fact that only BGP can be detected in cell media (44).

## VII. Regulation of BGP Production

### A. Regulation by 1,25-(OH)$_2$D$_3$ in Cell Culture

To date, the best characterized response of bone cells to 1,25-(OH)$_2$D$_3$ is the increased synthesis of BGP (50). In the ROS 17/2 line, administration of 1,25-(OH)$_2$D$_3$ increases intracellular BGP levels to sixfold above basal levels within 12 hours (50) (Fig. 6). A corresponding sixfold increase in the rate of BGP secretion is seen by 15 hours. Since there is substantial BGP synthesis in the absence of 1,25-(OH)$_2$D$_3$ (Fig. 6), BGP synthesis is modulated by rather than dependent upon vitamin D. This regulatory mechanism contrasts with that of the cytosolic Ca$^{2+}$ binding protein, whose synthesis is absolutely dependent upon vitamin D.

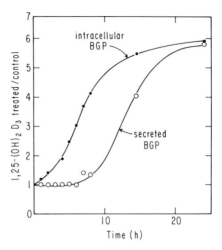

Fɪɢ. 6. Stimulation of BGP synthesis and secretion by 1.25-(OH)₂D₃. The media of confluent 60-mm culture plates were exchanged for the same media or media containing 1 ng/ml of 1,25-(OH)₂D₃ at time zero. Two experimental and two control plates were terminated at each time point and analyzed for intracellular and media levels of BGP. Each point is the average experimental value divided by the average control. From Price and Baukol (50), used with permission.

The BGP synthesis response is dose dependent and saturatable, with a half-maximal response at a 1,25-(OH)₂D₃ concentration of $10^{-10}$ $M$ (50). While the total concentration of 1,25-(OH)₂D₃ in rat serum is approximately equal to the concentration required for half-maximal BGP response in cell culture, it should be noted that the BGP response in the cell culture system was determined in the absence of serum and, consequently, the absence of vitamin D binding protein. There is considerable circumstantial evidence that the biologically relevant concentration of 1,25-(OH)₂D₃ is that of the unbound hormone rather than the hormone bound to vitamin D binding protein (51). Recent studies have shown that a far higher dose of 1,25-(OH)₂D₃ is consequently required for half-maximal stimulation of BGP synthesis in 100% serum than in serum-free media (52).

The action of 1,25-(OH)₂D₃ on BGP synthesis appears to be exerted at the transcriptional level. As would be expected for a transcriptionally regulated process, the BGP response is blocked completely by the inhibitors α-amanitin and actinomycin D (Fig. 7) (53). Preliminary investigations using the cDNA probe for BGP further show that 1,25-(OH)₂D₃ treatment produces the expected increase in the level of BGP message (personal observations). The transcriptional burst which follows 1,25-(OH)₂D₃ administration appears to be confined to the first 15

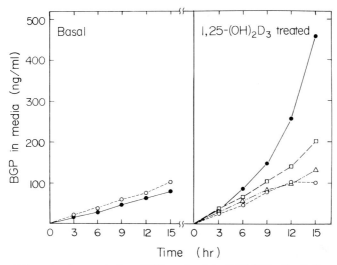

Fig. 7. Effect of actinomycin D on BGP synthesis by ROS 17/2 cells. Cells were grown in microtiter dishes with daily changes of Coon's F-12 media containing 2% fetal calf serum. At time zero, actinomycin D ± 1 ng/ml 1,25-$(OH)_2D_3$ was added to recently confluent monolayers in serum-free media. Each point represents the average radioimmunoassay data from three microtiter wells. (●), No inhibitor; (□), 0.005 $\mu M$ actinomycin D; (△), 0.05 $\mu M$ actinomycin D; (○), 0.5 $\mu M$ actinomycin D. From Pan and Price (53), used with permission.

hours of exposure to the hormone (53). Thus, treatment with transcriptional inhibitors at times up to 15 hours after 1,25-$(OH)_2D_3$ exposure truncates the BGP response to the expected degree while addition of inhibitors after 15 hours of exposure to the hormone does not alter the increased rate of BGP synthesis.

The lifetime of the BGP message in unstimulated or fully 1,25-$(OH)_2D_3$-stimulated cells appears to be quite long. This is indicated by the fact that 15 hours of exposure to transcriptional inhibitors affects neither basal (Fig. 7) nor fully stimulated (53) BGP synthesis. In addition, withdrawal of 1,25-$(OH)_2D_3$ by multiple exchanges with hormone-free media does not reduce BGP synthesis in fully stimulated cells over a subsequent 48-hour period (unpublished observations). Thus, the bone cell imprints a level of BGP synthesis response during its initial 15 hours of exposure to 1,25-$(OH)_2D_3$ and then retains this response without further BGP transcription.

This transcriptional burst model for the regulation of BGP synthesis by bone cells raises the interesting question of what prevents additional BGP message synthesis at 1,25-$(OH)_2D_3$ exposure times longer than 15 hours. A related question is what reestablishes sensitivity to

1,25-(OH)$_2$D$_3$ in the previously stimulated cell. It is the author's opinion that the answer to both questions will lie in a better understanding of the ROS 17/2 cell line. If, as has been postulated, the ROS 17/2 cells represent a mixed population of stem cells and differentiated cells, it could be that only the differentiated cells can give the increased BGP synthesis response. After the 1,25-(OH)$_2$D$_3$-induced transcriptional burst, the differentiated cell would become refractory to further stimulation, perhaps for its lifetime. The reacquisition of 1,25-(OH)$_2$D$_3$ responsiveness in the cell culture would then depend upon the rate at which stem cells grow and differentiate to 1,25-(OH)$_2$D$_3$-responsive, BGP-producing cells.

## B. Regulation by 1,25-(OH)$_2$D$_3$ in Animals

BGP in serum provides a convenient index of regulation of BGP synthesis by 1,25-(OH)$_2$D$_3$ in animals. As discussed below, serum BGP arises exclusively from new synthesis and is cleared by kidney filtration with a $t_{1/2}$ of 5 minutes (12). Because of the rapid turnover of serum BGP, a change in the rate of BGP secretion from bone cells should be reflected in altered serum levels of BGP within a few minutes.

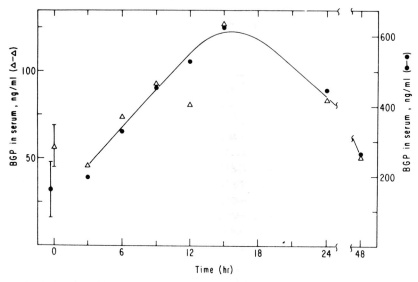

FIG. 8. Serum BGP response to 1,25-(OH)$_2$D$_3$ in 47-day-old (●) and 11-month-old (△) rats. Animals received a single intravenous injection of 350 ng 1,25-(OH)$_2$D$_3$ per 180 g of body weight at time zero. Each time point represents the average serum BGP level of 4 rats. From Price and Baukol (54), used with permission.

As can be seen in Fig. 8, the amount of serum BGP increases three-to fourfold after intravenous administration of $1,25\text{-}(OH)_2D_3$ to either young or old rats (54). Twelve hours are required for this response, a time course identical to that seen for the BGP response in ROS 17/2 cells (Fig. 8). Since the basal level of serum BGP in the young rats is 300 ng/ml, while that in the older rats is 100 ng/ml, it is evident that the degree to which serum BGP levels are increased by $1,25\text{-}(OH)_2D_3$ is independent not only of the age of the rat, but also of the initial level of serum BGP. The half-maximal serum BGP response is achieved by the administration of 80 ng of $1,25\text{-}(OH)_2D_3$ per 180 g of body weight (54). While this $1,25\text{-}(OH)_2D_3$ dose is considered pharmacologic, it should be noted that the notion of physiologic $1,25\text{-}(OH)_2D_3$ dosages is based solely on the serum $Ca^{2+}$ response of vitamin D-deficient animals. In vitamin D- and $Ca^{2+}$-replete rats of the same age and sex as the rats used in the BGP study, half-maximal response of the duodenal $Ca^{2+}$ binding protein also required 80 ng of $1,25\text{-}(OH)_2D_3$ per 180 g of body weight (55).

Serum BGP also is elevated in humans treated therapeutically with $1,25\text{-}(OH)_2D_3$ (56). In 10 patients with X-linked hypophosphatemia, there was an average 1.9-fold increase in serum BGP after 7–12 months of treatment with 10–72 ng/kg/day of $1,25\text{-}(OH)_2D_3$. A comparable 2.4-fold average increase was also found in 6 patients with autosomal recessive vitamin D dependence treated for 1 week with 13–27 ng/kg/day of $1,25\text{-}(OH)_2D_3$. While the degree to which $1,25\text{-}(OH)_2D_3$-elevated serum BGP in these patients is somewhat lower than the increase produced by $1,25\text{-}(OH)_2D_3$ in rats, the doses used in the human studies were lower than those used in the experiments in rats and may not have been sufficient to elicit the full BGP synthesis response.

The best evidence that the BGP synthesis response to $1,25\text{-}(OH)_2D_3$ is physiological comes from studies on the level of serum BGP in rats weaned onto a $Ca^{2+}$-deficient diet (57), a stress known to increase serum levels of $1,25\text{-}(OH)_2D_3$ by over 10-fold (58). As can be seen in Fig. 9, dietary $Ca^{2+}$ deficiency produced a fourfold increase in serum BGP only in the vitamin D-replete rat. In the vitamin D- and $Ca^{2+}$-deficient rat, serum BGP remained at the level of the $Ca^{2+}$-replete controls (57). When the vitamin D- and $Ca^{2+}$-deficient animals subsequently received 25 international units of vitamin $D_3$ daily, serum BGP levels increased to the elevated levels of the vitamin D-replete, $Ca^{2+}$-deficient rat within 2 days (59).

As is the case for the ROS 17/2 cells, BGP synthesis in the animal can occur in the absence of vitamin D. Bones of vitamin D-deficient chickens contain amounts of BGP 60% of normal (60), and vitamin D-deficient rats show serum BGP levels still 59% of normal (1). Since the

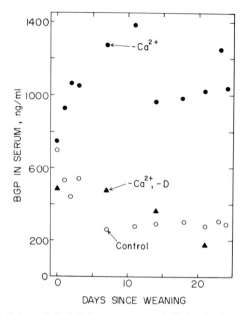

F<small>IG</small>. 9. Effect of dietary $Ca^{2+}$ deficiency on serum BGP levels. Rats were weaned onto a $Ca^{2+}$-deficient (●), a $Ca^{2+}$- and vitamin D-deficient (▲), or a normal (○) diet at 18 days of age. Each time point is the average serum BGP level in 4 rats. From Price *et al.* (57), used with permission.

unstimulated level of BGP synthesis is high, it seems probable that BGP plays a role in bone metabolism which is independent of vitamin D. This suggests that the physiological role of the $1,25$-$(OH)_2D_3$ regulation of BGP synthesis is to accelerate a normal BGP action in bone in order to adjust bone metabolism to stresses such as dietery $Ca^{2+}$ deficiency.

## VIII. P<small>LASMA</small> BGP

### A. R<small>ELATIONSHIP BETWEEN</small> P<small>LASMA</small> BGP <small>AND</small> BGP <small>IN</small> B<small>ONE</small>

With the development of sensitive radioimmunoassays for the detection of BGP came the discovery that BGP is in plasma at concentrations ranging from 8 ng/ml in human adults (9,14) to 200 ng/ml in weanling rats (10). The molecular weight of plasma BGP is identical to that for BGP extracted from bone (9,10,14). Plasma BGP also binds to added hydroxyapatite with an affinity equal to that for BGP extracted from bone (12), which indicates that the plasma protein has a full complement of $\gamma$-carboxyglutamate residues.

At the time BGP was first discovered in the circulation, it was unclear whether it was derived from new cellular synthesis or from the release of extracellular bone matrix BGP during bone resorption. This question has been resolved by analysis of plasma BGP in rats which have been given the vitamin K antagonist warfarin (12). In one investigation, normal rats received a single dosage of warfarin at the start of the experiment. Blood samples were removed at suitable intervals and the serum BGP in these samples was tested for the ability to bind to added hydroxyapatite. As can be seen in Fig. 10, plasma BGP loses the ability to bind to hydroxyapatite within 3 hours of warfarin administration. Since BGP in which all $\gamma$-carboxyglutamate residues have been thermally decarboxylated to glutamate also cannot bind from plasma to hydroxyapatite, it seems probable that the shift in plasma BGP affinity for hydroxyapatite after warfarin administration is best explained by the inhibition of the vitamin K-dependent $\alpha$-carboxylation of newly synthesized BGP. Since BGP isolated from the long bones of these rats at the end of the experiment, 8 hours after warfarin

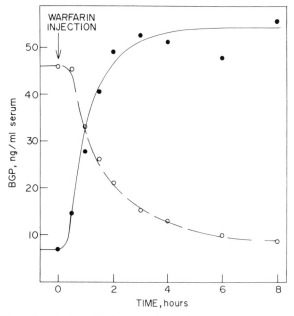

Fig. 10. Effect of warfarin on hydroxyapatite binding properties of serum BGP in 10-month-old rats. Serum samples were withdrawn at the indicated times after warfarin administration and tested for the ability to bind to hydroxyapatite. (●), Serum BGP not bound to hydroxyapatite; (○), serum BGP bound to hydroxyapatite. From Price *et al.* (12), used with permission.

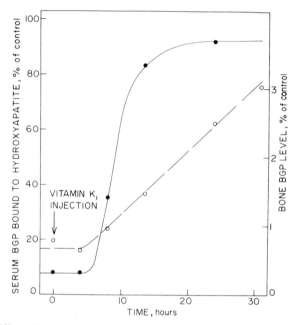

F<small>IG</small>. 11. Effect of vitamin K administration on BGP levels in 18-day-old rats which had been maintained from birth on warfarin. (●), Fraction of serum BGP which can bind to hydroxyapatite; (○), bone level of BGP as determined by radioimmunoassay of formic acid extracts of powdered femurs. Data are the average of determinations made on each of 6 animals killed at the indicated times. From Price *et al.* (12), used with permission.

administration, was fully γ-carboxylated and was able to bind to hydroxyapatite normally, it is evident that the abnormal plasma BGP in these animals could not have come from the release of extracellular bone matrix BGP during bone resorption.

In a second experiment, rats were given warfarin from birth in order to reduce bone content of BGP to 1% of normal, and then were given vitamin $K_1$. Within 12 hours serum BGP which can bind to added hydroxyapatite had returned to normal amounts, while the level of BGP in bone had only risen to 1.5% of normal (Fig. 11). Again, it is clear that the BGP in serum must arise from new cellular synthesis and subsequent secretion into plasma rather than from the release of bone matrix BGP during bone resorption.

The turnover of BGP in plasma is quite fast (12). One indication of this is the complete shift in the ability of serum BGP to bind to hydroxyapatite within 3 hours of warfarin administration. Since warfarin inhibits the γ-carboxylation of BGP at the microsomal level, this result indicates that the interval between new BGP synthesis within the cell and complete turnover of BGP in serum is only 3 hours. More direct evidence on the turnover of serum BGP has been obtained by following the level of BGP in serum after the injection of large amounts of purified BGP or the administration of [125]I-labeled BGP. These experiments concur in showing that the bulk of serum BGP is cleared with a half-time of 4–5 minutes. This rate of clearance is comparable to that of other small proteins, such as RNase (61), believed to be cleared from serum by glomerular filtration. Additional evidence that BGP is cleared from serum by the kidney is provided by the fact that most [125]I-labeled BGP initially accumulates in the kidney and by the observation that nephrectomy causes serum BGP concentration to rise rapidly (12).

The fact that serum BGP arises from new cellular synthesis and binds strongly to added hydroxyapatite has raised the possibility that BGP found in bone represents serum BGP bound to bone hydroxyapatite (9). Indeed, the level of BGP found in bone is essentially identical to that predicted upon the amount of BGP in plasma and the affinity of BGP for hydroxyapatite (9). It should be noted, however, that the affinity of BGP for hydroxyapatite used in this calculation was determined *in vitro* using purified BGP in 0.15 $M$ NaCl at pH 7.4 (38). The actual affinity of BGP for hydroxyapatite in serum is over 100-fold lower (12); at this affinity, the calculated level of BGP in bone would be far below the amount actually found. Additional evidence against the hypothesis that bone BGP arises from the equilibrium binding of serum BGP to hydroxyapatite in bone is provided by the observation that less than 7% of the [125]I-labeled BGP injected intravenously into a rat actually accumulates in bone (12).

An alternative model for the relationship between BGP in serum and bone is that BGP is secreted near mineralizing sites and so is thus at higher concentrations adjacent to hydroxyapatite than it is in serum. The BGP found in serum would then represent that fraction of newly synthesized BGP escaping from hydroxyapatite binding and diffusing away from the mineralizing site. This model accounts for the lack of significant serum BGP accumulation in bone. It also correctly predicts the increase in serum BGP upon warfarin administration which creates an abnormal BGP that cannot bind to hydroxyapatite (12) or upon ethylhydroxydiphosphate injection which competitively blocks the binding of BGP to hydroxyapatite (57).

An argument can be made that most, if not all, BGP in the extracellular bone matrix must be degraded to nonimmunoreactive fragments during osteoclastic bone resorption. As shown by the experiments outlined above, serum BGP contains no detectable component of BGP derived from osteoclastic resorption of the extracellular bone matrix. However, if all extracellular bone matrix BGP were released intact into serum during bone resorption, the estimated steady-state concentration in plasma of matrix-derived BGP would be 700 ng/ml, a concentration even greater than the 300 ng/ml concentration of BGP found typically in rat plasma. The estimate of steady-state concentration of matrix-derived BGP in plasma is based on the following argument. In a 100-g rat, bone levels of BGP are 3 mg/g undemineralized bone, and the quantity of bone resorbed is at least 0.5 g/day. If BGP were not degraded during resorption, 1.5 mg of BGP would be released from bone matrix to serum each day. In our experience, the infusion of 1.5 mg of BGP per day into 100-g rats produces a steady-state BGP concentration in serum of 700 ng/ml.

## B. PLASMA BGP IN METABOLIC BONE DISEASE

The assay of plasma BGP levels provides a specific measurement of bone metabolism in the diagnosis and treatment of patients with bone disease. As discussed above, plasma BGP arises directly from new cellular synthesis rather than from the release of BGP from the extracellular bone matrix during resorption. It is cleared rapidly by kidney filtration, with a half-time of 5 minutes, and thus provides a temporal resolution sufficient to detect transient changes in bone metabolism. The major tissue which contributes BGP to serum is probably bone. The only other tissue known to synthesize BGP, tooth dentine, almost certainly contributes very little BGP to plasma. Although the cells in bone that release BGP to plasma are almost certainly osteoblastic, the relationships between plasma BGP levels and the number and differentiated status of bone cell populations remain to be determined.

The major radioimmunoassay employed in the measurement of BGP in human plasma is based on the fact that antibody raised in rabbits against calf BGP cross-reacts completely with human BGP (9). The antigenic determinant recognized by this antibody requires the C-terminal 10 residues of BGP, a region shown by sequence analysis to be identical in the bovine and human proteins (15). The BGP detected by this radioimmunoassay in the plasma of normal adults and of patients with bone disease is identical to BGP isolated from human bone in molecular weight (Fig. 12) and in hydroxyapatite binding characteristics.

Plasma BGP content is elevated dramatically in patients with metabolic bone diseases characterized by increased bone turnover (Table I) and generally correlates with plasma alkaline phosphatase in such

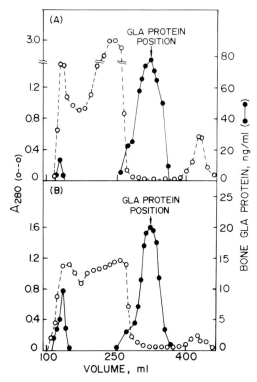

Fig. 12. Gel filtration of fetal calf serum (A) and plasma from a patient with Paget's disease of bone (B) on Sephadex G-100. Column, 2 × 150 cm; load, 10-ml plasma; eluent, 5 mM NH₄HCO₃, 4°C. (○), $A_{280}$; (●), BGP as determined by radioimmunoassay on 0.1 ml of effluent. Arrow indicates the elution position of purified calf BGP as determined in a subsequent chromatography on this column. From Price and Nishimoto (9), used with permission.

patients (14). Alkaline phosphatase can also arise from the liver, however, and so is elevated in patients with liver disease, while plasma BGP is not. Plasma BGP is affected by the treatment of bone disease and can therefore provide additional biochemical information in the management of such patients (62). For example, plasma BGP and alkaline phosphatase both fell by ~50% in patients with Paget's disease treated long-term with salmon calcitonin (62). In acute studies, plasma BGP and $Ca^{2+}$ fell within 2 hours of salmon calcitonin administration, while plasma alkaline phosphatase was unchanged. Additional investigations have shown that plasma BGP falls significantly after parathyroidectomy in women with primary hyperparathyroidism (62).

Clinical interpretation of plasma BGP determinations requires

TABLE I

RELATIONSHIPS BETWEEN BGP AND POSPHATASE (AP) IN HUMAN BLOOD[a,b]

| | BGP (ng/ml) | AP (IU/liter) | $r$ | $p$ |
|---|---|---|---|---|
| Normal adults ($n = 109$) | 6.78(0.20) | 26.7(1.3) | 0.10 | NS |
| Males ($n = 47$) | 7.89(0.32) | 28.1(2.1) | 0.40 | <0.005 |
| Females ($n = 62$) | 4.85(0.36) | 25.2(1.8) | −0.17 | NS |
| Paget's disease ($n = 13$) | 39.2(16)* | 587(181)* | 0.66 | <0.025 |
| Bone metastases ($n = 5$)[c] | 15.8(2.6)* | 132(26)* | 0.93 | <0.05 |
| Hyperparathyrodism | | | | |
| Primary ($n = 11$) | 16.5(1.7)* | 64(6.8)* | 0.16 | NS |
| Secondary ($n = 38$)[d] | 47.3(6.1)* | 56(8.5)* | 0.64 | <0.005 |
| Hypoparathyroidism ($n = 3$) | 2.40(0.92)* | — | — | — |
| Liver disease ($n = 11$) | 5.77(1.0) | 170(41)* | 0.10 | NS |
| Osteopenia ($n = 20$) | 9.05(1.8)* | 48(4.6)* | 0.64 | <0.01 |

[a] From Price et al. (14), used with permission.

[b] Except as indicated and in osteopenic group, all subjects are male. Results are mean ±SE.

[c] Squamous cell carcinoma of the lung (2), and adenocarcinoma of the colon (2) and of the breast (2).

[d] Chronic renal disease on hemodialysis.

* Significantly ($p < 0.50$–$0.0005$) different from normal controls.

knowledge of the bone cell activity correlating best with plasma BGP. For this objective, it is desirable to study bone histology in a patient group with very high plasma BGP content so that correlations between histology and BGP will show maximal statistical significance. Uremic bone disease was chosen for this investigation, since plasma BGP content is 7 times normal in the low bone turnover group and 120 times normal in the high bone turnover group. In these patients, plasma BGP correlated best with cellular and noncellular parameters of bone formation, such as volume of woven osteoid, surface of woven osteoid, and number of osteoblasts (63). There was little or no correlation, however, between plasma BGP levels in uremic bone disease and histologic parameters of bone mineralization, such as fractional labeling of osteoid and mineralization lag time (63). These results are consistent with the concept that the physiologic role of BGP is to inhibit mineralization (see below).

There has been some interest in the use of plasma BGP measurements to assess bone metabolic changes in postmenopausal osteoporosis. Initial studies showed that plasma BGP was high in women with osteopenia (14), a group composed primarily of individuals with osteoporosis. The increase was not great, and it has been necessary to determine plasma BGP as a function of age and kidney function with greater precision in order to better reveal the underlying correlations. Plasma BGP rises with renal impairment (64), but this effect is significant only at glomerular filtration rates below 20 ml/minute-1.73 m². Some investigators have reported no age dependence of serum BGP in women (14), while others have found a significant increase in plasma BGP with age (65,66). Further work will be necessary to establish whether these differences reflect differences in antisera preparations used. It is important to note that there is excellent agreement that in postmenopausal osteoporosis plasma BGP levels are increased. In all studies, plasma BGP levels are significantly elevated in patients with postmenopausal osteoporosis (66,67). This result indicates that bone turnover is increased in postmenopausal osteoporosis (67) and may be due to the rise of immunoreactive PTH in such patients (66).

## IX. DEVELOPMENTAL APPEARANCE OF BGP IN MINERALIZING TISSUES

Investigations into the developmental appearance of BGP in calcifying tissues have relied either on direct biochemical and immunochemical assays for BGP itself or on chemical analyses for γ-carboxyglutamic acid. These two approaches yield different pictures of the developmental appearance of BGP. Direct assays for BGP in demineralization extracts of calcifying tissues indicate that the protein itself does not appear in parallel with the accumulation of mineral, but rather 1–2 weeks later, at the approximate time that the initial mineral phase matures to hydroxyapatite. In contrast, chemical analysis of γ-carboxyglutamate in developing bone shows that the appearance of this amino acid does parallel the accumulation of mineral rather than subsequent mineral maturation. As will be discussed below in greater detail, the probable explanation for this difference between the developmental appearance of the bone Gla protein and of the amino acid Gla is that there is a significant amount of Gla in bone which is in a protein other than BGP. This other Gla-containing protein, matrix Gla protein (MGP), appears in parallel with the accumulation of mineral, while BGP appears 1–2 weeks subsequently.

The developmental appearance of BGP in rat (10) and human (13) bone is shown in Fig. 13. It is readily apparent that the first mineral phase in either species is essentially devoid of BGP. The overall amount of BGP per unit mineral rises rapidly with subsequent development in both species, reaching adult levels of this protein by 14 days

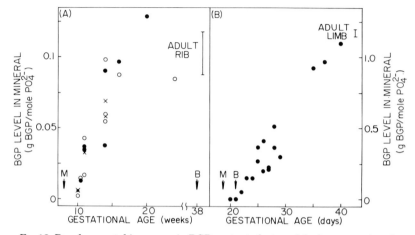

Fig. 13. Developmental increases in BGP content of mineral for human and rat bone.
Data were obtained by dividing the level of BGP in the extract of bone by the level of
phosphate in the same sample (grams of BGP mol of $PO_4$). (A), Human bone; (B), rat
bone; (●), limb bones; (○), rib bones; arrow M, approximate point at which mineralization is detectable; arrow B, approximate age of birth. From Price et al. (13), used with
permission.

of age in rats and by gestational age of 15 weeks in humans. The
general conclusion from both investigations is therefore that most
BGP appears in bone only after the initial accumulation of mineral.
Essentially identical results have been obtained in subsequent investigations on the developmental appearance of BGP in bovine and
chicken bone (28).

Since a given bone contains segments of recently mineralized matrix
as well as segments mineralized days or weeks previously, it is not
possible to deduce the precise temporal relationship between mineral
deposition and BGP appearance solely by measurement of the overall
content of BGP in whole long bones of animals at different stages of
growth. Two additional systems were therefore investigated to determine this relationship (13).

In one test, tibial bones of 2- and 4-week-old rats were divided into 1-
mm segments. Each of these segments was subsequently demineralized and the extract was assayed for BGP. In 2-week-old rats, the
segments at the proximal and distal growth plates contained less than
5% of the midshaft levels of BGP per unit of mineral, a result consistent with the fact that most new mineral is deposited at the growth
plate of these rats. By 4 weeks of age, segments previously located near
the growth plate have, by subsequent bone growth, become part of the
bone diaphysis, and the BGP levels of these segments have risen to

midshaft levels. Thus, the accumulation of BGP in a segment of growing bone is complete 2 weeks after initial mineralization.

In another test, the accumulation of mineral and of BGP was evaluated in the calcifying tissue induced in adolescent rats by implants of demineralized bone powder. This system has the advantage that the stages of induced endochondrial calcification and bone formation follow one another in a well-defined sequence throughout the implant (68). As can be seen in Fig. 14, the level of mineral at the implant site reaches half of its final level at postimplant day 11, while the level of BGP reaches half-maximal values at postimplant day 24. Again, it is

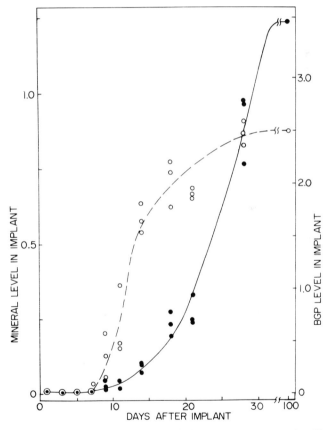

Fɪɢ. 14. Appearance of BGP and of mineral phosphate in demineralized bone matrix implants. Each BGP or phosphate point is from the analysis of the demineralization extract of one implant. (○), mmol of phosphate/gram of implant; (●), mg of BGP/gram implant determined by radioimmunoassay. From Price et al. (13), used with permission.

evident that mineral accumulation precedes BGP appearance by about 2 weeks.

Although it is not certain why BGP accumulates in calcifying tissues only 1–2 weeks after the accumulation of mineral, the available evidence suggests that this has to do with the maturation of initially deposited mineral to hydroxyapatite. Since serum BGP is within the adult range in newborn rats, it is clear that the 100-fold lower content of BGP in newborn rat bone is not due solely to the delayed developmental expression of the BGP gene. This conclusion is supported further by the identification of numerous cells which stain intensely with anti-BGP antibodies in the calvaria and tibia of 2- and 3-day-old rats (46). It therefore appears that BGP is in fact synthesized at a high rate by osteoblasts in the newborn rat bone, but fails to accumulate in the mineral phase to the expected degree. As discussed elsewhere, the accumulation of BGP in bone depends upon its ability to bind to hydroxyapatite strongly. Infrared spectral studies have established that the mineral phase in newborn rat bone is far less crystalline than that found in adult rat bone (69). It may be that this initial mineral phase is deficient in a binding domain required for a strong interaction with BGP. This hypothesis is supported by the fact that the kinetics of BGP accumulation in developing rat bone do correlate with the infrared spectral changes in bone mineral (10). *In vitro* BGP does not bind to amorphous calcium phosphate (3), a less ordered mineral phase sometimes used as a model for the initial mineral phase of bone.

Chemical analysis of γ-carboxyglutamate in developing bone has given a different picture of the appearance of vitamin K-dependent proteins with calcification. In developing chicken (70) and rat (10) bone and in the bone induced by demineralized bone powder in adolescent rats (71), whole bone Gla content rises at the time mineral first accumulates in bone and therefore long before the subsequent accumulation of BGP. For example, in newborn rats, Gla approaches 33% of adult content, while BGP concentrations are only at 1% of adult amounts (10). The amino acid Gla which appears in parallel with mineralization is primarily associated with the collagenous bone matrix which remains after either acid or EDTA demineralization. In contrast, BGP is extracted from bone by these demineralization procedures and is not associated with the matrix.

Two explanations have been advanced for the identity of the matrix-associated, Gla-containing component which appears in parallel with the accumulation of mineral in calcifying bone. Some investigators have suggested that his component is a high-molecular-weight precursor to BGP which has little or no immunologic activity in the radioimmunoassay used to detect the protein (28). With the cloning of the cDNA for BGP, however, it is now apparent that no high molecular precursors to BGP can exist (see above). The other possibility (10) is that bone contains another Gla-containing protein than BGP, one which precedes BGP in calcifying tissues and binds to the organic matrix of bone. A protein with these characteristics has in fact recently been discovered in denaturant extracts of demineralized bovine bone (23). This protein, termed matrix Gla protein (MGP), has five Gla residues per molecule and an apparent molecular weight on SDS–gel electrophoresis of 15,000 (23). Matrix Gla protein is associated with the matrix of demineralized bone (23) and is present in newborn rat bones at levels somewhat greater than those in adult rat bone (25). From the abundance of MGP in newborn rat bone and the Gla content of MGP, it has been calculated that MGP accounts for at least half of the matrix-associated Gla in newborn rat bone (24).

## X. EFFECTS OF WARFARIN ON BONE

### A. EFFECT OF WARFARIN ON BGP LEVELS IN BONE

Physiological investigations into the function of BGP have focused on bone metabolism in vitamin K-deficient animals (38–40). The rationale for this approach lies in the vitamin K dependence of the amino acid unique to BGP, γ-carboxyglutamic acid. In the absence of vitamin K, or when the action of vitamin K is antagonized with warfarin, the posttranslational conversion of glutamate to γ-carboxyglutamate cannot occur. As discussed above, the abnormal, non-γ-carboxylated BGP which is secreted from cells can neither bind to hydroxyapatite in the presence of serum nor accumulate in bone. When growing animals are made vitamin K deficient, the amount of BGP in bone falls as the original, high BGP content matrix is replaced through resorption and net growth with a new BGP-deficient matrix.

The primary experimental difficulty in maintaining animals in a vitamin K-deficient state is the tendency of such animals to hemorrhage due to the lack of vitamin K-dependent blood coagulation factors. This difficulty has been solved in two ways. The first approach was to isolate vitamin K-dependent blood coagulation factors from normal animals and use these to maintain blood coagulability in vitamin K-deficient animals (38). Rabbits were selected for these experiments because their ear veins provided an accessible site for frequent

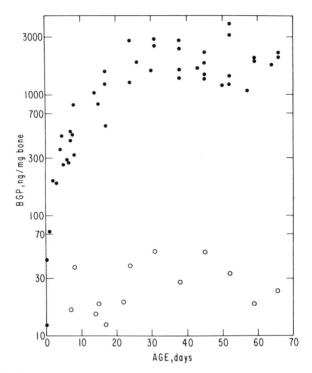

Fɪɢ. 15. BGP levels in bone from warfarin-maintained and control rats. Rats were maintained on warfarin (○) or control (●) protocols from birth to the indicated age and then killed. Femurs were dissected out and assayed for BGP by radioimmunoassay. From Price and Williamson (39), used with permission.

intravenous injections of blood coagulation factors. The second system evolved empirically from the chance observation that rats maintained on high dosages of warfarin together with the minimal dosage of vitamin K required to prevent bleeding have extremely low levels of BGP in bone (39). The rat vitamin K-deficiency protocol is simpler than the rabbit procedure, making it possible to test a greater number of possible BGP functions with this system. All measurements of bone strength and mineralization made in vitamin K-deficient rabbits have given the same picture as the studies in rats: In no instance has an abnormality in overall bone structure or mineralization been seen in either vitamin K-deficient model system (38,39).

The bone content of BGP in rats maintained from birth on the warfarin protocol is compared with those in control rats in Fig. 15. As discussed above, newborn rats show quite low levels of BGP in bone. Consequently, the effect of vitamin K deficiency is seen as a suppres-

sion of the normal developmental increase in BGP rather than as a net
decrease from the amounts in newborn bone. In rats started on the
vitamin K-deficiency protocol at weaning, BGP levels fall to 2% of
normal over the following 6 weeks as all of the high BGP content
matrix present at weaning is replaced by BGP-deficient matrix
through resorption and net bone growth.

As can be seen in Fig. 16, the overall weight gain of rats maintained
from birth in a vitamin K-deficient state is identical to that of control
animals. Long bones dissected from rats maintained for 3 months in a
vitamin K-deficient state were also indistinguishable from those of
control animals in length, weight, and total mineral content. Further
analysis showed that the mineral in hydrazine deproteinized bone

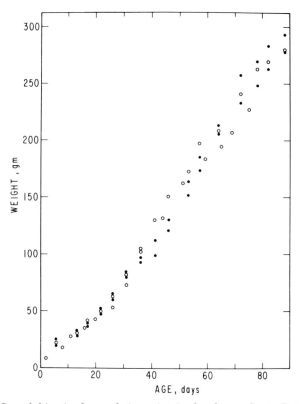

F<small>IG</small>. 16. Growth kinetics for warfarin-maintained and control rats. Rats were maintained from birth on the warfarin (○) or control (●) protocol. Each point represents the
average weight of a seven-animal group; there were two groups on each protocol. From
Price and Williamson (39), used with permission.

from warfarin-maintained and control animals is identical in X-ray diffraction pattern and in total surface area.

## B. EFFECTS OF WARFARIN ON THE GROWTH PLATE

The first evidence for an abnormality in warfarin-treated rats came from the analysis of a subgroup of rats whose growth kinetics are shown in Fig. 16 (40). Ten of the warfarin-treated and ten of the control rats were maintained on the respective treatment regimens until 8 months of age. The proximal tibias were then removed at necropsy and subjected to a battery of histomorphometric measurements. Microradiographs of these bones revealed a dramatic fusion of the growth plate

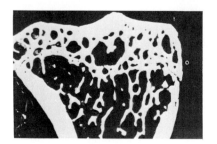
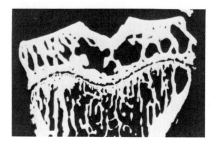

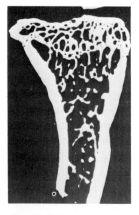
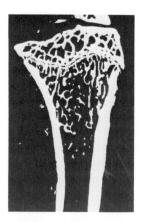

FIG. 17. Microradiographs of 100-μm-thick undecalcified frontal sections from the proximal tibia of warfarin-treated (left) and control (right) rats. Note the bony union of epiphysis and metaphysis in the tibia from the warfarin-treated animals (upper, ×10; lower, ×5). From Price et al. (40), used with permission.

TABLE II

PARAMETERS IN THE PROXIMAL TIBIA OF CONTROL AND WARFARIN-TREATED RATS AT 8 MONTHS OF AGE[a]

| | $\bar{x} \pm$ SD | | |
| | Control | Warfarin-treated | |
| Measurement | ($n = 10$) | ($n = 10$) | $p$ |
|---|---|---|---|
| Length of tibia (cm) | $4.16 \pm 0.13^b$ | $3.86 \pm 0.18^b$ | <0.05 |
| Width of growth cartilage ($\mu$m) | $111.50 \pm 22.90^c$ | 0 | |
| Rate of longitudinal growth ($\mu$m/day) | $9.69 \pm 3.75$ | 0 | |
| Size of degenerative cell ($\mu$m) | $12.79 \pm 1.60$ | 0 | |
| Rate of cartilage cell production (no./day) | $0.76 \pm 0.25$ | 0 | |
| Fraction of growth cartilage with epiphyseal/metaphyseal union | $0.16 \pm 0.07^c$ | $0.81 \pm 0.12^c$ | <0.001 |
| Occurrence of primary spongiosa[d] | $+(n = 10)$ | $0 (n = 5)$ | |
| | | $\pm (n = 5)$ | |

[a] From Price et al. (40), used with permission.
[b] $n = 7$.
[c] $n = 9$.
[d] +, Present; ±, partially present, 0, absent.

in the experimental rats (Fig. 17). Growth plates do not normally fuse in the rat and indeed remained open in the control animals. Parameters of bone growth (Table II) showed further that the fusion of the growth plate caused a cessation of longitudinal growth in the warfarin-treated rat. Since the length of the tibia in the warfarin-treated rats was only 10% shorter than that of the controls, it was apparent that growth plate mineralization had taken place relatively late in the 8 months of warfarin treatment. This conclusion is consistent with the observation that growth was not affected during the first 90 days of warfarin treatment (Fig. 16).

In order to define better the early stages of this warfarin effect, rats were started on the warfarin protocol at 3 months of age and maintained on warfarin for 1, 4, 7, or 10 weeks (72). Microradiographs of the proximal tibia from these animals revealed the presence of detectable growth cartilage mineralization after only 1 week of warfarin treatment. The mineralized fraction of growth cartilage increased with increasing time of warfarin treatment, from 2% at 1 week to 27% at 10 weeks of treatment. The first event in the development of this disorder appeared to be the abnormal intrusion of hydroxyapatite crystals from the existing bed of adjacent metaphyseal mineral into the normally unmineralized longitudinal septa of growth cartilage.

There are at least two possible explanations for a disorder character-ized by the mineralization of a structure not normally mineralized: unmasking of sites for the nucleation of hydroxyapatite crystals in the growth cartilage of the warfarin-treated rat, or failure to prevent the seeded growth of hydroxyapatite crystals from the mineralized areas of the metaphysis into the longitudinal septa of normally unmineralized growth cartilage. It is not possible to clearly differentiate between these alternatives, but the latter explanation appears to correspond best to the observed localization of abnormal hydroxyapatite deposits in the regions of growth cartilage septa closest to the mineralized areas of the metaphysis.

The excessive growth cartilage mineralization disorder in the war-farin-treated rat is almost certainly caused by the inhibition of the $\gamma$-carboxylation of a vitamin K-dependent bone protein. The identity of this protein, however, is open to question. To date, two vitamin K-dependent proteins have been isolated from bone, the $M_r$ 5800 BGP and the $M_r$ 15,000 MGP. Either of these proteins could prevent miner-alization of the growth cartilage in a process requiring $\gamma$-carboxyla-tion. The better studied BGP is known to be a potent inhibitor of hydroxyapatite formation only if it is $\gamma$-carboxylated. The abnormal non-$\gamma$-carboxylated BGP synthesized in the warfarin-treated rat would therefore be incapable of retarding mineralization sufficiently to pre-vent growth cartilage calcification.

## C. Effect of Warfarin on the Bone Response to 1,25-(OH)$_2$D$_3$

The regulation of BGP synthesis by 1,25-(OH)$_2$D$_3$ strongly implies that increased BGP synthesis is one component of bone response to increased circulating 1,25-(OH)$_2$D$_3$. To explore the possible roles of BGP in this response, weanling rats were given sufficient 1,25-(OH)$_2$D$_3$ to stimulate a threefold increase in BGP synthesis (73). One group of animals was then treated concurrently with warfarin to block the $\gamma$-carboxylation of BGP, while the other group was given vitamin K alone.

As can be seen in Fig. 18, warfarin treatment markedly altered the bone response to 1,25-(OH)$_2$D$_3$. In agreement with earlier results, war-farin had no effect on rats of this age not given 1,25-(OH)$_2$D$_3$. Thus, it is probable that warfarin blocks a component of the bone response to 1,25-(OH)$_2$D$_3$. The agent responsible for this effect must therefore be

NO
1,25-(OH)₂D₃

DAILY 1,25-(OH)₂D₃
(125 ng per 100 g body weight)

NO
WARFARIN

WARFARIN-
MAINTAINED

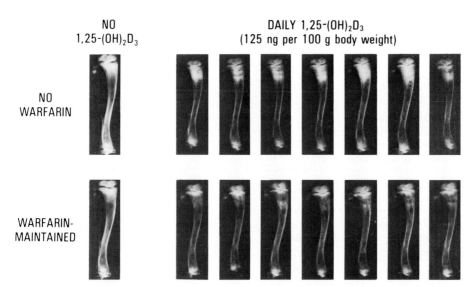

Fig. 18. Effect of warfarin on the radiological bone density of tibias from 1,25-(OH)₂D₃-treated and control rats. In this experiment, 28 weanling rats were divided into 4 treatment groups of 7 each and given subcutaneous injections of 1,25-(OH)₂D₃, warfarin, or vehicle for 11 days. All right tibias from the 7 animals in the 1,25-(OH)₂D₃ and the 1,25-(OH)₂D₃ plus warfarin treatment groups were compared with representative right tibias from the control and warfarin only groups. From Price and Sloper (73), used with permission.

regulated by 1,25-(OH)₂D₃ and be dependent upon vitamin K. These are properties characteristic only of BGP.

Since warfarin affects bone metabolism only in the 1,25-(OH)₂D₃-treated rat, discussion of physiological mechanisms might well begin with the bone response to 1,25-(OH)₂D₃. As can be seen in Fig. 18, treatment with 1,25-(OH)₂D₃ in the absence of warfarin markedly reduces the radiological bone density at the tibial midshaft compared with untreated controls. This effect is undoubtedly due to accelerated bone resorption in the 1,25-(OH)₂D₃-treated rat. Since warfarin does not modify this 1,25-(OH)₂D₃ effect (Fig. 18), it is apparent that there is no vitamin K-dependent component to 1,25-(OH)₂D₃-induced bone resorption in the diaphysis.

In contrast to the diaphysis, metaphyseal density on radiograph is changed little by treatment with 1,25-(OH)₂D₃ (Fig. 18). Radiological bone density measurements reflect primarily the quantity of mineral in a bone segment, however. A more detailed analysis of the metaphysis revealed a marked *increase* in the total hydroxyproline content (Table III) (74). Thus, 1,25-(OH)₂D₃ treatment causes a net increase in

TABLE III
EFFECT OF WARFARIN ON THE COMPOSITION OF THE PROXIMAL TIBIAL NETAPHYSIS[a]

|  | Untreated control ($n = 15$) | 1,25(OH)$_2$D$_3$ only ($n = 15$) | 1,25(OH)$_2$D$_3$ plus warfarin ($n = 13$) |
| --- | --- | --- | --- |
| Calcium, mg/segment | $8.4 \pm 0.5$ | $7.2 \pm 0.5$ | $4.3 \pm 0.4$ |
| 4-hydroxyproline, $\mu$mol/segment | $2.6 \pm 0.2$ | $4.3 \pm 0.3$ | $2.2 \pm 0.2$ |
| mg calcium per $\mu$mol Hyp | 3.2 | 1.7 | 2.0 |

[a] Results are mean ± standard deviation. The proximal tibial netaphysis was dissected from untreated control rats and from rats treated 11 days with 1,25(OH)$_2$D$_3$ or with 1,25(OH)$_2$D$_3$ plus warfarin. Each sample was then analyzed for total calcium and total 4-hydroxyproline content as described in Price and Sloper (73,74). From Price and Sloper (73,74), used with permission.

organic bone matrix in the metaphysis without a corresponding increase in the amount of bone mineral. The overall ratio of mineral to hydroxyproline, a measure of the density of bone mineralization, is therefore markedly reduced by 1,25-(OH)$_2$D$_3$ treatment (Table III). The effect of warfarin on this 1,25-(OH)$_2$D$_3$ effect is to reduce both the mineral and the organic matrix content of the metaphysis compared with the vitamin K-replete rat, causing dramatic reduction in radiological bone density (Fig. 18).

There are two general mechanisms by which concurrent warfarin treatment might reduce amounts of metaphyseal bone in the 1,25-(OH)$_2$D$_3$-treated rat. One possibility is that warfarin treatment accelerates 1,25-(OH)$_2$D$_3$-induced resorption of the proximal tibial metaphysis. This hypothesis would imply that the role of the vitamin K-dependent protein in this bone response to 1,25-(OH)$_2$D$_3$ is to retard or prevent bone resorption. The other possibility is that warfarin treatment decelerates bone formation in the metaphysis of the 1,25-(OH)$_2$D$_3$-treated rat. The latter hypothesis would suggest that the role of the vitamin K-dependent protein in this bone response is to accelerate bone formation.

To distinguish between these possibilities, metaphyseal bone was labeled with [$^3$H]tetracycline and the fate of the $^3$H label was monitored during subsequent treatment with 1,25-(OH)$_2$D$_3$ plus warfarin or with 1,25-(OH)$_2$D$_3$ alone (75). These investigations demonstrated that concurrent warfarin treatment reduces the amounts of label retained in the metaphysis of the 1,25-(OH)$_2$D$_3$-treated rat by 78% compared to 50% in the vitamin K-replete, 1,25-(OH)$_2$D$_3$-treated rat. Thus, concurrent warfarin treatment reduced the radiological bone density in the proximal tibial metaphysis by accelerating the rate of $1,25\text{-}(OH)_2D_3\text{-}$ induced metaphyseal bone resorption.

It follows that the role of the vitamin K-dependent protein in this bone response to $1,25\text{-}(OH)_2D_3$ must be to retard the rate of metaphyseal bone resorption. This could be accomplished either by direct inhibition of the metaphyseal osteoclast or by indirect action on the nature of the metaphyseal matrix which reduces its susceptibility to resorption. While it is not possible to rule out either hypothesis at present, the latter explanation is preferred by the author. Since BGP is the probable vitamin K-dependent protein responsible for this effect, a reasonable scenario would be that the increased BGP content induced by $1,25\text{-}(OH)_2D_3$ retards the rate of mineralization in the metaphysis and so results in a less densely mineralized matrix which is resistant to resorption. Warfarin treatment would lift the BGP block to mineralization and cause the formation of a more densely mineralized metaphysis which is correspondingly more susceptible to osteoclastic resorption.

## D. CHEMOTACTIC ACTIVITY OF BGP

The chemotactic activity of BGP was first observed in assays using peripheral blood monocytes (76). Other proteins found in bone were also comparably chemoattractic, including $\alpha_2$HS and peptides derived from type I collagen. The primary difficulty in ascribing physiological relevance to this observation has been the fact that 2.2–4.3 $\mu M$ BGP is needed for optimal response, while human bone itself has BGP concentrations of at most 17 $\mu$mol/liter solid bone. This solid-state concentration of BGP in bone can never correspond to a solution concentration. For example, the solid-state concentration of $Ca^{2+}$ in bone is over 12 mol/liter of bone. Even if the conditions at a resorbing surface are extraordinarily acidic and the diffusion of dissolved bone $Ca^{2+}$ is slow, it is unreasonable to expect that the concentration of $Ca^{2+}$ in the bone fluid between the osteoclast and a resolving bone surface can even achieve a steady-state concentration as high as 120 m$M$. If this should be the case, however, the corresponding concentration of BGP would be 0.17 $\mu M$, a concentration which is well below that needed for a chemotactic response.

Since the BGP in bone matrix is not in fact even released as an intact protein during bone resorption (see above), additional investigations have examined the chemotactic activity of BGP fragments that might be generated during the resorption process (77,78). The most potent fragment tested was the L-isomer of $\gamma$-carboxyglutamic acid, which is optimally active at $10^{-10}$ $M$ (77). The D-isomer of $\gamma$-carboxyglutamic acid and L-glutamic acid were without effect. Since the concentration of L-Gla in human bone is about $5 \times 10^{-4}$ $M$, it is very likely that a gradient in L-Gla could be generated at the site of bone resorption which would have a solution concentration near bone of at least the $10^{-10}$ $M$ needed to attract monocytes.

Since the monocyte cell population is believed to contain the precursors of macrophages and osteoclasts, it is possible that the recruitment of monocytes by L-Gla or BGP could play a role in the removal of dead bone by macrophages or in the resorption of bone by osteoclasts (76). Subsequent investigations have indeed shown that implants of dead bone powder from warfarin-treated rats are not removed by the phagocytic cells in the host rats as readily as are implants from control animals (79). It has been argued that the reduced rate of dead bone phagocytosis is due to reduced osteoclastic resorption rather than reduced macrophage phagocytosis. Reduced osteoclastic resorption is further assumed to be due to the reduced level of BGP in the bone from the warfarin-treated rat (79). Several lines of evidence, however, strongly argue against a primary role for BGP in osteoclastic bone resorption. Not only are the warfarin-treated rats not osteopetrotic (39,40), BGP is comparably abundant in dentine, a tissue which is not subject to resorption (4). It is the author's opinion that the reduced rate of phagocytosis of dead bone from the warfarin-treated rat is due to the reduced level of L-Gla rather than BGP. If this interpretation is correct, the acceleration of dead bone phagocytosis may represent a secondary function of all Gla-containing bone proteins, which include MGP and BGP.

## XI. SUMMARY

The author presently favors the hypothesis that BGP retards the mineralization of bone and dentine. This activity would be a function of the BGP concentration in the aqueous phase adjacent to the mineralizing front, a concentration maintained by continuous secretion of BGP from nearby osteoblasts and odontoblasts. The mechanism by which BGP inhibits mineralization would involve suppression of the formation of new hydroxyapatite crystals from the preexisting mineral phase.

One physiological function of BGP as a mineralization inhibitor would be to reduce the flux of serum $Ca^{2+}$ and phosphate to bone. The increased rate of BGP synthesis and secretion which is induced by $1,25\text{-}(OH)_2D_3$ would, by inhibiting mineralization, reserve for serum that fraction of $Ca^{2+}$ which would otherwise be incorporated into bone. As discussed, basal levels of BGP production in bone and dentine probably play a role in matrix formation rather than in serum $Ca^{2+}$ homeostasis. While it is not yet clear what biochemical processes are dependent upon the delayed mineralization of osteoid and predentine, the physiological function of delayed mineralization probably lies in the mechanical properties of each tissue.

In this model, serum BGP would represent that fraction of bone cell synthesis which escapes from the aqueous phase near the mineralization front. The total quantity of BGP in serum would reflect the number of cells secreting BGP, accounting for the observation that serum BGP levels correlate with the number of osteoblasts in bone (63). Since secretion of BGP is the presumed mechanism by which the mineralization of bone matrix is retarded, serum BGP levels should reflect the amount of osteoid rather than the rate of mineralization. Therefore, this model for BGP function would also account for the observed correlation between serum BGP and the volume of osteoid rather than the rate of mineralization.

In the present review, the author has emphasized the role of BGP as an inhibitor of mineralization, a hypothesis first advanced 9 years ago (3). The function of a hypothesis is to foster fruitful experiments, and it has been the author's objective in presenting this model to provide a framework for future experimental tests.

## REFERENCES

1. Price, P. A. (1983). Osteocalcin. *In* "Bone and Mineral Research Annual" (W. A. Peck, ed.), Vol. 1, pp. 157–190. Excerpta Medica, Amsterdam.

2. Hauschka, P. V., Lian, J. B., and Gallop, P. M. (1975). Direct identification of the calcium binding amino acid, $\gamma$-carboxyglutamate, in mineralized tissue. *Proc. Natl. Acad. Sci. U.S.A.* **72**, 3925–3929.

3. Price, P. A., Otsuka, A. S., Poser, J. W., Kristaponis, J., and Raman, N. (1976). Characterization of a $\gamma$-carboxyglutamic acid-containing protein from bone. *Proc. Natl. Acad. Sci. U.S.A.* **73**, 1447–1451.

4. Linde, A., Rhown, M., and Butler, W. T. (1980). Noncollagenous proteins of dentine. *J. Biol. Chem.* **255**, 5931.

5. Linde, A. (1984). Non-collagenous proteins and proteoglycans in dentinogenesis. *In* "Dentin and Dentinogenesis" (A. Linde, ed.), Vol. 2, pp. 55–92. CRC Press, Boca Raton, Florida.

6. Lian, J. B., Prien, E. L., Jr., Glimcher, M. J., and Gallop, P. M. (1977). The presence of protein-bound $\gamma$-carboxyglutamic acid in calcium-containing renal calculi. *J. Clin. Invest.* **59**, 1151–1157.

7. Levy, R. J., Lian, J. B., and Gallop, P. M. (1979). Atherocalcin, a $\gamma$-carboxyglu-

tamic acid-containing protein from atherosclerotic plaque. *Biochem. Biophys. Res. Commun.* **91**, 41–49.

8. Lian, J. B., Skinner, M., Glimcher, M. J., and Gallop, P. M. (1976). Presence of γ-carboxyglutamic acid in the proteins associated with ectopic calcification. *Biochem. Biophys. Res. Commun.* **73**, 349–355.

9. Price, P. A., and Nishimoto, S. K. (1980). Radioimmunoassay for the vitamin K-dependent protein of bone and its discovery in plasma. *Proc. Natl. Acad. Sci. U.S.A.* **77**, 2234–2238.

10. Price, P. A., Lothringer, J. W., and Nishimoto, S. K. (1980). Absence of the vitamin K-dependent bone protein in fetal rat mineral. Evidence for another γ-carboxyglutamic acid-containing component in bone. *J. Biol. Chem.* **255**, 2938–2942.

11. Patterson-Allen, P., Brantigan, C. E., Gundeland, R. E., Asling, C. W., and Callahan, P. X. (1982). A specific radioimmunoassay for osteocalcin with advantageous species crossreactivity. *Anal. Biochem.* **120**, 1.

12. Price, P. A., Williamson, M. K., and Lothringer, J. W. (1981). Origin of the bone γ-carboxyglutamic acid-containing protein found in plasma and its clearance by kidney and bone. *J. Biol. Chem.* **256**, 12760–12766.

13. Price, P. A., Lothringer, J. W., Baukol, S. A., and Reddi, A. H. (1981). Developmental appearance of the vitamin K-dependent protein of bone during calcification. *J. Biol. Chem.* **256**, 3781–3784.

14. Price, P. A., Parthemore, J. G., and Deftos, L. J. (1980). A new biochemical marker for bone metabolism. *J. Clin. Invest.* **66**, 878–883.

15. Poser, J. W., Esch, F. S., Ling, N. C., and Price, P. A. (1980). Isolation and sequence of the vitamin K-dependent protein from human bone. Undercarboxylation of the first glutamic acid residue. *J. Biol. Chem.* **255**, 8685–8691.

16. Price, P. A., Poser, J. W., and Raman, N. (1976). Primary structure of the γ-carboxyglutamic acid-containing protein from bovine bone. *Proc. Natl. Acad. Sci. U.S.A.* **73**, 3374–3375.

17. Hauschka, P. V., and Gallop, P. M. (1977). Purification and calcium-binding properties of osteocalcin, the γ-carboxyglutamic-containing protein of bone. *In* "Calcium Binding Proteins and Calcium Function" (R. H. Wasserman, R. A. Corradino, E. Carafoli, R. H. Kretsinger, D. H. MacLennan, and F. L. Siegel, eds.), pp. 338–347. Elsevier, Amsterdam.

18. Price, P. A. (1982). The vitamin K-dependent protein of bone. *AAOS Symp. Heritable Disorders Connect. Tissue* pp. 208–220.

19. Price, P. A., Otsuka, A. S., and Poser, J. W. (1977). Comparison of γ-carboxyglutamic acid-containing proteins from bovine and swordfish bone: Primary structure and $Ca^{++}$ binding. *In* "Calcium Binding Proteins and Calcium Function" (R. H. Wasserman, R. A. Corradine, E. Carafoli, R. H. Kretsinger, D. H. MacLennan, and F. L. Siegel, eds.), pp. 333–337. Elsevier, Amsterdam.

20. Carr, S. A., Hauschka, P. V., and Biemann, K. (1981). Gas chromatographic mass spectrometric sequence determination of osteocalcin, a γ-carboxyglutamic acid-containing protein from chicken bone. *J. Biol. Chem.* **256**, 9944.

21. Hauschka, P. V., Carr, S. A., and Biemann, K. (1982). Primary structure of monkey osteocalcin. *Biochemistry* **21**, 638.

22. Otawara, Y., Hosoya, N., Moriuchi, S., Kasai, H., and Okuyama, T. (1981). The $NH_2$-terminal amino acid sequence of a γ-carboxyglutamic acid-containing protein from rat femur cortical bone. *Biomed. Res.* **2**, 442.

23. Price, P. A., Urist, M. R., and Otawara, Y. (1983). Matrix Gla protein, a new γ-carboxyglutamic acid-containing protein which is associated with the organic matrix of bone. *Biochem. Biophys. Res. Commun.* **117**, 765–771.

24. Price, P. A., Williamson, M. K., and Otawara, Y. (1985). Characterization of matrix Gla protein, a new vitamin K-dependent protein which is associated with the organic matrix of bone. *In* "The Chemistry and Biology of Mineralized Tissues" (W. T. Butler, ed.), pp. 159–163. EBSCO Media, Birmingham.

25. Pan, L. C., and Price, P. A. (1985). Regulation of the bone Gla protein by 1,25-dihydroxyvitamin $D_3$: Progress in the molecular cloning of rat bone Gla protein. *In* "The Chemistry and Biology of Mineralized Tissues" (W. T. Butler, ed.), pp. 317–319. EBSCO Media, Birmingham.

26. Steiner, D. F., Quinn, P. S., Chan, S. J., Marsh, J., and Tager, H. S. (1980). Processing mechanisms in the biosynthesis of proteins. *Ann. N.Y. Acad. Sci.* **343**, 1–16.

27. Watson, M. E. E. (1984). Compilation of published signal sequences. *Nucleic Acids Res.* **12**, 5145–5164.

28. Hauschka, P. V., Frenkel, J., DeMuth, R., and Gundberg, C. M. (1983). Presence of osteocalcin and related higher molecular weight 4-carboxyglutamic acid-containing proteins in developing bone. *J. Biol. Chem.* **258**, 176–182.

29. Poser, J. W., and Price, P. A. (1979). A method for decarboxylation of γ-carboxyglutamic acid in proteins. *J. Biol. Chem.* **254**, 431–436.

30. Nishimoto, S. K., and Price, P. A. (1979). Proof that the γ-carboxyglutamic acid-containing bone protein is synthesized in calf bone. *J. Biol. Chem.* **254**, 437–441.

31. Price, P. A., Williamson, M. K., and Epstein, D. J. (1981). Specific tritium incorporation into γ-carboxyglutamic acid in proteins: The pH dependence of γ-proton exchange. *J. Biol. Chem.* **256**, 1172–1176.

32. Price, P. A. (1984). Decarboxylation of γ-carboxyglutamic acid residues in proteins. *In* "Methods in Enzymology" (F. Wold and K. Moldave, eds.), Vol. 107, pp. 548–551. Academic Press, New York.

33. Price, P. A. (1984). Specific tritium labeling of γ-carboxyglutamic acid residues in proteins. *In* "Methods in Enzymology" (F. Wold and K. Moldave, eds.), Vol. 107, pp. 544–548. Academic Press, New York.

34. Price, P. A., Nelson, C., and Williamson, M. K. (1984). Chemical modification of γ-carboxyglutamic acid, the vitamin K-dependent amino acid which binds $Ca^{2+}$. *Anal. Biochem.* **136**, 119–126.

35. Price, P. A. (1983). Quantitative determination of γ-carboxyglutamic acid in proteins. *In* "Methods in Enzymology" (C. H. W. Hirs and S. N. Timasheff, eds.), Vol. 91, pp. 13–17. Academic Press, New York.

36. Delmas, P. D., Stenner, D. D., Romberg, R. W., Riggs, B. L., and Mann, K. G. (1984). Immunochemical studies of conformational alterations in bone γ-carboxyglutamic acid containing protein. *Biochemistry* **23**, 4720–4725.

37. Hauschka, P. V., and Carr, S. A. (1982). Calcium-dependent α-helical structure in osteocalcin. *Biochemistry* **21**, 2538–2547.

38. Price, P. A., Epstein, D. J., Lothringer, J. W., Nishimoto, S. K., Poser, J. W., and Williamson, M. K. (1979). Structure and function of the vitamin K-dependent protein of bone. *In* "Vitamin K Metabolism and Vitamin K-dependent Proteins" (J. W. Suttie, ed.), pp. 219–230. Univ. Park Press, Baltimore.

39. Price, P. A., and Williamson, M. K. (1981). Effects of warfarin on bone. Studies on the vitamin K-dependent protein of rat bone. *J. Biol. Chem.* **256**, 12760–12766.

40. Price, P. A., Williamson, M. K., Haba, T., Dell, R. B., and Jee, W. S. S. (1982). Excessive mineralization with growth plate closure in rats on chronic warfarin treatment. *Proc. Natl. Acad. Sci. U.S.A.* **79**, 7734–7738.

41. Poser, J. W., Sunberg, R. T., Francis, S. L., and Benedict, J. J. (1982). The bone Gla protein as an inhibitor of seeded crystal growth. *Calcif. Tissue Int.* **34**, S26.

42. Lian, J. B., and Friedman, P. A. (1978). The vitamin K-dependent synthesis of γ-carboxyglutamic acid by bone microsomes. *J. Biol. Chem.* **253**, 6623.

43. Lian, J. B., and Heroux, J. M. (1979). *In vitro* studies of osteocalcin biosynthesis in the embryonic chick bone cultures. *In* "Vitamin K Metabolism and Vitamin K-dependent Proteins" (J. W. Suttie, ed.), pp. 245–254. Univ. Park Press, Baltimore.

44. Nishimoto, S. K., and Price, P. A. (1980). Secretion of the vitamin K-dependent protein of bone by rat osteosarcoma cells. Evidence for an intracellular precursor. *J. Biol. Chem.* **255**, 6579–6583.

45. Majeska, R. J., Rodan, S. B., and Rodan, G. A. (1980). Parathyroid hormone-responsive clonal cell lines from rat osteosarcoma. *Endocrinology* **107**, 1497.

46. Beresford, J. N., Gallagher, J. A., Poser, J. W., and Russell, R. G. G. (1984). Production of osteocalcin by human bone cells *in vitro*. Effects of 1,25-$(OH)_2D_3$, 24,25-$(OH)_2D_3$, parathyroid hormone, and glucocorticoids. *Metab. Bone Dis. Rel. Res.* **5**, 229–234.

47. Bronckers, A. L. J. J., Gay, S., DiMuzio, M. T., and Butler, W. T. (1985). Immunolocalization of γ-carboxyglutamic acid-containing protein in developing rat bones. *Collagen Rel. Res.* **5**, 17–22.

48. Dimuzio, M. T., Bhown, M., and Butler, W. T. (1983). The biosynthesis of dentine γ-carboxyglutamic acid containing protein by rat incisor odontoblasts in organ culture. *Biochem. J.* **216**, 249–257.

49. Bronckers, A. L. J. J., Gay, S., DiMuzio, M. T., and Butler, W. T. (1985). Immunolocalization of γ-carboxyglutamic acid containing proteins in developing molar tooth germs of the rat. *Collagen Rel. Res.,* in press.

50. Price, P. A., and Baukol, S. A. (1980). 1,25-Dihydroxyvitamin $D_3$ increases synthesis of the vitamin K-dependent bone protein by osteosarcoma cells. *J. Biol. Chem.* **255**, 11660–11663.

51. Bouillon, R., and Van Baelen, H. (1981). Transport of vitamin D: Significance of free and total concentrations in the vitamin D metabolites. *Calcif. Tissue Int.* **33**, 451–453.

52. Hardisty, T. K., Haddad, T. G., and Price, P. A. (1985). Influence of serum and of vitamin D-binding protein on the response of osteosarcoma cells to 1,25-dihydroxyvitamin $D_3$. Submitted.

53. Pan, L. C., and Price, P. A. (1984). Effect on transcriptional inhibitors on the bone γ-carboxyglutamic acid protein response to 1,25-dihydroxyvitamin $D_3$ in osteosarcoma cells. *J. Biol. Chem.* **259**, 5844–5847.

54. Price, P. A., and Baukol, S. A. (1981). 1,25-Dihydroxyvitamin $D_3$ increases serum levels of the vitamin K-dependent bone protein. *Biochem. Biophys. Res. Commun.* **99**, 928–935.

55. Buckley, M., and Bronner, F. (1980). Calcium-binding protein biosynthesis in the rat: Regulation by calcium and 1,25-dihydroxyvitamin $D_3$. *Arch. Biochem. Biophys.* **202**, 235.

56. Gundberg, C. M., Cole, D. E. C., Lian, J. B., Reade, T. M., and Gallop, P. M. (1983). Serum osteocalcin in the treatment of inherited rickets with 1,25-dihydroxyvitamin $D_3$. *J. Clin. Endocrinol. Metab.* **56**, 1063–1067.

57. Price, P. A., Williamson, M. K., and Baukol, S. A. (1981). The vitamin K-dependent bone protein and the biological response of bone to 1,25-dihydroxyvitamin $D_3$. *In* "The Chemistry and Biology of Mineralized Connective Tissues" (A. Veis, ed.), pp. 327–335. Elsevier, Amsterdam.

58. Rader, J. I., Baylink, D. J., Hughes, M. R., Safilian, E. F., and Haussler, M. R. (1979). Calcium and phosphorus deficiency in rats: effects on PTH and 1,25-dihydroxy vitamin $D_3$. *Am. J. Physiol.* **236**, E118–E122.

59. Price, P. A., Williamson, M. K., and Baukol, S. A. (1982). The vitamin K-dependent bone protein and the vitamin D-dependent biochemical response of bone to dietary calcium deficiency. *In* "Vitamin D: Chemical, Biochemical, and Clinical Endocrinology of Calcium Metabolism" (A. W. Norman, K. Schaefe, D. V. Herrath, and H. G. Grigoleit, eds.), pp. 351–361. De Gruyter, Berlin.

60. Lian, J. B., Glimcher, M. J., Hauschka, P. V., Gallop, P. M., Cohen-Solal, L., and Reit, B. (1982). Alterations of the γ-carboxyglutamic acid and osteocalcin concentrations in vitamin D-deficient chick bone. *J. Biol. Chem.* **257**, 4999.

61. Baynes, J. W., and Wold, F. (1976). Effect of glycosylation on the *in vivo* circulating half-life of ribonuclease. *J. Biol Chem.* **251**, 6016.

62. Deftos, L. J., Parthemore, J. G., and Price, P. A. (1982). Changes in plasma bone Gla protein during treatment of bone disease. *Calcif. Tissue Int.* **34**, 121–124.

63. Malluche, H. H., Faugere, M.-C., Fanti, P., and Price, P. A. (1984). Plasma levels of bone Gla protein reflect bone formation in patients on chronic maintenance dialysis. *Kidney Int.* **26**, 869–874.

64. Delmas, P. D., Wilson, D. M., Mann, K. G., and Riggs, B. L. (1983). Effect of renal function on plasma levels of bone Gla protein. *J. Clin. Endocrinol. Metab.* **57**, 1028–1030.

65. Delmas, P. D., Stenner, D. D., Wahner, H. W., Mann, K. G., and Riggs, B. L. (1983). Increase in serum bone γ-carboxyglutamic acid protein with aging in women. *J. Clin. Invest.* **71**, 1316–1321.

66. Epstein, S., McClintoch, R., Bryce, G., Poser, J., Johnston, C. C., Jr., and Hui, S. (1984). Differences in serum bone Gla protein with age and sex. *Lancet* **xx**, 307–310.

67. Delmas, P. D., Wahner, H. W., Mann, K. G., and Riggs, B. L. (1983). Assessment of bone turnover in postmenopausal osteoporosis by measurement of serum bone Gla protein. *J. Lab. Clin. Med.* **102**, 470–476.

68. Reddi, A. H., and Anderson, W. A. (1976). Collagenous bone matrix-induced endochondral ossification and hemopoiesis. *J. Cell Biol.* **69**, 557.

69. Termine, J. D., and Posner, A. S. (1966). Infrared analysis of rat bone: age dependency of amorphous and crystalline mineral fractions. Science 153, 1523–1525.

70. Hauschka, P. V., and Reid, M. L. (1978). Timed appearance of calcium-binding protein containing γ-carboxyglutamic acid in developing chick bone. *Dev. Biol.* **65**, 426–434.

71. Hauschka, P. V., and Reddi, A. H. (1980). Correlation of the appearance of γ-carboxyglutamic acid with the onset of mineralization in developing endochondral bone. *Biochem. Biophys. Res. Commun.* **92**, 1037.

72. Lee, W. S. S., Haba, T., and Price, P. A. (1983). Time course of growth plate mineralization in chronically warfarin-treated rats. *Calcif. Tissue Int.* **35**, 658.

73. Price, P. A., and Sloper, S. A. (1983). Concurrent warfarin treatment further reduces bone mineral levels in 1,25-dihydroxyvitamin D₃-treated rats. *J. Biol. Chem.* **258**, 6004–6007.

74. Price, P. A., and Sloper, S. A. (1984). The effect of warfarin administration on the bone response to 1,25-dihydroxyvitamin D₃. *In* "Endocrine Control of Bone and Calcium Metabolism" (D. V. Cohn, T. Fujita, L. T. Potts, Jr., and R. V. Talmadge, eds.), pp. 69–72. Excerpta Medica, Amsterdam.

75. Price, P. A., Sloper, S. A., Williamson, M. K., Dev, P. K., and Lee, W. S. S. (1984). Warfarin treatment accelerates resorption in the metaphysis of 1,25-dihydroxyvitamin D₃-treated rats. *Calcif. Tissue Int.* **36**, 523.

76. Malone, J. D., Teitelbaum, G. L., Griffin, G. L., Senior, R. M., and Kahn, A. J. (1982). Recruitment of osteoclast precursors by purified bone matrix constituents. *J. Cell Biol.* **92**, 227–238.

77. Malone, J. D., Teitelbaum, S. L., Hauschka, P. V., and Kahn, A. J. (1982). Presumed osteoclast precursors (monocytes) recognize two or more regions of osteocalcium. *Calcif. Tissue Int.* **84,** 511.

78. Mundy, G. R., and Poser, J. W. (1983). Chemotactic activity of γ-carboxyglutamic acid containing protein in bone. *Calcif. Tissue Int.* **35,** 164–168.

79. Lian, J. B., Tassinari, M., and Glowacki, J. (1984). Resorption of implanted bone prepared from normal and warfarin-treated rats. *J. Clin. Invest.* **73,** 1223–1226.

VITAMINS AND HORMONES, VOL. 42

# Hormone Secretion by Exocytosis with Emphasis on Information from the Chromaffin Cell System

## HARVEY B. POLLARD, RICHARD ORNBERG, MARK LEVINE, KATRINA KELNER, KYOJI MORITA, ROBERT LEVINE, ERIK FORSBERG, KEITH W. BROCKLEHURST, LE DUONG, PETER I. LELKES, ELI HELDMAN, AND MOUSSA YOUDIM

*Laboratory of Cell Biology and Genetics, National Institute of Arthritis, Diabetes, and Digestive and Kidney Diseases, National Institutes of Health, Bethesda, Maryland*

## I. Introduction

Exocytosis is the general mechanism by which many hormones, transmitters, enzymes, and other special proteins and peptides are secreted from cells. Exocytosis means that the chemical species to be secreted is stored in a secretory vesicle which, upon the appropriate stimulus, fuses with the cell membrane and deposits the vesicle contents outside the cell. The handmaiden of this process is usually calcium. Indeed, in many cases the ultimate signal for exocytosis seems to be an increase in the intracellular free calcium ion concentration. But the details of how calcium and other factors promote the necessary vesicle movements, specific membrane contacts, and fusion events leading to secretion have posed a fascinating mystery to cell biologists for years.

For many reasons, the chromaffin cell is the very best vantage point from which to examine the hormone secretion process. From a biochemical viewpoint, the chromaffin cell has no peer, since the adrenal medullary tissue is readily available whenever abatoires exist, subcellular fractionation is simple, and the cells are easily cultured. More interestingly, William Douglas used this tissue to first demonstrate that external calcium was required for secretion and Kirshner, Arqueros, and Viveros first showed that vesicle contents but not vesicle membranes were released during secretion. Thus, this tissue has been a chemical guidepost to exocytosis for all the rest of cell biology. Many excellent reviews have been written in recent years describing these exciting studies in detail, and we will refer to them subsequently.

For these reasons, one might expect that what is true of exocytosis in chromaffin cells is also true of the same process in other cells. However, the whole field of cell biology and biochemistry of secretion from chromaffin (and other) cells is in a dramatic state of flux and, as will be obvious soon, there are very few things that are known with certainty even in the chromaffin cell.

Finally, by way of an apologia for the fact that what follows is not precisely limited to the secretion process, it is important to realize that "exocytosis" is an umbrella term. It refers to much more than just the secretion process, in the same way that the firing of a gun involves much more than the simple emergence of the bullet from the barrel. In the case of the cell, hormone release cannot be studied in isolation from events in the nucleus, synthesis and packaging in the endoplasmic reticulum and Golgi, or involvement of the cytoskeleton in location and dislocation of granules. The fact is that each preliminary event presupposes the ultimate secretion events (and beyond) as well as all intervening events. This is, in a way, a trivial description of all true "systems," but is often ignored. The critical problems confronting us as we attempt to understand exocytosis are how the system synchronizes and targets events and interactions, and how specificity is achieved. This review will attempt to focus on these critical problems in hormone secretion as viewed from the perspective of the chromaffin cell.

## II. Ultrastructure of Secretion from Chromaffin Cells

Chromaffin cells in the adrenal medulla are joined and electrically coupled into cords of cells surrounded in the intact gland by an abundant fenestrated capillary bed. The cells receive innervation from cholinergic endings of the splanchnic nerve and secrete catecholamines physiologically into the blood in response to acetylcholine. Other agents affecting release are nicotonic cholinergic agonists and membrane-depolarizing agents such as high external potassium and electrical stimulation. While much of our knowledge of the catecholamine release process is derived from work on intact glands, more recent studies on isolated chromaffin cell cultures have provided new insights into the cell biology of secretion by exocytosis.

Current procedures for preparing isolated cells from intact gland (Kilpatrick *et al.*, 1980; Fenwick *et al.*, 1978; Waymire *et al.*, 1983) generate suspensions of single cells which contain chromaffin cells, endothelial cells (Banerjee *et al.*, 1985), and some cortical cells with a viability of greater than 90%. The chromaffin cells can be grown as plated cells on coated plastic surfaces or as floating cells in suspension culture. Plated preparations contain more endothelial cells than suspension cultures due to the greater plating efficiency of the latter cells. Plated chromaffin cells can adhere as an aggregate of many cells to underlying endothelial cells or flatten directly onto the substratum and acquire a neuronal-like appearance with extended fine processes. Chromaffin cells maintained in suspension cultures aggregate into clumps reminiscent of the intact gland. Both preparations are suitable for structural studies. Functional differences between the two culture conditions may exist, but remain to be determined (see Section V,A for more details).

### A. Structure of Chromaffin Cells and Granules

The ultrastructure of chromaffin cells has been studied since the beginning of biological electron microscopy (Lever, 1955). Images of chemically fixed chromaffin tissue reveal a deceptively simple-looking cell 15–20 $\mu$m in diameter, which contains the usual complement of cellular organelles in addition to numerous dense core granules. Based on the dense core granule appearance, two populations of chromaffin cells have been observed. One type, the norepinephrine-containing cells, has granules with retracted very dark staining cores. This is due to the retention of an osmiophilic norepinephrine–glutaraldehyde complex during processing (Coupland *et al.,* 1964). The second cell type, the epinephrine-containing cells, has a lighter staining, more disperse dense core in their granules. Beyond this, studies of granule fine structure have been of limited consequence in understanding granule function. Granule structure is dependent on fixation conditions (Wood *et al.,* 1971) such that the expected spherical or round granule shape can appear as dumbbell- (Coupland, 1965), comma- (Wasserman and Tramezzini, 1963), or pear-shaped structures. In addition to varying effects on granule structure, chromaffin cells themselves exhibit fixation effects, the most notable being the appearance of exocytotic figures in the absence of secretogogue. It is also known in other systems that fixatives induce secretion and exocytosis prior to fixation (Smith and Reese, 1980). This may explain in part the pleomorphism of granule and cell appearance in chemically fixed preparations.

A new and very different view of chromaffin cells is obtained with quick-freezing methods. Quick-frozen cells are free of aldehyde-induced exocytotic artifacts in that they have smooth plasma membrane contours along the narrow intercellular clefts separating neighboring cells (see Fig. 1a). Granules within quick-frozen cells are round with a uniform density and lack the differences in stain density seen in norepinephrine- and epinephrine-containing granules of aldehyde-fixed cells. Based on size, two types of granules are observed, large granules with a diameter of about 0.3 $\mu$m and small granules with a diameter of 0.15 $\mu$m. The most interesting feature of the fine structure of quick-frozen granules is the observation of small unit membrane-bounded vesicles within ~60% of the dense core granules (Fig. 1b). These intragranular vesicles are true independent vesicles in that they are free of cytoplasm and are released by exocytosis along with granule contents in stimulated cells. Granules usually have only one intragranular vesicle (IGV), but as many as five have been observed in large granules. The loss of IGVs with chemical fixation probably occurs by the insertion of IGV membrane into the granule membrane which further explains the pleomorphism of granule shapes previously described. Curiously, however, IGVs can be chemically "fixed" in isolated granules and may be the structural basis of the pockets observed by Karen Helle in earlier studies of isolated granules (Helle *et al.,* 1971). The content, biogenesis, and function of the IGV are presently under study. The existence of these structures may explain the biochemical heterogeneity of the granule suggested by recent nuclear magnetic resonance studies on isolated granules (Pollard *et al.*, 1979; Sen and Sharp, 1981; Sen *et al.*, 1979; Daniels *et al.*, 1978).

## B. EXOCYTOSIS

Catecholamines and granule contents are secreted by exocytosis. Morphological evidence showing granule membrane incorporation into the plasma membrane (DeRobertis and Vaz Ferreira, 1957) and biochemical evidence describing the corelease of granule contents in the same proportion as that found in isolated granule lysate (summarized in Viveros, 1975) provide the strongest support for exocytotic secretion. Exocytosis occurs in the intact gland both at sites where the plasma membrane is exposed to extracellular medium and at sites on the plasma membrane juxtaposed to a neighboring cell (Grynszpan-Winograd, 1971). This finding suggests that, unlike secretory nerve ending where specialized regions of membrane called active zones support release, the chromaffin cell is capable of supporting exocytosis over its entire surface.

A sequence of ultrastructural events used to define exocytosis has been proposed (Palade and Bruns, 1968) with the support of a plethora of studies on secretion in cells using chemical fixation. However, recent studies on secreting *Limulus* amoebocytes (Ornberg and Reese, 1981), mast cells (Chandler and Heuser, 1980), and chromaffin cells (Schmidt *et al.*, 1983; our own studies) using quick-freezing methods has led to slight modifications to this earlier sequence, the consequences of which, however, are quite profound and may be related to events in chromaffin cells.

The initial step of exocytosis, the approach step, involves the relative movement of the secretory granule toward the plasma membrane for subsequent interaction. In secreting amoebocytes the plasma membrane moves inward, presumably mediated by some contractile elements, and results in the formation of pedestal-shaped depressions in the plasma membrane upon which the granule rests. We have preliminary observations of similar invaginations in the plasma membrane of nicotine-stimulated chromaffin cells. These data are important in that they support the hypothesis of an active cytoskeletal mechanism for bringing the fusing membranes into contact (see Section IV). An alternative hypothesis for the role of the cytoskeleton in secretion has been that it forms a mechanical barrier to granule movement when the cell is at rest. Upon stimulation the cytoskeleton is imagined to undergo a transition from a gel state to sol state, thus allowing granule mem-

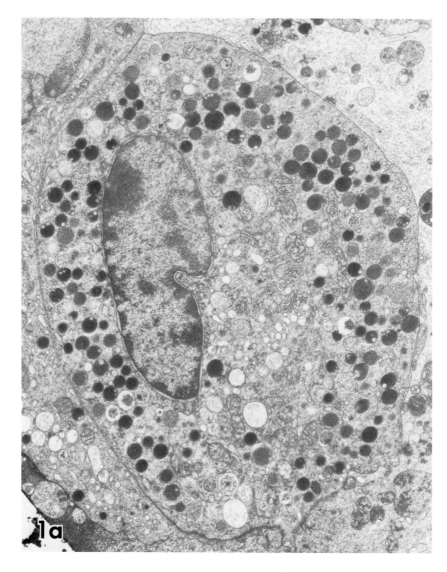

brane and plasma membrane to interact. Selective active and passive functions of the cytoskeleton cannot be excluded, especially coincident ones in different parts of the cell.

The second step of exocytosis, the contact step, refers to the molecular interactions occurring within the apposition of the granule membrane and the plasma membrane. In fixed cells, this apposition has been observed as an expansive joining of two trilaminar unit mem-

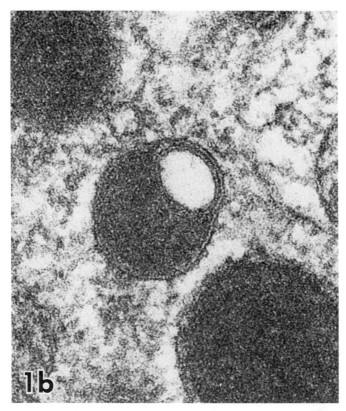

Fɪɢ. 1. (a) Ultrastructure of cultured bovine chromaffin cells preserved by a quick-freezing method. Granules are often observed to contain intragranular vesicles. (b) Bilayer structure of intragranular vesicles preserved by a quick-freezing method.

branes to form a pentalaminar contact. In freeze-fracture views this pentalaminar contact is free of intramembranous particles (Smith *et al.*, 1973). However, in quick-frozen cells, the apposition is neither expansive nor free of intramembranous particles or protein as reported (Schmidt *et al.*, 1983). Instead the structures resembling pentalaminar fusion are quite small or punctate in character and probably involve a few tens of lipid molecules at most. Within these constraints, a number of molecular intermediaries have been suggested as precursors for hole formation. These include proteins (See Section V for details), inverted lipidic micelles (Cullis *et al.*, 1983), and domains of fusogenic lipid (Bear and Friend, 1982).

The final step of exocytosis, the pore formation or "fission" step, is a rapid punctate event brought about by as yet unknown instabilities within the apposition region (see Section V for more details). The membrane elimination schemes proposed for fixed tissue probably do not occur, since the initial premise of an expansive pentalaminar contact is not correct. One can only speculate about processes leading to formation of a hole: weakened molecular interactions within the bilayers of the punctate fusion caused by nonbilayer structures; enzymatic protease or lipase activities; and/or intramembranous tension induced by cytoskeletal elements or increased osmotic pressure. Once formed, the hole quickly widens in a very rapid explosive step, presumably due to the tremendous osmotic force generated by water movements associated with the dissolving of the granule core. This is particularly evident in studies by Ornberg and Reese (1981) on *Limulus* amoebocytes and is probably quite relevant to chromaffin cell secretion. Because the lifetime of the pore is short, numerous questions regarding exocytotic pore formation remain. The most fundamental of these questions are as follows: (1) Is membrane conserved or are pieces of apposed membranes shed during pore formation and widening? (2) How do molecules in the membrane change position to allow pore enlargement while still preserving membrane integrity? While much more has to be done to answer these and other questions, any further elucidation of this dynamic process will depend on a coincidence of biochemical and ultrastructural analysis of a type as yet to be determined.

## C. MEMBRANE RECYCLING AND GRANULE BIOGENESIS

Immediately after exocytosis the cell has the tasks of granule membrane recovery and the biogenesis of replacement granules. Several investigators have attempted to measure the rate of removal of granule membrane protein from the chromaffin cell plasma membrane following exocytosis. The results seem to indicate that recycling is quite rapid, since proteins which are exposed to the external spaces following exocytosis are removed 15–30 minutes after stimulation. This suggests that granule membrane pinches off from the plasma membrane within that time (Dowd *et al.*, 1983; Phillips *et al.*, 1983). Patzak *et al.* (1984), using antibody labels to two different granule proteins, reported that both proteins disappeared at similar rates, suggesting that specific membrane conservation mechanisms are involved in recovery.

At the ultrastructural level, membrane retrieval is not so well characterized. Clathrin-coated pits have been identified budding from regions of the granule membrane incorporated into the plasma membrane after exocytosis (R. Ornberg, unpublished observation). From this observation it is tempting to assume that the compensatory membrane recycling sequel to exocytosis follows a structural route analogous to the other constitutive membrane uptake processes, i.e., endocytosis, receptor-mediated endocytosis.

In other systems these constitutive processes start with the budding of receptor-laden coated pits from the plasma membrane to form either a coated vesicle (Goldstein *et al.*, 1979) or a coat-free receptosome (Pastan and Willingham, 1983). These structures in turn transfer their contents to lysosomes. The receptors are collected for mass transport by the clathrin coat, but are spared from lysosomal digestion by a shuttle step back to the plasma membrane. This occurs after the ligand has undergone a pH-dependent dissociation from the receptor as the endosome acidifies (Tycho and Maxfield, 1982). In chromaffin cells, the endosomes consisting of granule membrane may also move to the stacked cisterns of the Golgi apparatus (Farquhar, 1981) for subsequent reuse (i.e., biogenesis).

The real meaning and complexity of biogenesis of chromaffin granules can be appreciated by recourse to a still valid review on biogenesis by Winkler (1977) and data summarized by Winkler and Westhead (1980) and Winkler and Carmichael (1982). We do not intend to reanalyze this information here, except to note that the membrane contains a variety of enzymes, including dopamine $\beta$-hydroxylase (dopamine $\beta$-monooxygenase), a proton pumping $Mg^{2+}$-ATPase, cytochrome $b_{561}$ (chromomembrin B), a catecholamine carrier, a nucleotide carrier, a calcium carrier, phosphatidylinositol kinase, NADH:(acceptor) oxidoreductase (NADH dehydrogenase), adenylate cyclase, a complement of phospholipids, cholesterol, and sialic acid-containing gangliosides. Loosely associated proteins may include $\alpha$-actinin, actin, and a spectrin-like protein. The list may even be more extensive based on the analysis by Abbs and Phillips (1980).

The contents are similarly complex and must obviously be loaded (or reloaded) into already complex and specific membrane vesicles. The contents include catecholamines, nucleotides (primarily ATP but minor amounts of others), calcium, chromogranins (acidic, immunologically related soluble proteins), glycoproteins and proteoglycans (Kiang *et al.*, 1982), and diverse enkephalin-containing peptides and proteins (Viveros *et al.*, 1979; Livett *et al.*, 1981, 1982; Udenfriend and Kilpatrick, 1983).

The mechanism of assembly of chromaffin granules in chromaffin cells is as obscure as is the process elsewhere in the field of cell biology. Therefore, we will concentrate in the next section on assembly from the standpoint of the lower molecular weight component, catecholamine, and the better understood biosynthetic enzymes.

III. Biosynthesis and Packaging of Catecholamines in Granules

As iterated in the previous section, we possess an exhaustive list of chemical and biochemical components of chromaffin granules (e.g., Winkler and Carmichael, 1982). In truth, our ideas are vague or non-existent about how many of these substances came to be in the granule. This is certainly true for the major granule protein, chromogranin A, the enkephalins and non-enkephalin-related peptides, the glyco-saminoglycans, and a host of others. For that reason, we have left out detailed discussion of these factors.

By contrast, we do know a little about the transport of catechol-amines, ATP, and $Ca^{2+}$ into granules, and about the biosynthetic en-zymes which both make the catecholamines and are to some extent structural components of the granule. Therefore, studying these bio-synthetic enzymes accomplishes two tasks at once insofar as the as-sembly problem is concerned. Accordingly, we have devoted the major-

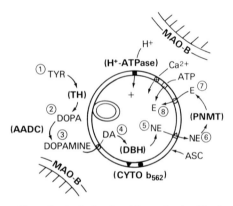

Fig. 2. Schematic outline of catecholamine biosynthesis. The large round structure represents a chromaffin granule. Tyrosine (1), derived from the diet, enters the chromaf-fin cell. It is converted by tyrosine hydroxylase (TH) to dihydroxyphenylalanine (2, dopa), which is rapidly converted to dopamine (3) by the enzyme aromatic-amino-acid decarboxylase (AADC). Dopamine enters the chromaffin granule via a membrane trans-port site (○), driven by an $H^+$-ATPase (■). Dopamine (4) is converted to norepinephrine (5, NE) by the enzyme dopamine $\beta$-hydroxylase (DBH, ▲). The conversion may be medi-ated by the membrane protein cytochrome $b_{562}$ (CYTOb$_{562}$, ●). Norepinephrine leaves the granule (6, NE) through a transport site (△), where it is methylated to epinephrine (7, E) by phenyl-*N*-methyltransferase (PNMT). The newly synthesized E is taken back up into the granule (8, E), driven by the $H^+$-ATPase. The granule membrane also has sites for uptake of calcium (⊗) and ATP (□). Monoamine oxidase B (MAO-B) has low affinity for catecholamines and thus permits efficient biosynthesis. It is associated with mitochondria.

ity of this section to these enzymes and transport systems and to related proteins and processes.

The currently accepted hypothesis for catecholamine synthesis in chromaffin cells, as illustrated in Fig. 2, is that cytosolic tyrosine is hydroxylated by tyrosine hydroxylase (TH; tyrosine 3-monooxygenase) in the soluble compartment of the cell. The dopa formed is immediately decarboxylated to dopamine by aromatic-L-amino-acid decarboxylase, and the dopamine then transported into the granules. Intragranular dopamine $\beta$-hydroxylase (DBH) synthesizes norpinephrine, believed to leak out of the granule and so become available for phenyl-$N$-methyltransferase (PNMT) -dependent conversion to epinephrine. Norepinephrine leakage from the granule is probably rate-limiting for the PNMT reaction. Epinephrine is then taken up into the granule for final storage in preparation for secretion. This whole scheme is quite complex.

Nonetheless, a way around the complexity may reside in the possibility that, like DBH, portions of TH (Treiman *et al.*, 1983) and PNMT (Joh and Goldstein, 1973; Van Orden *et al.*, 1977) may be associated with the external surface of the granule. Although these localization data are largely immunocytochemical studies whose validity can be questioned (Winkler and Carmichael, 1982), some kind of multienzyme complex of this sort might be capable of the quite efficient catecholamine synthesis we know takes place. These hypotheses point to directions of future work.

A. TYROSINE HYDROXYLASE: THE INITIAL ENZYME IN
   CATECHOLAMINE SYNTHESIS

Tyrosine hydroxylase (TH; tyrosine 3-monooxygenase, EC1.14.16.2) is a tetrameric mixed-function oxygenase enzyme with a molecular size of $\sim$240,000 Da in its oligomeric form of four 60,000-Da subunits (for review, see Kaufman, 1974; Kuhn and Lovenberg, 1983). The solubility characteristics of TH are a matter of some debate. Limited proteolysis has sometimes been used to generate a "soluble" species, while others have found ways to render intact TH readily soluble. Indeed, the major phosphorylated protein on isolated chromaffin granule membranes appears to be TH, as described in detail in a later section of this review. The active enzyme catalyzes the hydroxylation of tyrosine in the presence of molecular oxygen and $BH_4$ (Kaufman, 1963), which is oxidized to quinoid-dihydrobiopterin (q-$BH_2$). q-$BH_2$ can be reduced back to $BH_4$ by quinoid dihydrobiopterin reductase (DHPR), which requires NAD(P)H as the electron donor. The reaction apparently proceeds by a semiordered sequential mechanism (Joh *et al.*, 1969) whereby $BH_4$ and tyrosine are randomly added, followed by oxygen, with the liberation of L-dopa preceding liberation of q-$BH_2$.

The regulation of tyrosine hydroxylase *in vivo* is a complex process that is still not totally understood. Indeed, the importance of the enzyme seems pointed up by the fact that no aspect of its regulation seems free of controversy. Early studies developed the argument that the intracellular concentration of $BH_4$ in central nervous system (CNS) catecholamine neurons and adrenal medullary chromaffin cells was subsaturating for TH and played an important role in limiting TH activity *in vivo* (Kuczenski and Mandell, 1972; for review, see Lovenberg *et al.*, 1978; Levine *et al.*, 1981a). More recently, the question of the intracellular concentration of $BH_4$ and its rate-limiting role has been reexamined in both the CNS (Levine *et al.*, 1981b) and the adrenal medulla (Abou-Donia and Viveros, 1981). It is likely that the level of $BH_4$ in the cell is an important component of the overall regulatory process of TH, especially in conjunction with protein phosphorylation regulatory mechanisms, to be discussed below and in later parts of this review.

It was originally thought that the level of free tyrosine inside catecholamine-producing cells was sufficient to support catecholamine synthesis even when TH was in an activated state (for review, see Lovenberg *et al.*, 1978). However, more recent studies have suggested that under conditions which are known to activate TH, the rate of uptake of tyrosine across the blood–brain barrier and thus into catecholamine neurons may affect the rate of catecholamine biosynthesis (Wurtman *et al.*, 1980). However, the effects of circulating tyrosine on adrenal chromaffin cell catecholamine formation has not been thoroughly examined.

One of the best studied regulatory mechanisms for TH activity is protein phosphorylation. It was initially found in brain and adrenal extracts that endogenous TH could be activated *in vitro* when exposed to cyclic AMP-dependent phosphorylating conditions (Lovenberg *et al.*, 1975; Morganroth *et al.*, 1975). More recently, it has been shown that TH can be activated by a calcium–phospholipid-dependent protein kinase (protein kinase C; Takai *et al.*, 1979). A calcium–calmodulin-dependent kinase system has also been proposed to activate TH in selected areas of the brain (Yamauchi *et al.*, 1981). Whether this control system is actually operative in adrenal chromaffin cells is a matter of some controversy. TH in a phosphorylated state has been detected in a number of laboratories (Lentendre *et al.*, 1977; Joh *et al.*, 1978; Yamauchi and Fujisawa, 1979; Vulliet *et al.*, 1980). It also has been recently shown (Haycock *et al.*, 1982a) that TH can be phosphorylated at two distinct sites after stimulation of the cell by acetylcholine (ACh). This process apparently induces the phosphorylation of the different sites by different mechanisms. One phosphorylation site is dependent on the cyclic AMP-dependent phosphorylation system, whereas phosphorylation of the other site is mediated by a calcium-cAMP independent phosphorylation system (Haycock *et al.*, 1982b).

The end result of phosphorylation on TH kinetics *in situ* is also very controversial. It has been shown by several laboratories (Lovenberg *et al.*, 1975; Morganroth *et al.*, 1975; Vulliet *et al.*, 1980) that activation of TH *in vitro* by exposure to phosphorylating conditions results in a decrease in the $K_m$ of the enzyme for the cofactor $BH_4$, while there was no change in the $V_{max}$ of the enzyme under optimal cosubstrate conditions. It was also shown that phosphorylation conditions cause an increase in the $K_i$ of the enzyme for dopamine, so that the phosphorylated enzyme would presumably be less influenced by competitive feedback inhibition (Ames *et al.*, 1978). However, there have been reports that the $V_{max}$ of TH for the pterin cofactor can be elevated by phosphorylating conditions (Hoeldtke and Kaufman, 1977; Joh and Reis, 1975). The reason for these differences is yet to be resolved. In either event, the kinetic activation of TH provides more dopamine as the cells endeavor to synthesize more catecholamines.

It is often generally stated that tyrosine hydroxylase is the rate-limiting step in catecholamine biosynthesis. Indeed, it is probable that this is the case for dopamine synthesis in chromaffin cells. However, it is worth recalling that the situation is more complex for norepinephrine and epinephrine, since vesicular transport and storage mechanisms may contribute to regulating the rate of norepinephrine and epinephrine biosynthesis. It is to the details of the vesicular transport mechanism that we will now turn our attention.

B. Catecholamine Transport in Chromaffin Granules

The enzyme responsible for the conversion of dopamine to norepinephrine, dopamine $\beta$-hydroxylase, is located entirely within chromaffin granules so that the precursor dopamine must cross the granule membrane to reach the enzyme (Belpaire and Laduron, 1968; Laduron, 1975). The subsequent step in epinephrine synthesis requires norepinephrine efflux from the chromaffin granules to reach the cytosolic enzyme, phenyl-*N*-methyltransferase (Wurtman and Axelrod, 1966; Ciaranello *et al.*, 1973). The product of this enzyme, epinephrine, is then reaccumulated in chromaffin granules for eventual secretion by exocytosis. Therefore, implicit in all of these functions is a bidirectional transport mechanism for catecholamines.

The uptake arm of catecholamine flux in chromaffin granules has been studied by far in the greatest detail. Kirshner (1962) and Carlsson *et al.* (1963) showed that preparations of chromaffin granules contained a catecholamine transporter that required ATP. Taugner (1971) extensively characterized catecholamine flux across chromaffin granules, showing that the catecholamine pump appeared to be on the granule membrane and that uptake was associated with ATP hydrolysis and was relatively specific for the l-catecholamine stereoisomer (Taugner, 1971, 1972). Taugner suggested that catecholamine uptake was carrier mediated, a conclusion also reached by Slotkin (1973).

Taugner's experiments additionally characterized bidirectional flux across the granule and granule membrane (Taugner, 1971, 1972) using crude ghost preparations. Ghosts are essentially chromaffin granule membranes, or granules which are depleted of their intracellular contents by lysis and then allowed to reseal. The technique has been subsequently further modified by several groups (Phillips, 1974a,b; Njus and Radda, 1979; Johnson *et al.*, 1981). Phillips showed that catecholamine transport was MgATP dependent, proceeded with high affinity for several substrates, and was inhibited by reserpine (Phillips, 1974a,b). Other investigators confirmed a role for MgATP (Hoffman *et al.*, 1976).

What, then, was the specific function of MgATP? Radda and colleagues are principally responsible for our current understanding of the link between ATP hydrolysis and catecholamine uptake (Bashford *et al.*, 1975a,b, 1976). They based their observations on those of Von Euler and Lishajko (1969), who showed that catecholamine fluxes across vesicles from splenic nerve were particularly sensitive to mitochondrial uncouplers. They took advantage of the development of assays for energy states across mitochondrial membranes defined using fluorescent probes (Azzi *et al.*, 1969; Brocklehurst *et al.*, 1970), in particular 1-anilinonaphthalene-8-sulfonic acid (ANS). Radda's group then proceeded to show that the activity of the chromaffin granule ATPase was associated with enhanced fluorescence of the probe (the ANS response) as well as catecholamine uptake. The fluorescent enhancement was blocked by low concentrations of mitochondrial uncouplers, which also abolished catecholamine uptake into granules. The conclusion was that the ATPase pumped protons into the granules. An inward-directed proton pump would be expected to make the granule transmembrane electrical potential inside positive ($\Delta\Psi$) and increase internal proton concentration ($\Delta pH$). A combination of $\Delta\Psi$ and $\Delta pH$

could then provide the driving force for transport, according to the formula for proton electromotive force, $\Delta\bar{\mu}_{H^+} = \Delta\Psi + F\,\Delta pH$.

Indeed, the predictions concerning the proton pumping role of the ATPase have been borne out by several groups. In fact, separate changes in $\Delta\Psi$ and $\Delta pH$ have been predictably generated and measured, depending on the incubation conditions. When granules were incubated with permeant anions, the addition of MgATP generated an $H^+$ influx which was neutralized by influx of anions. The $H^+$/anion influx caused a drop in intragranular pH (Casey et al., 1977). The membrane potential induced by MgATP (Pollard et al., 1976b) was much smaller because of influx of anions along with positive charges (Johnson and Scarpa, 1979). Therefore, $\Delta pH$ can be changed with only a small change in $\Delta\Psi$. As expected, the converse has also turned out to be true. When intact granules were incubated without permeant anions, addition of MgATP generated an inside positive membrane potential without change of the internal pH (Casey et al., 1977; Holz, 1978; Johnson and Scarpa, 1979). The pH did not change presumably due to the relatively small number of entering positive charges responsible for the inside positive membrane potential, especially in comparison to the large buffering capacity of the matrix. Thus, $\Delta\Psi$ can be varied without changing $\Delta pH$.

Although the original experiments were done by measuring increases in ANS fluorescence, other direct techniques have since been developed for measurement of both $\Delta pH$ and $\Delta\Psi$ in chromaffin granules. For measurements of $\Delta\Psi$, the lipid-soluble anion thiocyanate has been useful (Pollard et al., 1976b; Holz, 1978; Johnson and Scarpa, 1979), while the lipid-soluble cation triphenylmethylphosphonium has also been employed (Holz, 1979). The voltage-sensitive dye 3,3'-dipropyl-2,2"-thiadicarbocyanine has been used by Ogawa and Inouye (1979) and Salama et al. (1980). These measurements of $\Delta\Psi$ in the absence of permeant ions indicated that addition of MgATP generated a membrane potential of +50 to +70 mV inside positive, with a resting potential of -70 mV inside negative at pH 6.9.

Measurements of $\Delta pH$ have been obtained in intact granules using the distribution of the base methylamine or by [31]P nuclear magnetic resonance (NMR). Both general types of methods, with modifications, yield an approximate resting intragranular pH of 5.7 (Johnson and Scarpa, 1976; Pollard et al., 1976b, 1979; Casey et al., 1977; Njus et al., 1978). Several of these experiments showed a fall of ~0.4 pH units over 30 minutes upon addition of MgATP in the presence of a permeant ion. The pH change was inhibited by uncouplers (Casey et al., 1977; Pollard et al., 1979).

Many of the techniques used for measurement of ΔpH as well as ΔΨ in intact granules have also been useful in chromaffin granule ghosts. For example, the distribution of thiocyanate in ghost preparations emphasized that MgATP generated a maximum membrane potential only in the absence of permeant ions (Phillips and Allison, 1978; Johnson *et al.*, 1979, 1981; Knoth *et al.*, 1980). Likewise, these same investigators as well as others showed that ΔpH was generated with MgATP in ghosts only when permeant ions were included in the medium, as measured by distribution of the weak base methylamine. Thus, much information gathered over just several years has solidified the concept that the ATPase in both ghosts and intact granules is responsible for generation of ΔpH and ΔΨ.

But what combination of these properties drives catecholamine transport? An electroneutral mechanism, one driven by ΔpH, was proposed initially (Bashford *et al.*, 1976; Johnson and Scarpa, 1976). In this scheme, a neutral amine enters the chromaffin granule and is then reprotonated and trapped via the action of the proton pumping ATPase. Essentially this mechanism is similar to trapping of weak bases on the more acidic side of a membrane. Indeed, several investigators have demonstrated that artificially imposed pH gradients can be generated across chromaffin granule ghosts and that these gradients can drive catecholamine uptake (Johnson *et al.*, 1978, 1981; Ingebretsen and Flatmark, 1979). These groups also found that dissipation of the pH gradients with ionophores or ammonium chloride blocked catecholamine uptake, as would be predicted.

However, ΔΨ might also be expected to drive catecholamine transport. This contention was tested in the absence of permeant anions so that ΔpH was not affected. In intact granules, there was a clear correlation between ΔΨ and catecholamine uptake, with inhibition of uptake induced by the uncoupler FCCP (Holz, 1978; Johnson and Scarpa, 1979). Ghosts suspended without permeant ions also accumulated catecholamines when an inside positive membrane potential was generated (Johnson *et al.*, 1979, 1981; Knoth *et al.*, 1980). The MgATP-generated membrane potential in ghosts was also sensitive to FCCP.

Thus, both ΔpH and ΔΨ can separately mediate catecholamine uptake in ghosts and granules. Maximal uptake, however, may indeed require generation of both ΔpH and ΔΨ concurrently (Johnson *et al.*, 1979). However, the fact that ΔΨ alone can generate amine uptake suggests that there must be some concomitant efflux of positive charge for electroneutrality to be maintained (see Njus *et al.*, 1981, for further review). Several models have been proposed to account for maintenance of electroneutrality in the granule or the ghost. The choice of models is directly dependent on the calculated number of exiting protons and the charge of the catecholamine transported inside (Knoth *et al.*, 1980; Njus *et al.*, 1981; Johnson *et al.*, 1981; Ramu *et al.*, 1983).

Several groups have suggested what the number of exiting protons might be (Knoth *et al.*, 1980, 1981; Njus *et al.*, 1981; Johnson *et al.*, 1981; Ramu *et al.*, 1983), using models that are based on stoichiometric measurements of catecholamine and proton exchange in ghosts. The models predict that one more proton should exit than the charge of the catecholamine that is transported inside, since exit of positive charge is necessary to account for influx of positive charge generated by the ATPase. For electroneutrality to exist, influx and efflux of positive charges must therefore take into account the charge of the transported catecholamine. This catecholamine must have one less positive charge than the number of effluxing protons, due specifically to the inward proton pumping of the ATPase. Thus, the number of predicted effluxing positive charges is directly dependent on the charge of the transported catecholamine.

It has not been possible to measure directly the charge of the transported species, but several indirect approaches have been taken. Studies from Njus' laboratory (Knoth *et al.*, 1980, 1981) have suggested that since catecholamines are predominantly positively charged at the chromaffin cell pH, a positively charged amine is transported inside in exchange for two positive charges. This contention was also supported by the apparent pH-dependent $K_m$ values of dopamine and serotonin uptake in chromaffin granule ghosts (Knoth *et al.*, 1981). These measurements, however, could not distinguish between binding and transport of the catecholamine species at each pH. Ramu *et al.* (1983) provided contrasting chemical evidence that the neutral catecholamine instead might be the species transported into the chromaffin granule. Their experiments used a novel, permanently positively charged catecholamine analog, dimethylepinephrine. Dimethylepinephrine competitively inhibited catecholamine transport, but was itself not transported into granules, thus providing evidence for the identification of the transported catecholamine as the neutral species. It may be argued that a negative result, no matter how controlled, must remain indirect. However, Scherman and Henry (1981) have also come to the conclusion that the neutral species is the true substrate based on extensive pH titration data. A series of models showing $H^+$ and catecholamine transport are illustrated in Fig. 3.

Nearly all of the evidence concerning catecholamine transport has focused on uptake or catecholamine accumulation. But norepinephrine efflux and its regulation are also integral granule transport functions

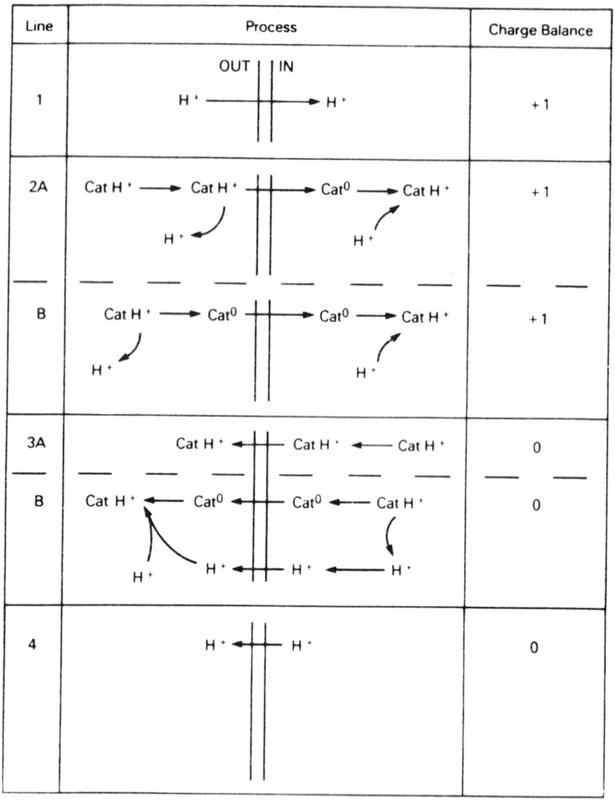

FIG. 3. Electrodissipative models for catecholamine transport by chromaffin granules. Each line corresponds to an event in the model, beginning (line 1) with ATPase-driven H⁺ transport, which causes an increment in internal charge of $+1$. Line 2 depicts alternative mechanisms by which an uncharged catecholamine can penetrate the granule membrane. Line 3 shows how charge can be dissipated, either by exchange or by a combination of exchange and H⁺ extrusion. Line 4 illustrates how net accumulation of catecholamines and charge dissipation can be accomplished by H⁺ extrusion.

due to the presumptive cytosolic location of the methylating enzyme phenyl-*N*-methyltransferase, necessary for epinephrine biosynthesis (Wurtman and Axelrod, 1966; Ciaranello *et al.*, 1973). Taugner, in her original observations, observed catecholamine efflux from intact granules (Taugner, 1971). Ramu *et al.* (1981) found that in intact granules catecholamine transport was coupled to efflux and that efflux was also MgATP dependent, but did not seem to involve the granule ATPase. A model of catecholamine transport incorporating both catecholamine efflux and influx and the assumption that the substrate for transport is the neutral species (Ramu *et al.*, 1983) is shown in Fig. 3, lower panel.

The transport site has also received considerable attention. Reserpine binds to this site and a reserpine analogue, [2-$^3$H]dihydrotetrabenazine, has been used to detect the site (Scherman *et al.*, 1983). The transporter in its uptake mode has broad substrate specificity (Slotkin and Kirshner, 1971; Da Prada *et al.*, 1975; Johnson *et al.*, 1982; Njus *et al.*, 1981), although very little is known about the efflux site (Ramu *et al.*, 1981). The physical properties of the actual site have just recently been appreciated. Using a photoaffinity labeling technique, Gabizon *et al.* (1982) have tentatively identified the transporter or portion of the transporter as a polypeptide with a molecular weight of 45,000. By contrast, Scherman *et al.* (1983) believe it to be 70,000. Continued efforts to isolate and reconstitute the transporter will likely provide further insight into how catecholamine transport is coupled to energy transduction and how many proteins are involved in the process.

The membrane ATPase has also received considerable attention. As mentioned above, the chromaffin granule ATPase seems to pump protons into the granule. Apps and Schatz (1979) showed that even though it differed in pharmacologic responses from classical mitochondrial $F_1$-ATPase, the granule ATPase was closely similar to the $F_1$-ATPase proteins characteristic of mitochondria. For example, treatment of the chromaffin granule with chloroform or dichloromethane solubilized most of the activity, just as with $F_1$-ATPase of mitochondria (Apps, 1982). The ATPase from chromaffin granules had three major subunits as well as a DCCD-binding proteolipid (Apps *et al.*, 1980), just like the mitochondrial enzyme complex. However, chromaffin granule membrane ATPase did not interact with aurovertin, in which the $\beta$ subunit is important. Cidon and Nelson (1983), on the other hand, have concluded that the $F_1$-type activity associated with the granule membrane is a contaminant from mitochondria and that a separate, novel, anion-sensitive ATPase is actually responsible. More work is clearly needed on this important enzyme to resolve this controversy.

The next step in catecholamine synthesis is the conversion of newly transported dopamine to norepinephrine by dopamine $\beta$-hydroxylase (DBH).

C. Synthesis of Norepinephrine by Dopamine
   $\beta$-Hydroxylase

Dopamine $\beta$-hydroxylase (3,4-dihydroxyphenylethylamine, ascorbate:oxygen oxidoreductase, dopamine $\beta$-monooxygenase, DBH, EC 1.14.17.1) is a copper-containing mixed-function oxidase catalyzing the conversion of dopamine to norepinephrine utilizing an electron donor and molecular oxygen.

DBH is found in the chromaffin granules of the adrenal medulla (Skotland and Ljones, 1979; Flatmark, 1982) and in the synaptic vesicles of adrenergic neurons (Helle and Serck-Hanssen, 1981; Geffen, 1981; Winkler, 1982). In these secretory vesicles, DBH exists in a membrane-bound form as well as a soluble form. The differences between the membranous and soluble DBH have been subjects of recent intense investigations, and many controversies still exist regarding the structural, biosynthetic, and functional relationships of the two forms of the enzyme.

The assay for DBH *in vitro*, in addition to $O_2$ and copper, also requires an electron donor such as ascorbate as well as fumarate, catalase, and a pH of 5.5–6.0 for optimal activity. These conditions may be quite relevant to the function of the enzyme *in vivo*. For example, the interior of the chromaffin granule has a pH in this range (see previous section), and ascorbate may be of importance to the enzyme in the intact cell (Levine *et al.*, 1985). The importance of fumarate is not known, but the enzyme generates $H_2O_2$, and $H_2O_2$ would inactivate the enzyme if not for the presence of catalase. *In vivo,* the chromaffin cell has high levels of catalase activity, mainly soluble but also associated with the chromaffin granule (Pazoles *et al.*, 1980).

The importance of DBH to the exocytosis process, however, lies not only in the fact that DBH catalyzes a step in the synthesis of the hormone to be secreted, but also in the fact that it is a principal structural component of the chromaffin granule itself.

In bovine chromaffin granules, dopamine $\beta$-hydroxylase is a major constituent (25%) of the membrane proteins and a minor component (4%) of the intragranular soluble proteins (Hortnagl *et al.*, 1972; Helle *et al.*, 1978). Dopamine $\beta$-hydroxylase activity is distributed equally between the membranes and the soluble lysate of the bovine chromaffin granules, and it has therefore been calculated that the membranes should contain about four times more DBH per milligram protein than the lysate (Winkler, 1976).

tein in the membrane (Slater *et al.*, 1981; Helle *et al.*, 1982).

It is generally believed that the membranous and soluble dopamine $\beta$-hydroxylases have very similar molecular properties. Nonetheless, the fate of these two forms of the enzyme is clearly different in the adrenal medullary cells. The soluble form of the enzyme is released during exocytosis of the granule contents and the membranous enzyme is reinternalized after the exocytosis of the granule contents (Viveros *et al.*, 1969; Silver and Jacobowitz, 1979; Phillips *et al.*, 1983). The soluble enzyme from bovine adrenal is a tetrameric glycoprotein which is made up of identical subunits of 72,500 (Aunis *et al.*, 1973; Ljone *et al.*, 1976; Wallace *et al.*, 1973; Craine *et al.*, 1973). Two of the subunits are joined by disulfide bonds and the two dimers are then held together by noncovalent interactions (Craine *et al.*, 1973). The membranous form of DBH has also been reported to possess similar subunit structure (Slater *et al.*, 1981; Aunis *et al.*, 1974; Blakeborough *et al.*, 1981). However, the membranous enzyme has been suggested to contain a hydrophobic domain which can be responsible for anchoring the protein in the membrane (Slater *et al.*, 1981; Helle *et al.*, 1982).

The two forms of dopamine $\beta$-hydroxylase have displayed identical immunological activities as determined by polyclonal antibodies made against either form (Hortnagl *et al.*, 1972, 1974). Using charge shift crossed immunoelectrophoresis, however, Bjerrum *et al.* (1979) have differentiated between an amphiphilic membranous and a more hydrophilic soluble DBH. Furthermore, the membranous form can be converted into the soluble form by limited proteolysis. These results therefore strongly suggested that the soluble DBH has a compact structural domain and that an extra domain in the membranous form is a small hydrophobic tail which can insert this compact structure into the membrane. This suggestion was supported by a recent report on the heterogeneity in subunit composition of both forms of DBH. On sodium dodecyl sulfate–polyacrylamide gel electrophoresis, the soluble enzyme had a major subunit of 70,000 Da and a small amount of 75,000-Da subunit (Saxena and Fleming, 1983). The membranous DBH, however, contained stoichiometric amounts of the 70,000 and 75,000 subunits, perhaps indicating that the higher molecular subunit might contain the hydrophobic domain.

The orientation of dopamine $\beta$-hydroxylase in membranes has been investigated using proteolysis and radiolabeling studies of intact and lysed chromaffin granules (Konig *et al.*, 1976; Abbs and Phillips, 1980; Blakeborough *et al.*, 1981). These studies generally indicated that DBH was exclusively exposed to the matrix side of the granule membrane. In contrast to these studies, Zaremba and Hogue-Angeletti (1981) found that proteolysis of intact chromaffin granules cleaved membranous DBH, generating a slightly lower molecular weight enzyme. Furthermore, these authors found DBH to be labeled when intact chromaffin granules were iodinated in the presence of lactoperoxidase and concluded that the hydrophobic tail of the membrane-bound DBH might be transmembranous in character. A more recent study, however, showed that membranous DBH is not accessible to lactoperoxidase-catalyzed iodination of the intact chromaffin granules (Duong and Fleming, 1983). Differences in apparent orientation of the membranous enzyme could be due to the lack of two critical controls in the earlier studies. These controls were whether the granules were completely intact and whether complete inhibition of the labeling reagents occurred prior to DBH isolation.

Other kinds of biochemical studies have also supported the conclusion that structural differences exist between the soluble and the membranous form of dopamine $\beta$-hydroxylase (Fleming and Saxena, 1982; Saxena and Fleming, 1983). On gel filtration chromatography, the molecular weight of soluble DBH was estimated to be 480,000 rather than the 280,000 estimated from its known structure, while membranous DBH had a much larger apparent molecular weight of over 1,000,000. These results indicated that soluble DBH was asymmetric in solution. On the other hand, the membranous DBH was apparently aggregated in solution. The basis of this difference in state might be due to the extra hydrophobic region, or be related to phospholipid, predominantly phosphatidylserine, or to entirely other reasons. This form of the enzyme, however, can be reconstituted into artificial phospholipid vesicles and then converted into the soluble form upon limited chymotryptic digestion of the vesicles (Saxena and Fleming, 1983).

The carbohydrate compositions of the membranous and soluble dopamine $\beta$-hydroxylase have also been investigated. Fischer-Colbrie *et al.* (1982) found that the carbohydrate contents of both forms of the enzyme were 5% of the total weight of each enzyme and that their compositions were identical. They concluded that the glycosylation of the enzyme could not be responsible for the membrane binding properties of DBH. Composition analysis might not be sufficient to detect subtle differences between the glycosylated moieties of the two forms of the enzyme, and more detailed studies can be anticipated. Recently, Hogue-Angeletti *et al.* (1983) have reported the development of monoclonal antibodies to both forms of DBH, and it will be therefore interesting to see the result from this work.

Genetic analysis is yet another nascent approach to study the relationship of membranous and soluble DBH. Two groups have independently reported the cloning of genes for catecholamine biosynthetic enzymes isolated from rat pheochromocytoma (PC 12) cell line (Joh *et al.*, 1981; O'Malley *et al.*, 1983). From these studies, the structural information on the two forms of DBH might be expected to become more specific.

The existence of membranous and soluble forms of dopamine $\beta$-hydroxylase has also raised the possibility of a biosynthetic relationship between the two forms. Recent studies have suggested that the membranous form might be the posttranslational precursor of the soluble enzyme. For example, immature bovine adrenal medullary vesicles in microsomal and Golgi fractions have been found to contain predominantly the membranous DBH (Helle and Serck-Hanssen, 1981). Furthermore, in a recent study on the biosynthesis of the two forms of DBH in PC 12 cells, Sabban *et al.* (1984) demonstrated that DBH was initially synthesized as a single polypeptide with a molecular weight of 67,000 on membrane-bound polysomes. After posttranslational modification, the mature DBH was found to consist of two subunit forms (77,000 and 73,000). The higher molecular weight form was found in the crude membrane fractions, whereas the lower molecular weight form was soluble. An analysis of pulse-chase experiments indicated that the membranous DBH was initially synthesized and then converted into the soluble enzyme. The same group later reported that DBH was completely converted into the soluble form in monensin-treated PC 12 cells (Sabban *et al.*, 1984). Since monensin causes a pileup of Golgi vesicles, the authors suggested that the processing of the 77,000 to the 73,000 subunit form of DBH occurred prior to exit of newly synthesized DBH from the Golgi into secretory vesicles. This conclusion may be in question, however, in view of further recent study on the two forms of DBH in PC 12 cells. McHugh *et al.* (1984) have reported that the membranous form of the enzyme contained both the 77,000 and 73,000 subunits in stoichiometric amounts and that the soluble form had only the lower molecular weight subunit. This observation confirms the results of earlier studies on the heterogeneous subunit structure of the purified membranous bovine chromaffin granule DBH (Fleming and Saxena, 1982; Saxena and Fleming, 1983). In any event, it will have to be borne in mind that chemical events in PC 12 cells may not be directly correlated with homologous chemical events in chromaffin cells.

D. Synthesis of Epinephrine by Phenylethanolamine
   N-Methyltransferase

Phenylethanolamine *N*-methyltransferase (EC 2.1.1.28, PNMT), also referred to as norepinephrine *N*-methyltransferase, is the terminal enzyme in the epinephrine biosynthetic pathway, catalyzing the methylation of norepinephrine at the nitrogen moiety to form epinephrine (Axelrod, 1962). S-Adenosylmethionine provides the methyl group for the reaction (Kirshner and Goodall, 1957). In mammals, the adrenal medulla contains by far the largest concentration of PNMT in the body (Pendleton *et al.*, 1978), although it is now clear that in lower concentrations the enzyme enjoys a wide tissue distribution. In the rat, PNMT activity has been found in heart (Axelrod, 1962; Pendleton *et al.*, 1978), lung [Pendelton *et al.*, 1978; Padbury *et al.*, 1983 (sheep)], spleen (Pendleton *et al.*, 1978), skeletal muscle (Pendleton *et al.*, 1978), retina (Hadjiconstantinou *et al.*, 1983; Osborne and Nesselnut, 1983), and in the brain (Axelrod, 1962; Pendleton *et al.*, 1978; Saavedra *et al.*, 1974; Hokfelt *et al.*, 1974; Van der Gugten *et al.*, 1976), the most prominent areas being cell bodies in two areas of the medulla oblongata and in many nuclei of the hypothalamus. The significance of the presence of PNMT in the adrenal medulla is clearly to provide epinephrine for the reaction to stress that constitutes the hormonal "fight or flight" response. The medulla oblongata and hypothalamic PNMT probably synthesize epinephrine for neurotransmission. Whether PNMT in other tissues is due to epinephrine-secreting endocrine activity of cells or neurotransmission is not known.

In chromaffin cells, the enzyme is generally thought to exist as a glycosylated 31,000–40,000 monomer (Joh and Goldstein, 1973; Connett and Kirshner, 1970; Park *et al.*, 1982; Baetge *et al.*, 1983), although Joh and Goldstein (1973) have reported the existence of dimeric and tetrameric forms. Recently, translation of poly(A) RNA from bovine adrenal medulla and immunoprecipitation with PNMT antibody confirm that the monomeric protein has an $M_r$ of 31,000 in the absence of posttranslational modification (Park *et al.*, 1982). Reports of higher molecular weights may reflect the influence of glycosylation or other posttranslational modification on the accuracy of the methods used for $M_r$ determination. In addition, variously charged isozymes of the monomer have been reported to exist in bovine adrenal (Joh and Goldstein, 1973). The basis of the charge heterogeneity is not clear, but may be a result of microheterogeneity of glycosylation (Joh and Goldstein, 1973; Park *et al.*, 1982). PNMT is considered a soluble, cytosolic protein (Axelrod, 1962; Kirshner and Goodall, 1957; Dunn and Holz, 1983), although two reports suggest possible particulate localization. Joh and Goldstein (1973) have shown that 20% of the activity can be found in the pellet after homogenization and 100,000 $g$ centrifugation; and Van Orden and colleagues (1977) reported that PNMT is localized in association with chromaffin granules by electron microscopy. The subcellular localization of PNMT as well as of the other catecholamine biosynthetic enzymes is of particular importance, since the precise movement and availability of catecholamines within the cell during their biosynthesis is an important problem.

The cellular regulation of PNMT has been most extensively studied in the rat adrenal medulla and brain. During development, there is an appearance of the enzyme in peripheral autonomic ganglia and adrenal medulla at distinct developmental time periods. The medulla oblongata and adrenal PNMT persist throughout life, the adrenal medullary enzyme requiring glucocorticoids for its continued expression. The appearance of the superior cervical ganglion enzyme is transient. For an extensive review of developmental control of PNMT expression, see Bohn (1983).

In the adult animal, it has been suggested that PNMT is subject to dual regulation *in vivo* by both glucocorticoids and cholinergic innervation (Ciaranello, 1977). Originally, the unique anatomical proximity of the adrenal cortex, the main endogenous source of glucocorticoid hormones, led to speculation that corticosteroids were important in medullary function (West, 1951). Then Wurtman and Axelrod (1965, 1966) demonstrated the dependence of epinephrine synthesis in the adrenal on glucocorticoids. A decline in PNMT activity is induced by hypophysectomy and can be reversed by ACTH or high concentrations of dexamethasone and depends on protein synthesis (Wurtman and Axelrod, 1965, 1966). The levels of PNMT activity in adult hypothalamus, medulla oblongata, and superior cervical ganglion are also reported to be regulated by glucocorticoid administration. Moore and Phillipson (1975) demonstrated a rise in PNMT activity in these neuronal areas in rat after dexamethasone treatment.

In the intact adult animal, the enzyme also seems to be under regulatory control by transsynaptic stimulation of the PNMT-containing cells. This is demonstrated by the increases in PNMT activity found after heat or immobilization stress (Tessel and Burgess, 1980; Saavedra, 1980), treatments which cause medullary stimulation and, therefore, epinephrine release. Similarly, pharmacological stimulation of the nervous input to the adrenal or brain with reserpine (Molinoff *et al.*, 1970) or 6-hydroxydopamine (Fety and Renaud, 1983) also produces an increase in enzyme activity. Ciaranello (1978) has shown that glucocorticoid-induced increases in PNMT proceed via an inhibition of enzyme degradation, whereas increases caused by innervation are due to a higher rate of PNMT synthesis. He also proposes that the rate of degradation of PNMT is altered by glucocorticoid-induced changes in the synthesis and levels of *S*-adenosylmethionine which serves to stabilize the enzyme against degradation *in situ* (Ciaranello *et al.*, 1978).

*In vitro* systems potentially allow for clearer resolution of the factors and mechanisms important in regulation of PNMT activity and expression. Although there have been numerous *in vitro* regulatory studies on TH and DBH with PC 12 and related cells, the lack of PNMT expression in these lines precludes their use for studies on PNMT regulation. The recent availability of primary cultures of adrenal medullary cells has allowed investigation into PNMT regulation. Bovine adrenal medullary cells maintained in culture retain their initial (day 1 of culture) content of catecholamines [epinephrine (60–70%) and norepinephrine (30–40%)], DBH, and TH (Waymire *et al.*, 1977; Hersey and DiStefano, 1979; Kilpatrick *et al.*, 1980; Wilson and Viveros, 1981). In contrast, the concentration of PNMT declines with time (Waymire *et al.*, 1977). This drop has been attributed to withdrawal of the cells from endogenous glucocorticoids in culture. Upon addition of

5 µg/ml of cortisol, Hersey and DiStefano (1979) found the drop in PNMT activity delayed by 3–4 days, but not prevented. PNMT levels did not increase during culture. This is analogous to the situation in rat *in vivo* where exogenous administration of glucocorticoids does not increase the PNMT activity in the adrenal above normal (Pohorecky and Wurtman, 1968). This regulation of PNMT levels *in vitro* in bovine-cultured cells may be equivalent to glucocorticoid control of PNMT in the rat *in vivo* outlined above. The inevitable drop in PNMT activity seen even in the presence of dexamethasone in culture may be due to the withdrawal of cholinergic input, which is clearly necessary for PNMT maintenance *in vivo*. Alternatively, other unknown regulatory factors normally provided by the adrenal cortex may be missing in culture (see also Kelner and Pollard, 1985).

Other studies on the regulation of catecholamine biosynthetic enzymes have been performed *in vitro* with nerve growth factor (NGF). Addition of NGF to dissociated rat adrenal medullary cells causes neurite outgrowth and a concomitant increase in TH activity (Tischler *et al.*, 1982). DBH and PNMT were not tested. *In vivo*, NGF increases the activity of adrenal TH and DBH (Unsicker *et al.*, 1980). When NGF-treated or untreated cells were exposed *in vitro* to $10^{-5}$ M dexamethasone they did not contain storage granules typical of epinephrine, implying that PNMT may not have been increased (Unsicker *et al.*, 1980). Neurite outgrowth was, however, inhibited by this treatment. More studies investigating coincident regulation of the enzymes in the catecholamine biosynthetic pathway ought to be pursued, particularly in view of the current hypothesis regarding the similarity of these enzymes and their possible structural as well as biosynthetic roles in granule function.

Until this point in our review, we have considered assembly of the granule and its contents from a biosynthetic viewpoint exclusively. However, coincident with this anabolic parade is a catabolic system for catecholamines, mediated by monoamine oxidase (MAO). In many tissues, the continued existence of a catecholamine is tenuous because MAO tries to oxidize any catecholamine which comes within its reach. The adrenal medulla's solution to this problem is the subject of the next section of this review.

E. METABOLISM OF CATECHOLAMINES BY MONOAMINE OXIDASE

The amine neurotransmitters, epinephrine (E), norepinephrine (NE), dopamine (DA), serotonin (5-HT), and other amines with false neurotransmitter or sympathomimetic actions [e.g., octopamine, tyramine, phenylethylamine (PEA), and tryptamine] are considered as classic substrates for the ubiquitous mitochondrial MAO [amine:oxygen oxidoreductase, deaminating, flavin containing; EC 1.4.3.4). Inhibition of MAO *in vivo* with an irreversible inactivator (e.g., tranylcypramine) caused an increase in concentration of the above amines, with a concomitant decrease of their deaminated metabolites in the aminergic neurons (see Youdim *et al.*, 1985b, for review). Thus, a role has been assigned to MAO for maintaining the cytoplasmic concentrations of amines within the neuron at a low level (Tipton *et al.*, 1975; Youdim and Finberg, 1982, 1984). The function of MAO in catecholamine metabolism of adrenal medulla, however, has been uncertain even though substantial enzyme activity has been described (Tipton *et al.*, 1975).

In the normal adrenal gland, MAO activity per milligram protein is higher in the cortex than the medulla [as found for the pig and the dog (Youdim and Holzbauer, 1976)]. For the rat, experiments on regenerated adrenal glands after demedullation have indicated that MAO activity per milligram protein is probably similar in the cortex and medulla (Youdim and Holzbauer, 1976). Data for bovine adrenal gland are not available.

As in other tissues, adrenal medullary MAO is mainly associated with mitochondria (Holzbauer *et al.*, 1973; Tipton *et al.*, 1975), although some activity can be sedimented in the microsomal fraction (Youdim *et al.*, 1985a). While strong association of MAO with the outer mitochondrial membrane has hampered its purification, the enzymes from brain, liver, adrenal gland, and other tissues have been purified to homogeneity. It is now generally accepted that MAO in peripheral tissue and brain is a flavoprotein, containing ~1 mol of covalently bound FAD per 100,000 Da (see Finberg and Youdim, 1983, for review). The flavin is attached to a cysteine residue in the enzyme by a thioether bond at the eighth position of the isoalloxazine moiety of enzymes in liver (Kearney *et al.*, 1971; Walker *et al.*, 1971) and brain (Salach *et al.*, 1976). In contrast to earlier studies, it is now agreed that MAO does not contain a metal cofactor, but it has two essential sulfhydryl groups (Finberg and Youdim, 1983). The minimum molecular size of the active enzyme has been determined to be in the region of 100,000, with two subunits of 55,000–65,000 (Finberg and Youdim, 1983), one of which contains the flavin.

In spite of the relatively active adrenal medullary MAO (Tipton *et al.*, 1975), one can detect relatively little evidence of catecholamine deamination in this tissue. Indeed, tranylcypramine, a nonselective inhibitor of MAO, has no apparent influence on NE or E accumulation either in adrenal gland, in partially purified chromaffin granules, or in isolated chromaffin cells (M.Y., unpublished data; see also Ungar and

Phillips, 1983). Such a result can be accounted for either by the chromaffin cells' having relatively low MAO activity or by the cells' having an enzyme form that has a poor affinity for the catecholamines. Indeed, Tipton *et al.* (1975) reported that in comparison to other amines (5-HT, DA, and tyramine), norepinephrine and especially epinephrine were poor substrates of bovine adrenal medulla MAO, with $K_m$ values in the range of 900–1500 $\mu M$.

This problem was recently solved by utilizing recently developed pharmacologic and biochemical information about MAO forms in tissues. In short, there are two types of MAO, A and B, which can be distinguished on the basis of sensitivity to specific inhibitors and substrate specificity (see Table I). Chromaffin cells contain only the B form (Youdim *et al.*, 1984). Youdim *et al.* (1984) were able to differentiate MAO activity in adrenal medulla tissue into type A (30%) and type B (70%) according to Johnston's (1968) criteria, using clorgyline as the inhibitor of type A. As shown in Table II, mitochondria MAO prepared

TABLE I

SUSBSTRATES AND INHIBITORS OF MONOAMINE OXIDASE TYPE A AND TYPE B[a]

| Type A | Type B | Both forms |
|---|---|---|
| Substrates | | |
|   Epinephrine | $\beta$-Phenylethylamine | Tyramine |
|   Norepinephrine | Benzylamine | Dopamine |
|   5-Hydroxytryptamine | Tryptamine | Kynuramine |
|   Octopamine | | |
|   Metaepinephrine | | |
|   Metanorepinephrine | | |
| Irreversible inhibitors | | |
|   Clorgyline | 1-Deprenyl | |
|   MB9303 | Pargyline | |
|   LY51641 | AGN1135 | |
| Reversible inhibitors | | |
|   Amphetamine | Tricyclic uptake blockers | |
|   Harmaline | MD780236 | |
|   MD780515 | | |
|   FLA336 | | |
|   RO-11-1163 | | |
|   K-511 | | |
|     (5-Fluoro-$\alpha$-methyltryptamine) | | |
|   $\beta$-Carbolines | | |

[a] The above list is an abridged list of substrates and inhibitors of MAO (see Youdim and Finberg, 1982; Youdim and Finberg, 1984).

TABLE II

MICHAELIS CONSTANTS AND RELATIVE $V_{max}$ OF MAO IN ISOLATED BOVINE ADRENAL
MEDULLARY CHROMAFFIN AND ENDOTHELIAL CELLS AND PHREOHROMOCYTOMA
CELLS (PC12)[a]

| Substrate | Chromaffin cells | | Endothelial cells | | PC 12 cells | |
|---|---|---|---|---|---|---|
| | $K_m$ ($\mu M$) | $V_{max}$ | $K_m$ ($\mu M$) | $V_{max}$ | $K_m$ ($\mu M$) | $V_{max}$ |
| Tyramine | 280 | 100 | 400 | 100 | 227 | 100 |
| Serotonin | 385 | 35 | 230 | 63 | 170 | 60 |
| Phenylethylamine | 25 | 60 | 250 | 8 | 235 | 6 |
| Norepinephrine | 1110 | 20 | 430 | 38 | 400 | 35 |
| Dopamine | 400 | 65 | 416 | 61 | | |

[a] Maximum velocity ($V_{max}$) is expressed relative to tyramine, which is 100.

from isolated cultured bovine chromaffin cells could deaminate monoamines with different efficiencies and relative $V_{max}$ values. Nonhydroxylated amines such as phenylethylamine and kynuramine had significantly lower $K_m$ values than hydroxylated amines such as tyramine, dopamine, serotonin, and norepinephrine. In the chromaffin cell, the $K_m$ of MAO for norepinephrine is nearly three times that of serotonin (type A substrate) and 50 times that of phenylethylamine (type B substrate). Furthermore, the relative $V_{max}$ for norepinephrine, as compared to tyramine, dopamine, and phenylethylamine, is significantly lower (Table II) (Youdim et al., 1985b,c). These observations, together with the fact that clorgyline is a poor inhibitor of tyramine, phenylethylamine, and serotonin deamination in these cells ($IC_{50}$ = $10^{-8}$ $M$), indicate that the MAO in the chromaffin cell is primarily the B form of the enzyme.

The identification of MAO type A in the adrenal medulla homogenates can now be attributed to the existence of this enzyme form in the capillary endothelial cells (Table II) isolated by differential plating during culture of chromaffin cells (Banerjee et al., 1985).

In retrospect, it is now apparent that the physiology of the chromaffin cell demands the presence of the type B MAO activity. As previously discussed, chromaffin cells synthesize and store the highest concentrations of catecholamine in the body. It has been presumed by many investigators that MAO was probably not particularly important in the process of catecholamine metabolism in the chromaffin cells, since little deamination occurred. In light of the recent findings, a more accurate explanation would be that the MAO present in the chromaffin cell is the wrong sort, namely, MAO type B, and thus little deamination of catecholamines can occur. Indeed, an adrenal medulla as we now know it might be impossible if it contained MAO-A.

The existence of MAO type B as the sole form of the enzyme in chromaffin cells at first glance appears to be unusual. However, an analogous situation exists in the human platelet which can store the highest concentration of serotonin in the body without being deaminated (Garrick and Murphy, 1982). Although both cell types contain primarily MAO type B, the kinetic and substrates specificity studies indicate that the two cells may contain different variants of the B form of the enzyme. No matter what the physiological importance of these enzyme variants, it is clear that both platelet and chromaffin cells must respectively conserve serotonin and catecholamines (Youdim *et al.*, 1984b), and these properties apparently depend on their altered MAO activity.

Since sympathetic neurons and chromaffin cells both originate from the neural crest, it is curious that the MAO activities are different. The nerve endings contain primarily the A form of the enzyme (Gordis and Neff, 1971a,b; Neff and Fueutes, 1976; Jarrott and Iversen, 1971; Ashkenazi *et al.*, 1983), which maintains the cytoplasmic pool of catecholamines at a low level. This is the reason why MAO inhibitors can elevate neuronal amines. To date, however, no cultured tissue of neural origin, except chromaffin cells, has been described with predominantly MAO type B activity (Donelly *et al.*, 1976; Hawkins and Breakefield, 1978). Consistent with this observation are studies on the PC 12 cell. PC 12 cells are pheochromocytoma cells, apparently derived from chromaffin cells, and share many properties with chromaffin cells (Lee *et al.*, 1977). Interestingly, PC 12 cells have close similarity to noradrenergic nerve endings in that the MAO activity in PC 12 cells is primarily type A (Youdim *et al.*, 1985c) (Table II).

IV. Movement of Chromaffin Granules in Cytoplasm

The cytoplasm of cells is composed of a three-dimensional meshwork of cytoskeletal elements including microfilaments, microtubules, and intermediate filaments (Lazarides and Weber, 1974; Fuller *et al.*, 1975; Osborn *et al.*, 1977). In chromaffin cells, direct interactions between chromaffin granules and cytoskeletal elements (microtubular system) have been observed by stereo electron microscopy of cells embedded in water-soluble media (Kondo *et al.*, 1982). Since chromaffin granules must move from one region of the cell to another, first as part of diverse reactions of synthesis and later toward the membrane for secretion, we presume there must be quite specific mechanisms regulating granule–cytoskeletal interactions. Indeed, the weave of the cytoskeletal network seems so fine that without specific mechanisms it would otherwise be hard to understand how large granules or other organelles could change position in the cell.

## A. ACTIN AND SECRETION

Actin and its associated contractile protein, myosin, have been widely noted in chromaffin cells (Phillips and Slater, 1975; Burridge and Phillips, 1975; Trifaro and Ulpian, 1976; Creutz, 1977; Hesketh *et al.*, 1978, 1981; Trifaro *et al.*, 1978; Lee *et al.*, 1979; Aunis *et al.*, 1980b; Lee and Trifaro, 1981). Actin per se, according to some, may actually be associated with the granule membrane (summarized in Winkler and Carmichael, 1982). However, Zinder *et al.* (1978) showed that the band comigrating with authentic actin on one-dimensional SDS gels of highly purified chromaffin granule membranes was not actin by fingerprint analysis of peptides from the protein in the band. By contrast, a band comigrating with actin on gels of purified plasma membranes from chromaffin cells was indeed actin by this stringent criterion. The reason for this difference may lie with the relative purity of granule membranes analyzed by the different groups. The fact that actin becomes depleted from purified granule membranes, however, does not mean that no association occurs *in vivo*. Indeed, studies with less pure granule membrane preparations may point to real physiological situations.

Consistent with this concept is the fact that actin can be found to interact with granule membranes when mixed experimentally. Burridge and Phillips (1975) found that simple mixing of muscle F-actin with granule membranes led to formation of a complex. Wilkins and Lin (1981) also reported that they could detect stable oligomers of actin on granule membranes, using as an assay binding of radiolabeled cytochalasin B. They suggested that these oligomers might be nuclei for the subsequent assembly of actin filaments.

Fowler and Pollard (1982a,b), however, found that F-actin could interact with highly purified granule membranes. The technique they used was low shear, falling ball viscosimetry in which the chromaffin granule membranes cross-linked F-actin and thus raised the viscosity of the solution. This interaction was inhibited by calcium. A titration of the inhibition revealed that 0.2 $\mu M$ free $Ca^{2+}$ inhibited cross-linking by 50%. Anticalmodulin and antisynexin drugs such as trifluoperazine had no influence on this activity. On the other hand, trypsin treatment of membranes blocked the cross-linking activity, indicating that the actin binding site might be protein in nature.

In other studies, $\alpha$-actinin has been detected in preparations of granule membranes (Jockusch *et al.,* 1977; Bader and Aunis, 1983). $\alpha$-Actinin is a component of Z-bands of muscle, implicated by some investigators in the interaction of actin with the organelle. It was thus a reasonable candidate for the F-actin binding site on granule membranes. However, the purified membranes used by Fowler and Pollard (1982a,b) were prepared under magnesium-free, low ionic strength conditions designed to elute out $\alpha$-actinin (Aunis *et al.,* 1980a). Aunis and Petrin (1984) have verified that $\alpha$-actinin is indeed removed, and have proposed that a spectrin-like protein (fodrin) may be the granule membrane component responsible for binding F-actin.

Perhaps the most important property of the actin binding site on granule membranes is its sensitivity to calcium, although the physiological significance remains uncertain. One might imagine that under resting conditions of cell calcium (0.1 $\mu M$), granules might be relatively immobilized in the cytoplasm. Upon elevation of cell calcium from external sources after stimulation, the interaction between F-actin and granules would become labile. Granules would then become free to interact with the cell membrane and undergo fusion processes (Pollard *et al.,* 1982).

Studies that would appear to be capable of testing such ideas have been reported by Friedman *et al.* (1980, 1985a) who used liposomal vectors to bypass the membrane permeability barrier and to gain access to the cytoplasm in intact cells (Lelkes and Friedman, 1985). DNase I, enclosed in liposomes, was introduced into chromaffin cells by fusing the DNase I containing liposome with acutely dissociated cells. DNase I binds to G-actin, changing the equilibrium between the polymeric (F) and monomeric (G) forms. The consequence of introducing DNase I into cells was that basal secretion increased significantly, but no changes occurred in the amount of catecholamines released upon exposure of the cells to acetylcholine. By contrast, introduction of heavy meromyosin (HMM) and the myosin subfragment (S-1) induced an augmentation of both basal and stimulated secretion (Friedman *et al.,* 1985a). An important control was that $N$-ethylmaleimide (NEM) treatment of HMM and S-1 partially suppressed these events, NEM-HMM being more effective. This may be due to its irreversible F-actin cross-linking ability.

These data tend to argue that some agents capable of binding actin might be able to dislodge granules from actin, thus freeing the granules for other activities in the cell. These molecules produced other effects, however. The liposome-mediated introduction of these macromolecules brought about changes in the transmembrane potential, as determined optically using a potential sensitive dye. $N$-Ethylmaleimide-treated molecules did not affect the resting membrane potential ($-55$ mV at $37°C$) or even induce a slight hyperpolarization. Introduction of Dnase I or of heavy meromyosin caused membrane depolarization to approximately $-20$ mV (Friedman et al., 1985b). In line with the notion of potential sensitive $Ca^{2+}$ channels operating on the plasma membranes, the calcium influx into the cells treated with the two above-mentioned proteins was found to increase significantly in comparison to control cells or cells incubated with liposomes containing buffer (Harish et al., 1984). These somewhat unexpected properties of actin binding proteins may indicate that cytoskeletal functions in chromaffin and perhaps other cells may include hitherto unanticipated processes.

## B. MICROTUBULES AND SECRETION

Microtubules have long been considered as possible structures involved in movement of organelles in cells. In addition to widely appreciated changes occurring in dividing cells, many biochemical and pharmacological studies on axonal transport have implicated microtubules in the movement of synaptic vesicles in neurons (Schliva, 1984; Reichardt and Kelly, 1983).

For microtubule function in chromaffin cells, it has been more a case of guilt by association rather than by specific demonstration of microtubule action in secretory processes. Tubulin is indeed present in chromaffin cells, as summarized by Poisner and Cooke (1975). However, colchicine has been found to block only nicotine-induced secretion, and that only by nonspecific action at the cholinergic receptor (Trifaro et al., 1972).

On the other hand, microtubules have been frequently observed to make close contact, en passant, with chromaffin granules in quick-frozen, cultured chromaffin cells (R. Ornberg, unpublished observation). Consistent with this observation are reports from Aunis' group (Bader et al., 1981) clearly showing the existence of microtubules by immunofluorescence, but lack of tubulin in chromaffin granule membranes. Zinder et al. (1978) also detected no tubulin in chromaffin granules by fingerprint analysis but found it readily in chromaffin cell plasma membrane preparations. Bernier-Valentin et al. (1983) detected tubulin binding sites on plasma membranes, mitochondrial membranes, and chromaffin granule membranes. These tubulin binding sites were all high-affinity sites, reversible, colchicine insensitive, and sensitive to tubulin concentrations well below the critical concentration needed for polymerization. Thus, microtubules could indeed structurally integrate the chromaffin cell, and Bader *et al.* (1981) have suggested that tubulin could mediate neurite outgrowth in cultured chromaffin cells. Conclusive evidence directly implicating tubulin in mechanisms of secretion, however, is yet to be collected.

## V. Membrane Contact and Fusion During Exocytosis: The Role of Calcium

The role of calcium in the regulation of secretion is one of the most hotly pursued topics in cell biology today. In the chromaffin cell, secretion requires external calcium. The calcium seems to enter the cytosol upon stimulation and then provokes a cascade of morphological changes causing vesicle contents such as catecholamines, ATP, enkephalins, DBH, chromogranin A, and other factors to leave the cell. Such questions of how calcium enters, how much is free, and over what time course it remains free are as yet unanswered with certainty.

The second aspect of calcium action is how calcium leads to exocytosis once it enters the cell. There are no end of hypotheses; and indeed, these proposals are not mutually contradictory. On the one hand, calcium may act directly on the plasma membrane and granule membrane to induce fusion. But there is really no compelling experimental reason to support or not support such a contention. On the other hand, there are decades of biochemistry to indicate that some specific protein could mediate calcium action. Recent candidates include calmodulin, actin, myosin, tubulin, synexin, protein kinase C, metabolic products of phosphatidylinositol and inositol phosphates, metalloendoproteases, and other as yet unspecified fusion factors.

Action of some of these proteins depends on elevation of the free calcium concentration, as does the concept of direct calcium action. By contrast, protein kinase C seems to depend on an increased sensitivity of the enzyme to ambient free calcium concentration. Does the calcium ion concentration change or not? Different proteins have different affinities for calcium, so that an accurate knowledge of the exact free calcium ion concentration within the cell becomes of critical importance. The disturbing aspect of this, however, is the fact that the calcium concentration at the surface of the membrane may not ever be known with accuracy. With this caveat we begin this section of our review.

## A. CALCIUM ENTRY AND SECRETION

There is considerable evidence that calcium entry into the cell is necessary to activate the exocytotic process. Indeed, ACh or high $K^+$-stimulated secretion of catecholamines from chromaffin cells can be lowered to prestimulus levels if $Ca^{2+}$ is removed from the extracellular medium (Douglas, 1975). Inhibition of $Ca^{2+}$ entry by either D600 (Corcoran and Kirshner, 1983a) or by divalent cations such as $Mg^{2+}$ or $Ni^{2+}$ is accompanied by marked inhibition of catecholamine release (Schneider et al., 1981). These data and the fact that secretagogues induce pronounced $^{45}Ca^{2+}$ influx (Kilpatrick et al., 1982; Holz et al., 1982) suggest that the source of the $Ca^{2+}$ for the excytotic secretion is extracellular. Indeed, recent studies using the fluorescent probe quin 2 for the measurement of intracellular calcium concentration (Knight and Kesteren, 1983) demonstrated that stimulation of chromaffin cells with either high $K^+$ or ACh produced a transient elevation of intracellular calcium only when free calcium was present in the extracellular medium.

To explain the coupling between $Ca^{2+}$ entry and exocytotic secretion, it has been proposed that the elevated free cytosolic calcium might activate some $Ca^{2+}$-dependent process(es) which leads to the fusion of granules with the plasma membrane (Baker and Knight, 1984) and results in secretion of the granular contents. We will discuss these concepts elsewhere in this review (see Duncan, 1983, for a short summary) and will concentrate in this section on the question of whether elevation of cytosolic calcium is suffcent to activate the exocytotic machinery.

The notion that elevated cytosolic calcium levels promote intracellular processes which lead to secretion presumes that once the cytosolic free calcium has been increased, the secretion process will be turned on, provided that other necessary processes will not be inhibited. However, a close examination of the published data indicates that the elevation of the cytosolic calcium level alone might not be enough to activate the exocytotic machinery. We will therefore advance the argument that additional factors, rather than the total cytosolic free calcium alone, may govern the exocytotic release. In the following sections these data will be discussed in detail.

### 1. Kinetic Considerations

Holz et al. (1982) reported a close correlation between $Ca^{2+}$ uptake and catecholamine secretion from chromaffin cells at various extracellular calcium concentrations. Both these authors and Kilpatrick et al.

(1982) found that calcium entry preceded catecholamine secretion, and the rate of $Ca^{2+}$ entry was found to decline faster than the rate of the catecholamine secretion (Kilpatrick *et al.,* 1982). These findings are thus consistent with the view that an increased intracellular free calcium concentration activates some intracellular process(es) which is coupled to release and indicates that these processes might be slow relative to the calcium influx. If these interpretations were correct, one might expect that once the free cytosolic calcium concentration had been built up, then the calcium could be available for the activation of the exocytotic machinery, thus promoting secretion.

However, the experimental results are not exactly consistent with this view. Experiments were performed (Kilpatrick *et al.,* 1982) in which calcium uptake was stimulated by either nicotine or high potassium, and calcium uptake then blocked abruptly with either curare or D600, respectively. The results were that catecholamine release stopped abruptly upon addition of the inhibitors, even though the cellular calcium content, measured with $^{45}Ca$, dropped much more slowly. Such results would seem to argue that calcium influx is required throughout the entire period of stimulation to keep exocytosis working. Data collected by Knight and Kestenen (1983), however, using the intracellular fluorescent probe quin 2, seem at variance with this view. They found that the cytosolic calcium level reached its maximum within a few seconds following cell stimulation and that it declined to its resting levels within about four minutes. The time course of catecholamine secretion was briefer than that of the intracellular $Ca^{2+}$ transient. The authors explain this phenomenon by suggesting that the secretory process might require more than one $Ca^{2+}$ ion.

Of course, other explanations are possible, and we have also recently examined this problem with cultured chromaffin cells using the quin 2 probe (Heldman *et al.,* 1984). In these experiments cholinergic agonists were added and then simply removed 1 minute after stimulation. The result was that secretion indeed ceased, even though high cytosolic levels of free calcium persisted. The result was especially pronounced when the cells were depolarized by high $K^+$. In this case calcium levels in the cytosol reached basal levels only 8–16 minutes after stimulation, while release of catecholamines had terminated much earlier. We concluded that little correlation could be found between cytosolic levels of free calcium and the rate of catecholamine release (see also a later part of this discussion). On the contrary, the rate of calcium influx seemed better correlated with the release rate (Heldman *et al.,* 1984).

Another problem encountered with studying catecholamine release per se is that the published rates of release vary so widely from one laboratory to the next. For example, Holz *et al.* (1982) claimed that release induced by carbachol ceased 5 minutes after stimulation. By contrast, Kilpatrick *et al.* (1982) found that ACh-induced release continued for up to 30 minutes. Data collected by other groups (e.g., Trifaro and Lee, 1980; Levine *et al.*, 1983) fall in between these values, and it is clear that agonist differences do not seem to explain the variation.

It is our present impression that differences in culturing conditions may also be important factors in these discrepancies. For example, in a recent series of experiments, we found significant variations in response to cholinergic agonists in chromaffin cells prepared either acutely, cultured in a suspended condition, or plated. The differential effects of mere culture conditions on secretion rate make it difficult to determine which condition gives the more valid data. More disquieting are results like those of Ito (1983) who found that guinea pig chromaffin cells secreted catecholamines, DBH, and ATP at different rates. The question of which granular component should be measured thus also becomes important, and we are not prepared at present with a definitive answer.

An entirely different approach to the problem of calcium and the catecholamine release rate has been to study how calcium analogues such as manganese and barium behave. Manganese can substitute for extracellular calcium (Arqueros and Daniels, 1981; Corcoran and Kirshner, 1983b) when cells are stimulated with nicotine. Manganese, however, supports release that is much more delayed and prolonged in comparison to release supported by calcium, a property mirrored by the slow rate of manganese entry into chromaffin cells (Corcoran and Kirshner, 1983b). With calcium and manganese in the medium, the effects of the two cations are additive. Such a result would also tend to argue that the mechanisms of action for calcium and manganese might differ.

Barium, on the other hand, evokes a prompt, vigorous, and continuous release of catecholamines from chromaffin cells. This is in spite of its relatively poor capacity to promote such calcium-activated events as calmodulin-dependent phosphorylation, synexin-induced granule aggregation and fusion, or some mammalian actomysin or sarcoplasmic reticulum systems. These processes have all been proposed to be involved in some way in exocytosis. Barium, however, differs from manganese in that it enters the cell spontaneously. This fact reminds us once again of the concept that the rate of entry of calcium into the chromaffin cell rather than net accumulation may be an important, critical regulation factor for secretion.

## 2. *Release and Cytosolic Calcium Levels*

Having questioned the importance of the cytosolic calcium concentration for secretion in the previous section, it is nonetheless a strongly held view in the cell biology community that these calcium levels are important. Therefore, it seemed of interest to examine in more detail the actual data in chromaffin cells.

The resting level of the cytosolic free calcium was found to be about 100 n$M$ (Knight and Kesterner, 1983). At this level, the spontaneous release of catecholamines is low. During stimulation, cytosolic calcium increases to micromolar levels and promotes induced release. However, different secretagogues induce different rates and amounts of $Ca^{2+}$ flux and also result in different rates and amounts of released catecholamines. The critical question is whether there is any relationship between the amount of $Ca^{2+}$ that accumulates inside the cell and the amount of catecholamines which are secreted as a consequence of a specific stimulus. The amount of calcium that enters the cell during stimulation with veratridine is significantly lower than that which enters the cell following high $K^+$ or nicotine stimulation, especially at early time points (Kilpatrick *et al.*, 1982; Heldman *et al.*, 1984). However, veratridine induces greater release of catecholamines than does high $K^+$ (Kilpatrick *et al.*, 1982; Heldman *et al.*, 1984) or nicotine (Levine *et al.*, 1983). The calcium-selective ionophore ionomycin causes a much greater increase in $^{45}Ca^{2+}$ uptake in relation to catecholamine secretion than do other secretagogues (Kilpatrick *et al.*, 1982). Recently, we confirmed the above-mentioned results by measuring the intracellular calcium concentrations with quin 2 following various stimuli (Heldman, unpublished results). We also found that while nicotine and $K^+$ induced an equivalent rise of cytosolic free $Ca^{2+}$, veratridine produced a significantly smaller rise. When the amounts of catecholamines were compared released with these stimuli, we found that veratridine was much more effective and produced greater release of the amines. This is a general finding in the chromaffin cell literature. We noted, however, that the influx rates of $^{45}Ca^{2+}$ and of catecholamine release were actually slower upon veratridine stimulation than with $K^+$ or nicotine stimulation. On the other hand the amount of catecholamines released by veratridine was higher, even very early in the time course. One explanation for these results is that only a small portion of the accumulated calcium may be critical for inducing secretion. Similar disparate results have been observed with KCl and ACh.

Calcium influx and catecholamine secretion were studied as a function of $K^+$ concentration in the bathing medium by Kilpatrick *et al.* (1982). They found that the amount of $Ca^{2+}$ accumulated rose with concentration up to 90 m$M$ $K^+$, but the peak effect of the catecholamine release was at about 50 m$M$ $K^+$. Raising the extracellular $Ca^{2+}$ from 0 to 10 m$M$ caused an almost linear increase in the amount of $^{45}Ca^{2+}$ accumulated intracellularly. The maximum release of catecholamine under the same conditions, however, was at 2 m$M$ $Ca^{2+}$ (Kilpatrick *et al.*, 1982). Measurement of the cytosolic free $Ca^{2+}$ concentrations after $K^+$ or Ach stimulation revealed that although the intracellular $Ca^{2+}$ level was higher after $K^+$ stimulation, ACh produced greater release of catecholamines (Knight and Kestenen, 1983). Here again, the amount of calcium accumulated did not seem directly related to secretory rate.

The effect of temperature on catecholamine release and $^{45}Ca^{2+}$ influx has also been studied. The optimum temperature for carbachol-induced release was around 20°C (Knight and Baker, 1983b; compare Hiram *et al.*, 1984). At this temperature carbachol induced far greater release than did high $K^+$ or veratridine. We have confirmed these results in our own laboratory. In addition, we also found that the $Q_{10}$ for $^{45}Ca^{2+}$ influx was relatively small compared to that for release. Furthermore, we found that at 20°C $K^+$- and nicotine-stimulated cells accumulated similar amounts of $^{45}Ca$.

The results described in this section can be interpreted in two ways. One interpretation is that there is a minimum amount of $Ca^{2+}$ needed to trigger intracellular events leading to exocytotic secretion, and that once this level has been reached, additional calcium produces no further effect. A problem with this idea is that if $Ca^{2+}$ is indeed a second messenger triggering release, we should not expect different secretagogues to differ in effectiveness for release. The fact is that different secretagogues do show different efficiencies in evoking release.

The alternative interpretation of the above-mentioned results is that the total free calcium level inside the cell does not exclusively determine the amount of catecholamine to be released. Instead, a local $Ca^{2+}$ gradient, formed near or at the site where coupling between $Ca^{2+}$ and secretion occurs, may determine the rate and the amount of release. One simple experiment supporting this alternative is our recent observation that returning $Ca^{2+}$ to the medium of cells depleted of $Ca^{2+}$ produces a sharp rise in intracellular calcium and catecholamine release. Release in these cells, however, can be observed before calcium reaches its original resting level, as defined by quin 2 fluorescence. Thus, the change in $Ca^{2+}$ level and not its absolute intracellular concentration may be responsible for triggering exocytosis in this experimental paradigm. This is clearly a subject for more intense study.

### 3. *Sites for Ca²⁺ Entry and Their Relevance to Secretion*

It has been argued that in chromaffin cells $Ca^{2+}$ must enter the cell from the extracellular fluid in order to produce release. Indeed, simple calcium mobilization inside the cell alone does not seem to effect release. Oka *et al.* (1982) showed that muscarinic stimulation of bovine adrenal medullary cells produced intracellular calcium mobilization leading to $Ca^{2+}$ efflux but not release of catecholamines. Phospatidic acid can mimic the muscarinic action and produce a transient rise in intracellular calcium which also results in $Ca^{2+}$ efflux, but without noticeable release (Ohsako and Deguchi 1983). Since $Ca^{2+}$ entry seems to be the trigger that initiates release, and since it seems, as argued above, that its action is very proximal to its point of entry, it is very important to know all the possible sites for $Ca^{2+}$ entry and to find out whether they are all relevant to release.

Ungar and Phillips, in a recent review (1983), suggest three possible mechanisms: (1) the entry of $Ca^{2+}$ through an ACh receptor channel that is not cation selective; (2) the activation of a voltage-dependent $Ca^{2+}$ channel by depolarization; and (3) a $Ca^{2+}$ component of spike activity. Support to mechanism (1) was first given by Corcoran and Kirshner (1983a) who showed that D600 differentially affected nicotine- and veratridine-induced release. The nicotine-induced release was three times more sensitive to D600, suggesting that different populations of channels were stimulated by these secretagogues. This evidence was only suggestive, since D600 may affect the nicotinic receptors (Bregestovski *et al.*, 1980) and thus indirectly affect the channels "common" to nicotine and veratridine.

Recently, we found that nicotine-induced $Ca^{2+}$ uptake is not affected by high osmolality of the extracellular fluid, while the $K^+$-induced $Ca^{2+}$ influx was greatly affected, especially when NaCl was used to raise the osmolality (Heldman *et al.*, 1984). This very strongly suggested that two channel populations, the voltage-dependent and the receptor-associated channels, were two distinct entities, and that the receptor-associated channel was cation selective at least as far as $Na^+$ ions are concerned. However, both channels were apparently associated with capacity for supporting complete release. The evidence was that stimulation of one channel, while the other was desensitized, still evoked full release. The $Ca^{2+}$ channels on chromaffin cells have also been characterized by patch-clamp techniques and were found to be similar to those of muscle cells (Fenwick *et al.*, 1982). They seem to differ pharmacologically, however, from those in muscle cells, since the concentrations of D600 (Corcoran and Kirshner, 1983a) or nifedipine

(E. Heldman, unpublished data) needed to inhibit the $Ca^{2+}$ influx, and the subsequent release in chromaffin cells were 1000 times greater.

The relevance of mechanism (3), the calcium component of spike activity, to exocytotic secretion was reported by Kidokoro and Ritchie (1980); they found that the spike frequency induced by various concentrations of KCl corresponded well to TTX-sensitive adrenaline release. Both the spike activity and the release were abolished by cobalt, suggesting the involvement of $Ca^{2+}$ in the spike activity as well as in evoking release.

Calcium may also enter the cell via "passive channels" or "leaks" through the resting membrane. Sodium–calcium exchange might be involved in such transport although the $Na^+$–$Ca^{2+}$ exchange mechanism usually moves calcium out of the cell. The relevance of this $Ca^{2+}$ transport to exocytosis, however, is questionable. We have observed that basal release in resting cells does not increase appreciably when $Ca^+$-depleted cells are provided with calcium. Furthermore, blocking basal $Ca^{2+}$ entry into the cell by $La^{3+}$ does not affect basal release. Thus, it seems that the sites of $Ca^{2+}$ entry which are associated with the exocytotic process are specific, and only when flows occur through those sites can release be evoked.

Having thus introduced the concept that $Ca^{2+}$ somehow is involved with the stimulus-secretion coupling mechanism, we will now proceed to discuss proposals relating to how this can be specifically accomplished. There are many such proposals, and we have chosen to focus on those which seem to relate to fusion mechanisms or to signals which could be involved in regulating fusion.

## B. CALCIUM AND MEMBRANE FUSION

During granule assembly, and particularly during release of granule contents by exocytosis, fusion of granule membranes with other membranes must occur. By fusion we mean that two volumes enclosed by respective continuous bilayers approach one another, touch, and then undergo a change that results in a common lumen bounded by elements of both bilayers. During secretion, granule membranes fuse with plasma membranes. Frequently, the granule membrane residue of the first fusion lingers in the plasma membrane and acts as a target for a second granule fusion event. This is called compound exocytosis and occurs in many secretory systems, including chromaffin cells. In many ways this fusion event is the crux of the secretion problem, but is perhaps more poorly understood than any of the subjects we discuss in this review.

Membrane fusion in general can be divided into three distinct, consecutive stages: (1) compensation of the mutual repulsive forces between the two membranes by charge neutralization and/or dehydration, leading to the close approach of the fusing partners to within ~10–20 Å (Rand, 1981); (2) initial destabilization of the membrane architecture, which most probably commences at the two adjacent outer lipid monolayers and involves the transient formation of nonbilayer structures (Rand *et al.*, 1981) and/or lipidic particles (Verkleij, 1984); and (3) merging of the two membranes and reorganization of the bilayer structure. While we are uninformed about how these processes occur, it is evident that the fusion process can be studied by analyzing membrane–membrane interactions in simplified model systems. These include interaction between liposomes (Papahadjopoulos, 1978), between liposomes and planar lipid bilayers (Cohen *et al.*, 1984), between isolated secretory granules (Gratzl *et al.*, 1980a; Morris *et al.*, 1982a), between isolated secretory granules and liposomes (Nayar *et al.*, 1982; Bental *et al.*, 1984), and, more realistically, between isolated secretory granules and plasma membranes (Davis and Lazarus, 1976; Lelkes *et al.*, 1980; Konings and DePotter, 1981).

## 1. *Liposome–Liposome Interactions*

The advancement of reliable fusion assays, which monitor either the mixing of the vesicle contents (Wilschut *et al.*, 1980) or of the membrane components (Struck *et al.*, 1981) during the fusion process, has greatly enhanced our knowledge about the requirements in the process for specific phospholipids and fusogens, such as divalent metal ions, polypeptides, or proteins. The concomitant development of a suitable mathematical model (Nir *et al.*, 1980) has allowed us to dissect in such kinetic experiments the respective contributions of the initial vesicle aggregation and of the subsequent fusion events.

Phosphatidylcholine liposomes are generally not fusogenic except for very small ones, which fuse spontaneously at temperatures below the phase transition of their constituent lipids (Lichtenberg *et al.*, 1981). By contrast, liposomes composed of negatively charged phospholipids, e.g., phosphatidic acid or phosphatidylserine, can be induced to fuse by calcium concentrations ranging from 0.1 to 2 m$M$, depending on the size of the vesicles. Smaller liposomes have lower thresholds, presumably because of the greater lability of the highly curved membranes in contact with each other (Wilschut *et al.*, 1981). Small unilamellar vesicles, composed solely of phosphatidic acid, are the most fusogenic species, requiring ~100 $\mu M$ $Ca^{2+}$, whereas the threshold for inducing fusion between similarly sized liposomes, composed of phosphatidylserine, was found to be ~1.25 m$M$. Other negatively charged phospholipids of biological interest, such as phosphatidylglycerol, cardiolipin, or phosphatidylinositol, were also found to be fusogenic, albeit to a lesser degree. The fusogenicity of the various acidic phospholipids, as determined by the calcium requirements, has been found to be in the order phosphatidic acid > phosphatidylserine > phosphatidylglycerol > cardiolipin, and phosphatidylinositol which is practically refractory to $Ca^{2+}$-induced fusion (Duzgunes et al., 1981a).

The initial aggregation of acidic liposomes, involving neutralization of the repulsive electrostatic forces residing at the phospholipid headgroups, can be achieved with divalent cations like $Ca^{2+}$, $Mg^{2+}$, $Mn^{2+}$, or $Co^{2+}$ at ~1 m$M$, or even with high concentrations (greater than 500 m$M$) of monovalent cations (Nir et al., 1983). However, true fusion of these liposomes is rather specific for calcium in the sense that the threshold concentrations for calcium are significantly lower than those for magnesium. This calcium specificity has been ascribed to the higher affinity of phospholipid headgroups for calcium. The consequence could be a higher degree of dehydration. Alternatively or additionally, calcium may form trans bonds in contrast to $Mg^{2+}$ which will form cis-bonds (Duzgunes and Paphadjopoulos, 1982). Interestingly, while $Mg^{2+}$ is by itself a less potent fusogen than $Ca^{2+}$, synergistic effects on the rate and extent of liposome fusion can be observed when both metal ions are added together at subthreshold concentrations (Hoekstra, 1982).

Upon increase in the vesicle size, e.g., from 250 Å to greater than 1000 Å, the threshold concentrations for $Ca^{2+}$ are increased, while the efficiency of $Mg^{2+}$ to support multiple vesicle fusion is drastically reduced. Concomitant with the increase in fusogen concentrations the kinetics of the fusion process are slowed down; both effects are probably an expression of the increased stability of the less curved membranes in contact with each other (Wilschut et al., 1981).

Extending this simple one-component model system to a more complex and realistic one, fusion of liposomes containing lipids of various compositions, including cholesterol, and in a variety of molar ratios has been investigated (Duzgunes et al., 1981b). Phosphatidylcholine, which by itself is refractory to fusion induced by multivalent cations, strongly inhibits fusion of liposomes bearing an overall net negative charge. As a matter of fact, fusion was completely abolished if the phosphatidylcholine contents exceeded 50%. In contrast, phosphatidylethanolamine, at concentrations up to 70% of the liposomal membrane lipids, was able to sustain and in some cases even to promote fusion of acidic liposomes (Uster and Deamer, 1981). The latter effect is presumably due to the tendency of phosphatidylethanolamine to form nonbilayer (hexagonal II) structures, which could promote the initial membrane destabilization required for the onset of fusion proper. Alternatively, the enhanced dehydration of the ethanolamine headgroup could provide the mechanism for the more intimate contact of the fusing membranes. Cholesterol has most recently been found to decrease the rate of aggregation of phosphatidylserine containing liposomes with a concomitant, significant increase in the rate of vesicle fusion (Braun *et al.*, 1985).

The fusion of liposomes with planar lipid bilayers calls for both acidic phospholipids and $Ca^{2+}$ concentrations in the millimolar range, similar to the interaction between liposomes. It requires an osmotic gradient across the black lipid films with the cis side, containing the vesicles, hyperosmotic to the trans side (Cohen *et al.*, 1980). These findings imply a chemiosmotic component in the fusion of small vesicles with planar membranes, similar to that postulated for exocytosis (Pollard *et al.*, 1984).

A number of soluble proteins [e.g., bovine serum albumin (Garcia, 1983)], polypeptides [e.g., polylysine (Gad, 1983)], and amphipathic peptides [e.g., mellitin (Eytan and Almary, 1983)] were shown to induce liposome–liposome fusion. These molecules seem all to act via similar mechanisms. First they form an initial electrostatic interaction with the negatively charged phospholipid headgroups, causing the vesicles to aggregate. Hydrophobic segments of these compounds then intercalate into the bilayer core and cause perturbation of the bilayer. In some manner this leads ultimately to fusion. Addition of synexin to liposome suspensions (Hong *et al.*, 1982) or of an unidentified calcium-binding protein from synaptic membranes to the planar black lipid membranes (Zimmerberg *et al.*, 1980) dramatically reduced the threshold for calcium-induced fusion of liposomes containing a net negative charge to ~10 $\mu M$. At present, it is not yet clear whether these calcium-binding proteins merely increase the local calcium concentrations at the lipid bilayer surface or whether calcium activates a novel type of protein to induce fusion. Clearly, mathematical analysis of kinetic experiments with these proteins is required to resolve these questions. Other calcium-binding proteins, such as prothrombin or calmodulin which do not exhibit calcium-induced membrane aggregating activities, have inhibitory effects on liposome fusion (Hong *et al.*, 1982). This suggests some degree of specificity for those proteins that do promote fusion in a calcium-dependent manner, such as synexin (see next section for details).

The involvement of integral membrane proteins in the fusion process is clear for enveloped viruses, which contain specific proteolytic/agglutinating and/or fusion proteins in their outer viral membranes

(White *et al.*, 1983). The fusion competence of these proteins is fully retained in reconstituted "virosomes," containing only the viral spike proteins in the lipid bilayers (Kawasaki *et al.*, 1983). In addition, it was recently shown that liposomes containing a membrane-bound $Ca^{2+}$-dependent ATPase exhibited enhanced fusogenicity, implying a possible structural role of this enzyme for membrane fusion *in situ* (Baydoun and Northcote, 1981).

## 2. *Granule–Granule and Granule–Liposome Interactions*

Granule–granule interactions have been investigated in numerous secretory systems and exhibit practically identical features (Gratzl *et al.*, 1980a, b). Such systems may model the granule–granule contact and fusion events occurring during compound exocytosis. At calcium concentrations between 0.1 and 100 $\mu M$, a small percentage of these granules (10%) will interact with each other, mostly forming fusion products comprising a couple of granules only. Magnesium by itself fails to induce fusion of secretory vesicles and inhibits $Ca^{2+}$-promoted fusion. At higher calcium concentrations (exceeding 2–3 m$M$), massive granule–granule fusion occurs, not unlike that observed for liposomes, with fusion products made up of many individual vesicles (Eckerdt *et al.*, 1981). The fusion at low calcium concentrations is inhibited by proteolytic enzymes (e.g., trypsin) and by fixation of the granules with glutaraldehyde, indicating the involvement of proteins associated with the cytoplasmic face of the granule membranes. Proteins also exist which promote granule–granule interactions in a calcium-dependent manner. These will be discussed in the next section.

These findings are surprisingly similar to some aspects of catecholamine release from digitonin-permeabilized chromaffin cells: At micromolar calcium concentrations only a limited amount of catecholamines ($\sim$10%) can be released (Wilson and Kirshner, 1983; Dunn and Holz, 1983), whereas at higher calcium concentrations (greater than 3 m$M$) the amount of catecholamines liberated increases dramatically to up to 50% of the total contents (Wilson and Kirshner, 1983). By contrast, chromaffin cells permeabilized by high voltage discharge were sensitive only to low concentrations ($\sim$1 $\mu M$) of calcium (Baker and Knight, 1978). Yet, another resemblance of the granule–granule interactions *in vitro* to release from permeabilized cells is seen in the calcium–magnesium antagonism.

Chromaffin granules interact with liposomes, and this system has been viewed as a model for similar interactions with plasma membranes. Nayar and co-workers (1982) found by electron microscopy that after incubation for 5 minutes with a 5:1 excess of liposomes containing acidic phospholipids, addition of calcium caused appearance of nonbilayer, lipidic structures in the granule membranes. These experiments, performed at high calcium concentrations (1–5 m$M$), resulted in leaky fusion between the granules and the liposomes. In extension of these studies, Bental *et al.* (1984) followed the kinetics of the interactions of liposomes with chromaffin granules and granule ghosts employing a fluorescence resonance energy-transfer assay. Liposome–granule ghost fusion was additionally verified electronmicroscopically by transfer of liposome-encapsulated colloidal gold particles into the resealed granule ghosts. Both studies found that liposomes containing negatively charged phospholipids, especially cardiolipin, fused avidly with the granule membranes. In the study by Bental *et al.* (1984), the liposome:granule ratio was the reverse of that used by Nayer *et al.* (1982), producing essentially nonleaky fusion events. Bental *et al.* (1984) found that immediately upon mixing, spontaneous fusion between the liposomes and the granule membranes occurred at quite low calcium concentrations (less than $10^{-8}M$). Calcium in the millimolar range enhanced the initial rates and the overall extent of fusion, concomitant with an augmented leakiness of the fusion process.

These studies, showing a calcium-independent fusion process and its sensitivity to low pH, temperature, and proteolytic enzymes, may suggest the existence of a putative fusion factor (protein) located on the cytoplasmic face of the granule membrane. Such a concept is reminiscent, in some respects, of the viral fusion proteins (White *et al.*, 1983). Clearly, liposomes are not the natural target membranes for chromaffin granules. However, this approach appears to be useful for isolating and characterizing the putative fusion protein(s) involved in the interactions between the granules and liposomes, and presumably in exocytosis as well. It is also an interesting intermediate state for eventual studies with entirely biological systems.

## 3. Granule–Plasma Membrane Interactions in Vitro

The *in vitro* preparation most closely resembling exocytosis *in situ* combines isolated secretory granules and plasma membranes. Originally initiated for the *in vitro* study of exocytotic fusion during insulin release from pancreatic islet cells (Davis and Lazarus, 1976), the system has been adopted for granules and plasma membranes isolated from bovine adrenal chromaffin cells (Lelkes *et al.*, 1980; Konings and DePotter, 1981) as well as for a preparation of sea urchin plasma membranes with intact granules attached to them (Whitaker and Baker, 1983).

Lelkes and co-workers (1982) found low rates of fusion between intact granules and isolated plasma membrane vesicles. The plasma membrane vesicles were loaded with the fluorescent, nonpermeant dye carboxyfluorescein; fusion was ascertained by monitoring the rate of transfer of the dye into the granule interior upon fusion. Concomitantly up to 10% of the acetylcholinesterase, a typical marker for the plasma membrane fraction, became associated with the granules. The granule–plasma membrane interactions were independent of the calcium concentration (in the range between $10^{-6}$ and $2 \times 10^{-3}$ $M$) and were enhanced in a dose-dependent fashion upon addition of $10^{-5}$ to $5 \times 10^{-4}$ $M$ ACh. Since the plasma membranes spontaneously form vesicles which are overwhelmingly (greater than 90%) oriented right-side out, this physiologically "wrong" orientation might be at least one explanation for the low fusion yields.

These findings have recently been confirmed and extended by Bental (1983). The fusion assay involved labeling of the plasma membranes with rhodamine isothiocyanate and mixing with chromaffin granules. The same amount of catecholamine release, however, was observed upon incubating the granules with either granule ghosts or with right-side out erythrocyte ghosts, casting serious doubts on the specificity of this system to serve as a model for exocytosis.

In contrast to these findings, Konings and DePotter have reported quite different results. Monitoring the release of granule contents as an indication for fusion between granules and plasma membranes, fusion in their experiments depends on micromolar calcium concentrations (Konings and DePotter, 1981). The authors describe the concomitant and quantitative release of the soluble granule contents in an all or none fashion (Konings et al., 1982), a role for sialic acid-containing substrates (Konings and DePotter, 1982), and the involvement of ATP and of protein phosphorylation (Konings and DePotter, 1983). At present there is no plausible explanation for the controversy in the findings of Konings and DePotter and of Lelkes and co-workers other than subtle differences in the preparational techniques. Alternatively, the preparation of Konings and DePotter may have preserved some unknown cytosolic components associated with the chromaffin granule membrane, which may turn out to be essential for exocytotic fusion to occur. In light of these findings we are at present left with a model system, the validity of which still remains to be verified, for granules and plasma membranes derived from chromaffin cells.

## C. SYNEXIN AND SYNEXIN-RELATED PROTEINS

As described in previous sections, elevation of the free calcium concentration and subsequent calcium action within the cell seem to be essential prerequisites for the membrane contact and fusion events leading to exocytosis. Therefore, to understand exocytosis one must understand how calcium can induce these essentially mechanochemical events. While calcium can act directly in a number of model systems, many biochemical processes depend on a calcium binding protein for specificity and sensitivity. In exocytosis, synexin, a widely distributed calcium binding protein, has been proposed as a likely mediator of membrane contact and membrane fusion. Indeed, in the presence of calcium this protein promotes just these events when added to isolated chromaffin granules, and for that reason it has attracted substantial attention.

## 1. *Properties of Adrenal Medullary Synexin*

Synexin from adrenal medulla is a 47,000-Da calcium binding protein that causes isolated chromaffin granules to aggregate to one another by pentalaminar membrane contact (Creutz, Pazoles and Pollard, 1978). The formation of such contacts may indeed be of physiological relevance, since secretion from chromaffin cells proceeds by both simple and compound exocytosis. In compound exocytosis, chromaffin granules make contacts with membrane vesicles of previous exocytotic events remaining on the plasma membrane. The advantage of this process in chromaffin and other cells may be that upon stimulation limited movement of granules is necessary, and the resulting tunnels of fused granules provide a pathway for controlled penetration of calcium into the depths of the cell.

The mechanism of synexin-dependent granule aggregation is a source of some controversy. Cruetz *et al.* (1979) found that the calcium titration curve for granule aggregation coincided with that for calcium-dependent polymerization of synexin to form $50 \times 100$ Å rods. They suggested that calcium acted on synexin to form active polymers, which themselves caused granules to aggregate. Consistent with this proposal was the observation that only calcium promoted both processes. The calcium-dependent polymerization of synexin has also been used as part of a synexin purification scheme by Morris *et al.* (1982b). However, these authors preferred the interpretation that calcium acted only on the granule membranes and that synexin promoted this calcium effect at a membrane site.

The site to which synexin binds on the granule membrane is similarly a source of controversy. Dabrow *et al.* (1980) found that treatment of granules with proteolytic enzymes could block synexin action, suggesting that the synexin receptor was a protein. However, Morris and Hughes (1979) and Hong *et al.* (1981) noted that synexin caused aggregation and perhaps fusion of phosphatidylserine vesicles in a calcium-dependent manner, thus throwing into question the existence of a protein receptor and suggesting instead that the receptor could be a lipid. In circumstantial support of this conclusion were findings, summarized by Cruetz et al. (1984), that synexin was among a series of proteins, termed "chromobindins" (Cruetz et al., 1982), that show affinity for the lipid fraction of chromaffin granules when bound to a Sepharose affinity column.

Pursuing the concept that the synexin receptor might be a lipid, Hong et al. (1982) used liposomes of defined composition to investigate the nature of synexin-induced aggregation and fusion. The specificity of synexin was manifest by the observation that calmodulin slightly inhibited phospholipid vesicle fusion induced by calcium, while other calcium binding proteins such as bovine prothrombin and its proteolipid fragment 1 had a strong inhibitory action. Synexin alone was able to lower the threshold for calcium-induced fusion of phosphatidic acid (PA) phosphatidylethanolamine (PE) (1:3) liposomes from 1 m$M$ Ca$^{2+}$ to 100 $\mu M$ Ca$^{2+}$, and subsequently to ~10 $\mu M$ Ca$^{2+}$ in the additional presence of 1 m$M$ Mg$^{2+}$. These authors felt that the mechanism of the fusion process depended on formation of anhydrous Ca$^{2+}$ complexes with acidic phospholipid headgroups and that synexin somehow promoted this effect.

In retrospect, the specific dependence of this liposome interaction on calcium and its potentiation by magnesium seem somewhat different from the observed action of synexin on intact chromaffin granules. In the first instance, synexin only induces aggregation of granules, not aggregation and fusion as it does in PA/PE (1:3) liposomes. Second, synexin action does not need magnesium to achieve its threshold for granule aggregation at ~6 $\mu M$ Ca$^{2+}$ (Creutz et al., 1978). Added magnesium neither potentiates nor inhibits calcium-activated synexin activity. Indeed, the critical variable affecting binding of synexin to chromaffin granule membranes, aside from calcium, is pH. Not unexpectedly, the $K_{1/2}$ for calcium dependence of synexin binding to granule membranes is ~5 $\mu M$ at neutral pH and rises as the pH declines (Creutz and Sterner, 1983).

However, one element in the study by Hong et al. (1982) was more reminiscent of the effects of synexin on native chromaffin granules. In a survey of a variety of phospholipids, the authors discovered that phosphatidylinositol (PI) profoundly inhibited fusion when it replaced phosphatidic acid in the PA/PE (1:3) liposomes. This was seen as a unique property of PI, possibly due to inositol blocking access of synexin to the phosphate group of the phospholipid. When viewed from the perspective of the synexin reaction with granules, however, it seems inescapable that phosphatidylinositol may be the bona fide lipid receptor for synexin rather than the other phospholipids. The possible importance of PI in secretion has been discussed in another part of this review and will not be emphasized here.

While calcium and synexin can only aggregate chromaffin granules, it is indeed possible to cause the granule aggregates to fuse. This is achieved by the addition of a small amount (5 $\mu M$) of arachidonic acid or other fatty acids, so long as the fatty acid has a cis unsaturated bond(s) (Creutz, 1981b; Creutz and Pollard, 1981). The relevance of this reaction to exocytosis *in vivo* rests in the fact that the fusion structures formed by treatment of granule aggregates with arachidonic acid are very similar to structures observed in secreting cells (Pollard *et al.*, 1982). Furthermore, arachidonic acid is rapidly produced by chromaffin cells stimulated to secrete catecholamines (Hotchkiss *et al.*, 1981; Frye and Holz, 1984). An important conclusion from these observations is that a phospholipase $A_2$-type activity may be important for secretion. Frye and Holz (1983), however, have shown that phospholipase inhibitors block both calcium uptake as well as secretion from intact cells, thereby rendering inhibitor studies uninterpretable (see also Wada *et al.*, 1983b).

The synexin-dependent granule aggregation reaction is also quite sensitive to phenothiazine drugs in a manner that distinguishes synexin from proteins such as calmodulin or processes such as local anesthesia. Trifluoperazine (TFP) blocks synexin-dependent granule aggregation at a concentration of ~4 $\mu M$ when the reaction is carried out in a high (400 $\mu M$) calcium concentration (Creutz *et al.*, 1982; Pollard *et al.*, 1983). Promethazine (PMTHZ), a phenothiazine with low affinity (300–500 $\mu M$) for calmodulin, was only slightly less potent. In chromaffin cells both drugs were similarly potent, with $ID_{50}$ values of ~1 $\mu M$ and doses below those observed to block $Ca^{2+}$ transport in some studies (Koenigsberg *et al.*, 1983; Baker and Knight, 1981), but not in others (Wada *et al.*, 1983a). TFP and PMTHZ also inhibited glucose-induced insulin release at similarly low doses, indicating some generality of the effect (Sussman *et al.*, 1983). These data thus provide some direct but obviously fragile support for the involvement of synexin-like processes in secretion.

## 2. Synexin-like or Synexin-Related Proteins

Since the initial discovery of synexin in 1978, there has been a virtual torrent of synexin-like or synexin-related proteins studied. As shown in Table III, there are at least eight in total. The etymology of

TABLE III
KNOWN SYNEXIN-LIKE OR RELATED PROTEINS

| Protein | Source[a] | MW | Action | Reference |
|---|---|---|---|---|
| Synexin | L,A,B,S | 47,000 | Aggregates granules, $K_{1/2}$ = 200 $\mu M$, Thr = 5 $\mu M$ | Creutz et al. (1978) |
| $\nu$-Synexin | ↑ L, ↓ A | 38,000 | Aggregates granules, at $[Ca^{2+}] < 1$ $\mu$m | Lee and Pollard (see text) |
| Synhibin | ↓ L, ↑ A | 67,000 | Inhibits synexin, $\nu$-synexin, calelectrins | Pollard and Scott (1982) |
| Synexin II | A, L | 56,000 | Aggregates granules in 800 $\mu M$ $Ca^{2+}$ | Odenwald and Morris (1983) |
| $\mu$-Synexin | L, A, M | 51,000 | Similar to 47,000 synexin, only form in muscle | Curetz (see text) |
| Calelectrin | torp | 34,000 | Aggregates granules, $K_{1/2}$ = 200 $\mu M$ | Walker (1982); Sudhoff et al. (1982) |
| Calelectrin | mam B, A | 32,500 | Same | Sudhoff et al. (1984) |
| Calelectrin | mam B, A | 67,000 | Same | Sudhoff et al. (1984) |

[a] L, Liver; A, adrenal medulla; B, brain; S, spleen; M, muscle; torp, *Torpedo marmorata;* mam, mammalian; thr, threshold; ↑ = increased; ↓ = decreased.

synexin, from the Greek word *synexos* for "meeting" or "coming together," has the functional connotation of proteins which, in the presence of calcium, cause chromaffin granules to agglutinate. However, the second synexin-related protein to be discovered, synhibin, was a 67,000-MW protein that "inhibited" synexin (Pollard and Scott, 1982). The inhibition seemed to be competitive with synexin. Synhibin is found in liver, but in much greater quantity in the adrenal medulla.

Synexin II is a 56,000-MW protein that has been found to be a minor contaminant of synexin preparations prepared from the adrenal medulla (Odenwald and Morris, 1983). Like synexin, it aggregates chromaffin granules in the presence of calcium. The relation of synexin II to standard synexin is in question.

Another synexin variant, $\mu$-synexin, is a 51,000-MW protein, found in adrenal, liver, and muscle tissue, that reacts with polyclonal antibodies to synexin and that aggregates chromaffin granules with a strict calcium dependence similar to that for authentic synexin (C. Creutz, personal communication, 1984). It is the only form of synexin found in muscle, hence its name, $\mu$-synexin.

Another granule-aggregating protein, $\nu$-synexin, is active at quite low calcium concentrations ($> 1$ $\mu M$) On the other hand, it is inhibited by increasing concentrations of calcium. Strontium and barium are inactive. This protein, having a molecular weight of 38,000, is found in both liver and adrenal. There is a greater portion of $\nu$-synexin than of synexin in the liver.*

A similar group of synexin-like activities has been reported from Whittaker's laboratory, but given a different name. These are the cale-lectrins. Initially, they were found in the electric organ of *Torpedo marmorata* and hence given this special name. The calelectrin from the electric organ was found to be a protein of 35,000 MW (Südhoff, 1982), with aggregation properties similar to that for synexin. Later, Sudhof *et al.* (1984) reported the discovery of calelectrins in mamma-lian tissues, including bovine liver and adrenal medulla, that were similar in properties to the *Torpedo* protein. In mammalian tissues, however, the aggregating activities were associated with molecular species of both 32,500 and 67,000 MW. Antibodies to each calelectrin species reacted with each of the other two proteins, regardless of ori-gin. In addition, like synexin, the calelectrins also caused phosphati-dylserine liposomes to aggregate, indicating a possible common mech-anism of action.†

It is our feeling that the synexin-like family of proteins will prove important for membrane contact and fusion processes, not only in ex-ocytosis, but elsewhere. Only further experimentation with these sub-stances will show whether this expectation is warranted.

Signal mechanisms for inducing or modulating fusion are discussed next. Such signals do not detract from or replace the calcium-depen-dent fusion mechanisms hitherto discussed. Instead, they may present possible higher orders of control.

### D. Protein Phosphorylation and Stimulus-Secretion Coupling

Protein phosphorylation plays a key regulatory role in many cellular processes. Examples include glycogen metabolism (for review, see Co-hen, 1982), smooth muscle contraction (for review, see Hartshorne and Siemankowski, 1981), ion transport (for review, see Tada and Katz, 1982), protein synthesis (see Hunt, 1983), DNA transcription (see Rose *et al.*, 1983), and photosynthesis (for review, see Bennett, 1983). It is becoming increasingly possible that protein phosphorylation may also play a role in exocytosis, although, as will be apparent in the adrenal medulla, the present evidence remains indirect.

* However, like synexin, $\nu$-synexin is inhibited by trifluoperazine and promethazine and granules aggregated by $\nu$-synexin are fused by arachidonic acid. Synhibin also blocks $\nu$-synexin.

† While calelectrins and synexins are immunologically distinct, synhibin also blocks calectrin activity (C. Creutz, pers. comm.).

The potential significance of protein phosphorylation in stimulus-secretion coupling in the adrenal medullary chromaffin cell was investigated by Amy and Kirshner (1981). They showed that nicotine stimulated the incorporation of $^{32}$P specifically into two endogenous proteins of 95,000 and 60,000 $M_r$ in intact bovine chromaffin cells preincubated with $^{32}$P$_i$. Enhanced incorporation of $^{32}$P into the same protein bands was also promoted by veratridine and the $Ca^{2+}$ ionophore ionomycin, both of which stimulate secretion in a $Ca^{2+}$-dependent manner, and also by $Ba^{2+}$, which stimulates secretion in $Ca^{2+}$-free media. The increase in phosphorylation of these two proteins was most rapid during the first minute of stimulation and occurred prior to detectable secretion. Nicotine-induced secretion and phosphorylation of the 95,000 and 60,000 $M_r$ proteins shows similar dependencies on extracellular $Ca^{2+}$ concentration. Using bovine adrenal medullary cells rendered permeable by exposure to intense electric fields and then incubated with [$\gamma$-$^{32}$P]ATP, Baker et al. (1982) showed that phosphorylation of a 59,000 $M_r$ protein paralleled catecholamine release from these cells with respect to time course, $Ca^{2+}$ dependence, and MgATP dependence. Phosphorylation of a comigrating protein was also detected in $^{32}$P$_i$-labeled intact medullary cells stimulated to secrete. Evidence has been presented by another group that the 59,000/60,000 $M_r$ protein is tyrosine hydroxylase, and that phosphorylation of this enzyme is related to the secretagogue-induced increase in catecholamine biosynthesis in adrenal chromaffin cells (Haycock et al., 1982a,b; Meligeni et al., 1982). It is difficult to imagine phosphorylation of this protein to be related to the exocytotic process per se, although it certainly cannot be excluded on present evidence.

Finally, Brooks et al. (1984) have reported that saponin permeabilized cells treated with ATP-$\gamma$-S[adenosine 5'-O-(3-thiotriphosphate)] do not release catecholamines when exposed to calcium and conventional ATP. They suggest that the secretory system is "locked" in the thiophosphorylated state, thus implicating a phosphorylated intermediate in secretion.

Studies such as these can only be considered qualitative and perhaps even potentially misleading for the following reasons. In fact, many proteins are labeled in these cells. Indeed, autoradiograms resemble the proverbial picket fence, and the changes we detect by eye affect only a few. If the pattern of protein phosphorylation is to be representative of that achieved intracellularly, then it is essential that protein kinase and phosphoprotein phosphatase activities be rapidly and completely inhibited during the preparation of the tissue for analysis of phosphoproteins. If, for example, a secretagogue were to cause an increase in the extent of phosphorylation of a particular protein, then this effect might never be detected if during the subsequent treatment of the tissue a phosphoprotein phosphatase were to reverse this effect.

One reasonable alternative approach has been to examine kinase reactions in subcellular fractions, hoping to isolate an important substrate or to resolve competing kinase or phosphatase reactions. Secretory granules isolated from the bovine adrenal medulla contain kinases that catalyze cyclic AMP and $Ca^{2+}$-dependent protein phosphorylation reactions. Burgoyne and Geisow (1981, 1982a) showed that chromaffin granule membranes incubated with [$\gamma$-$^{32}$P]ATP catalyzed the $Ca^{2+}$/calmodulin-dependent phosphorylation of proteins of 59,000, 58,000, 53,000, 43,000, and 27,000 $M_r$ and the $Ca^{2+}$-dependent phosphorylation of an 18,000 $M_r$ protein. The 59,000 and 43,000 $M_r$ proteins also were substrates for cyclic AMP-dependent phosphorylation. In another report, Burgoyne and Geisow (1982b) showed that the 43,000 $M_r$ protein appeared to be the subunit of pyruvate dehydrogenase from residual mitochondrial contamination of the granule fraction. The authors concluded that the majority of the substrates for endogenous protein kinase activity seemed to be on the cytoplasmic face of the granule membrane.

Treiman *et al.* (1983) have also investigated phosphorylation reactions catalyzed by chromaffin granule membranes. This group reported that cyclic AMP increased the phosphorylation of proteins with molecular weights of 249,400, 141,500, 81,800, 60,300, and 55,900. The 60,300 $M_r$ protein was a vesicle-bound form of tyrosine hydroxylase, and the 55,900 $M_r$ protein represented two forms of the regulatory subunit of type II cyclic AMP-dependent protein kinase, distinguishable by molecular weight (56,000 and 52,000). Phosphorylation of a 29,800 $M_r$ granule protein was stimulated by $Ca^{2+}$ and calmodulin. Treiman *et al.* stated that it was not possible to assess the significance of the discrepancies between their findings and those of Burgoyne and Geisow, but point out that the conditions of the phosphorylation assay and the method for isolation of chromaffin granules were among the important differences between the two studies. Although these differences need to be resolved, it is possible that phosphorylation of granule proteins could regulate the interaction of granules with the cytoskeletal and contractile elements of the cell or perhaps control the fusion event at the plasma membrane.

A $Ca^{2+}$-activated phospholipid-dependent protein kinase (protein kinase C) appears to be important in the release reaction of platelets (for review, see Nishizuka, 1984). The function of this enzyme in the secretory mechanism of the adrenal chromaffin cell has been suggested by two recent observations. First, this enzyme binds in a $Ca^{2+}$-dependent manner to an affinity column prepared from adrenal medullary chromaffin granule membranes (Creutz *et al.*, 1983). Second, a tumor-promoting phorbol ester, an analogue of diacylglycerol, activates protein kinase C (Castagna *et al.*, 1982) and thus increases the affinity of the enzyme for $Ca^{2+}$. The same phorbol ester shifts the $Ca^{2+}$ requirement of secretion from high-voltage permeabilized chromaffin cells to lower $Ca^{2+}$ concentrations (Knight and Baker, 1983a). The phorbol ester, however, did not affect the secretory properties of intact cells.

Thus, the investigation of the possible function of protein phosphorylation in the secretory process in the chromaffin cell is at a relatively early stage, and more results are needed before conclusions can be drawn. We will now proceed to a discussion of phosphatidylinositol metabolism and secretion in chromaffin cells. This is a particularly timely subject given the close connection in some systems (Nishizuka, 1984) between this lipid and the protein kinase C activity just discussed.

## E. Inositol Metabolism and Secretion

From the moment of interaction with agonist to the initiation of fusion and exocytosis, many discrete cellular processes and information transfer events probably occur. The term "second messenger" has been used to describe the putative chemical basis of the information transfer, and examples include the familiar cyclic nucleotides and, of course, calcium.

Another system that may be energetically poised to generate a second messenger consists of phosphatidylinositol (PtdIns) and its phosphorylated derivatives phosphatidylinositol 4-phosphate (PtIns4P) and phosphatidylinositol 4,5-bisphosphate (PtdIns4,5P$_2$). As early as 1953, Hokin and Hokin observed a large increase in phospholipid turnover in exocrine pancreas stimulated to secrete amylase, either by ACh or pancreozymin. Later, using adrenal medullary slices from guinea pig, Hokin *et al.* (1958) showed that the phospholipid turnover stimulated by ACh was primarily due to the turnover of phosphoinositides, even though these lipids constituted only a small portion of total membrane phospholipid.

The suggestion that PtdIns turnover might be an early event after receptor occupancy that could initiate diverse cellular response was first made by Durell *et al.* (1969) and Lapetina and Michell (1973). Michell (1975) reviewed the literature concerning receptor-initiated PtdIns turnover and noted that receptor stimulation which caused an elevation in intracellular $Ca^{2+}$ also activated PtdIns metabolism. He suggested that the breakdown of PtdIns, PtdIns4P, and/or PtdIns4,5P$_2$ preceded and might be responsible for the opening of Ca$^{2+}$ channels and the influx of Ca$^{2+}$ ions (Mitchell, 1975).

Currently, the most widely held hypothesis concerning function of PtdIns metabolism is that the breakdown of PtdIns4,5P$_2$ and perhaps PtdIns4P rather than PtdIns itself effects an increase in intracellular Ca$^{2+}$ (see review by Downes and Michell, 1982). Using cellular systems labeled to isotopic equilibrium with either [$^{32}$P]phosphate or [$^{3}$H]inositol, several investigators have shown a rapid loss after agonist interaction of PtdIns4,5P$_2$ and PtdIns4P (within 5 to 15 seconds), which often precedes the loss of label in PtdIns (Abdel-Latif *et al.*, 1977; Creba *et al.*, 1983; Rebecchi and Gershengorn, 1983; Putney *et al.*, 1983; Litosch *et al.*, 1983; Rendu *et al.*, 1983; Martin, 1983; Billah and Lapetina, 1982; Orchard *et al.*, 1984; Godfrey and Putney, 1984; Hasegawa-Sasaki and Sasaki, 1983; MacPhee and Drummond, 1984). The hydrolysis of PtdIns45P$_2$, PtdIns4P, and PtdIns is apparently due to specific phospholipase C molecules which attack one or more of the phosphoinositides (Irvine, 1982; Shukla, 1982; Low and Weglicki, 1983; Irvine *et al.*, 1984). The products are diacylglycerol, which is converted to phosphatidic acid (PA) by diacylglycerol kinase, and inositol 1-phosphate (Ins1P), inositol 1,4-bisphosphate (Ins1,4P$_2$), and inositol 1,4,5-trisphosphate (Ins1,4,5P$_3$) from the hydrolysis of PtdIns, PtdIns4P, and ptdIns4,5P$_2$, respectively (Downes and Michell, 1982). It is the products of phospholipase C action on PtdIns4,5P$_2$, diacylglycerol, and Ins1,4,5P$_3$, that currently generate the most interest regarding potential function as second messengers. (For discussion of the role of diacylglycerol and its relationship to protein kinase C, see the previous section.) The suggestion has been made that the concomitant loss of PtdIns and PtdIns4P after PtdIns4,5P$_2$ hydrolysis may be due to phosphorylation by PtdIns kinase and PtdIns4P kinase to replenish PtdIns4,5P$_2$ levels (Downes and Michell, 1982).

The rapid hydrolysis of PtdIns4,5P$_2$ and PtdIns4P after activation of a Ca$^{2+}$-mobilizing receptor is usually accompanied by a large and rapid increase in the water-soluble products Ins1,4P$_2$ and Ins1,4,5P$_3$ (Berridge, 1983; Berridge *et al.*, 1983; Rebecchi and Gershengorn, 1983; Akhtar and Abdel-Latif, 1980; Orchard *et al.*, 1984; Joseph *et al.*, 1984; Martin, 1983; Burgess *et al.*, 1984; Drummond *et al.*, 1984). Ins1,4,5P$_3$ and Ins1,4P$_2$ are then dephosphorylated to Ins1P by soluble or membrane-bound phosphomonoesterases (see Irvine, 1982). The conversion of Ins1P to *myo*-inositol by the enzyme inositol-1-phosphatase can be inhibited by 10 m$M$ Li$^+$, and thus Li$^+$ has been used to study the accumulation of Ins1P upon receptor stimulation (Berridge *et al.*, 1982).

Inositol 1:2-cyclic phosphate (the initial product of phospholipase C action on PtdIns, which is converted to Ins1P by 2-phosphohydrolase (Dawson and Clarke, 1972)), was once proposed to be a second messenger (Lapetina and Michell, 1973), and PA was once thought to be a calcium ionophore (Putney $et$ $al.$, 1980). Neither inositol 1:2-cyclic phosphate nor PA, however, are currently believed to physiologically mediate changes in intracellular $Ca^{2+}$. Rather, recent evidence suggests that $Ins1,4,5P_3$ may mobilize $Ca^{2+}$ from intracellular stores, thus making $Ins1,4,5P_3$ a second messenger while relegating $Ca^{2+}$ to a third messenger role (Streb $et$ $al.$, 1984; Joseph $et$ $al.$, 1984; Burgess $et$ $al.$, 1984; Suematsu $et$ $al.$, 1984; Dawson and Irvine, 1984; Prentki $et$ $al.$, 1984). In these studies, cells were permeabilized using a detergent (saponin) or by washing them with nominally $Ca^{2+}$-free solutions. The permeabilized cells were incubated in high-potassium buffers which contained an ATP regenerating system plus ATP. Free $Ca^{2+}$ declined to a steady-state concentration within 10 to 20 minutes of adding either the cells or ATP, at which point addition of micromolar concentrations of $Ins1,4,5P_3$ caused a rapid increase in $Ca^{2+}$ in the buffer. The lack of an effect of mitochondrial poisons on this $Ca^{2+}$ release plus the observation of Dawson and Irvine (1984) and Prentki $et$ $al.$ (1984) that $Ins1,4,5P_3$ could release $Ca^{2+}$ from microsomal fractions suggested that $Ins1,4,5P_3$ released $Ca^{2+}$ from the endoplasmic reticulum.

Although the idea that phosphoinositide turnover may act to mobilize intracellular $Ca^{2+}$ is gaining wider acceptance, results from some cellular systems need further expansion and interpretation to fit the model. The system of primary concern to this review, the bovine adrenal medullary chromaffin cell, behaves differently than one might expect if phosphoinositide turnover were really important in increasing intracellular $Ca^{2+}$. Phosphoinositide metabolism in adrenal chromaffin cells, however, has not been as extensively studied as it has in other cell systems (see review by Hawthorne and Swilen, 1982).

The first report of a metabolically active pool of phosphoinositides in adrenal chromaffin cells was made by Hokin $et$ $al.$ (1958). ACh ($10^{-5}$ $M$) presented to slices of guinea pig adrenal medulla stimulated both catecholamine secretion and [$^{32}P$]phosphate incorporation into phosphoinositides and phosphatidic acid. Since atropine ($10^{-5}$ $M$) blocked both catecholamine secretion and phosphate incorporation, Hokin $et$ $al.$ (1958) suggested that the phosphoinositides might generally control secretion from endocrine glands. They also noted that high concentrations of ACh ($10^{-4}$–$10^{-3}$ $M$) inhibited $^{32}P$ incorporation into the phospholipids.

With results similar to those obtained in guinea pig, Trifaro (1969a,b) found that ACh could stimulate $^{32}P$ incorporation into PtdIns and PA in bovine adrenal medulla slices. Since ACh had no effect on either the incorporation of [³H]glycerol or the actual amounts of PA and PtdIns, the effect was presumably due to an increase in the turnover rate of these phospholipids. In contrast to the results obtained in guinea pig adrenal medulla, however, two results of Trifaro's suggested that there was no correlation between $^{32}$P incorporated and catecholamine secretion in bovine adrenal medulla. First, the increase in $^{32}$P incorporation occurred after catecholamine secretion had peaked. Second, removing $Ca^{2+}$ from the incubation medium abolished ACh-stimulated catecholamine secretion, but did not affect $^{32}$P incorporation into PtdIns and PA. Thus, unlike many other systems where phosphoinositide metabolism had been correlated with an elevation in intracellular $Ca^{2+}$ leading to exocrine or endocrine secretion, phosphoinositide metabolism in bovine adrenal medullary cells could be disassociated from the $Ca^{2+}$-activated cellular response of catecholamine secretion.

Adnan and Hawthorne (1981) and Fisher *et al.* (1981) pharmacologically determined that the cholinergic receptor mediating catecholamine secretion from bovine adrenal medullary cells was nicotinic while the receptor mediating PtdIns turnover was muscarinic. Thus, as stated by Fisher *et al.* (1981), "In this experimental preparation, stimulated phospholipid labeling appears to be neither a prerequisite for nor a consequence of secretion." Two additional results of Fisher *et al.* (1981) support this statement. First, removing $Ca^{2+}$ from the medium blocked catecholamine secretion but had no effect on phospholipid labeling. Second, high $K^+$ stimulated secretion but had no effect on PtdIns turnover.

Fisher *et al.* (1981) also found that muscarinic stimulation did not affect $^{45}Ca^{2+}$ influx, whereas nicotinic stimulation increased $^{45}Ca^{2+}$ influx. This suggests that if PtdIns metabolism leads to an elevation of intracellular free $Ca^{2+}$ in these cells, it must mobilize $Ca^{2+}$ from an intracellular pool. Interestingly, several studies indicated that muscarinic receptor stimulation causes $^{45}Ca^{2+}$ efflux from bovine adrenal chromaffin cells (Ohsako and Deguchi, 1983; Oka *et al.*, 1982). Whether this $^{45}Ca^{2+}$ efflux represents an increase in intracellular $Ca^{2+}$ or release of $Ca^{2+}$ from a plasma membrane pool is unknown. Kao and Schneider (1985) have shown that exposure of chromaffin cells to muscarine leads to a brief increase in intracellular calcium concentration. However, Derome *et al.* (1981) have reported that muscarinic receptor stimulation can actually inhibit catecholamine secretion stimulated by ACh (Derome *et al.*, 1981). Therefore, PtdIns metabolism in bovine adrenal chromaffin cells may not be correlated either with secretion or with an increase in intracellular $Ca^{2+}$.

In considering the reasons for this, it is possible that PtdIns metabolism as measured in these cells is not accompanied by PtdIns4,5P$_2$ or
PtdIns4P metabolisms. This would be consistent with the idea that
PtdIns4,5P$_2$ breakdown forming Ins1,4,5P$_3$ is required to increase intracellular Ca$^{2+}$. In this light, it should be noted that Fisher et al.
(1981) reported no effect of muscarinic receptor stimulation on polyphosphoinositide (PtdIns4,5P$_2$ and PtdIns4P) metabolism.

With one exception, the studies mentioned to this point concerning
phosphoinositide metabolism in adrenal chromaffin cells were performed using either slices of medullary tissue or perfused glands. The
possibility that the observed effects occurred in cells other than the
chromaffin cells should not be neglected. Fisher et al. (1981) used primary cultures of partially purified bovine adrenal chromaffin cells in
the studies mentioned above. The use of primary cultures should reduce the risk of contaminating cells, but the possible occurrence of
some endothelial (Banerjee et al., 1985) or cortical cells (Kilpatrick et
al., 1980) remains.

The function of the considerable amounts of PtdIns, PtdIns4P, and
PtdIns4,5P$_2$ in bovine adrenal chromaffin cells (Chang and Sweeley,
1963) is unclear. It is interesting to note that the chromaffin-granule
membrane contains large amounts of PtdIns4P and the enzyme PtdIns
kinase, but that PtdIns4P kinase is lacking (Trifaro and Dworkind,
1975; Buckley et al., 1971; Phillips, 1973; Muller and Kirshner, 1975;
Lefebvre et al., 1976). PtdIns4P kinase is presumably restricted to the
plasma membrane. The function of this enzyme distribution is not
known. Further investigation using primary cultures of adrenal chromaffin cells should help clarify the role of the inositol phospholipids in
chromaffin cells and may determine whether the hypothesis that Pt-
dIns4,5P$_2$ metabolism is involved in Ca$^{2+}$ mobilization is general for
all cell types.

## F.  METALLOENDOPROTEASES AND SECRETION

Metalloendoproteases (MEPases) have recently come into consideration as possible regulators of secretion. Some MEPase inhibitors
block not only fusion of myoblasts (Couch and Strittmatter, 1983), but
even synaptic transmission at the neuromuscular junction (Baxter et
al., 1983). These inhibitors are characterized by common architectural
features: two or more hydrophobic amino acid residues with a blocked
C-terminal and an amide group at the N-terminal, e.g., CBZ-Gly-Leu-
amide (Morihara, 1974). Recently, an irreversible, specific MEPase
inhibitor and its fluorescent derivative was developed, which binds
selectively and with high affinity to the active site of MEPases

(Rasnick and Powers, 1978). Another fluorogenic oligopeptide is specific for MEPases and can conveniently be used to identify MEPase activity in subcellular fractions.

Strittmatter and co-workers have provided evidence for the involvement of metalloendoprotease (MEPase) activity in the fusion of myoblasts (Couch and Strittmatter, 1983, 1984) and in synaptic transmission at the neuromuscular junction (Baxter *et al.*, 1983). In the latter instance, the MEPase(s?) could be located on the presynaptic nerve terminal. In myoblasts, two different MEPases were demonstrated, one membrane bound, the other in the soluble cytoplasmic fraction (Couch and Strittmatter, 1984). In addition, MEPase activity was found in mast cells, in bovine adrenal chromaffin cells (Mundy and Strittmatter, 1983, 1985; Lelkes *et al.*, 1984), as well as in human polymorphonuclear neutrophils. In the latter two systems studied in this laboratory, the involvement of MEPases in the stimulus-secretion coupling was verified by pretreating the cells with specific MEPase inhibitors and substrates and measuring release of catecholamines and lysosomal enzymes, respectively.

In cultured chromaffin cells, MEPase inhibitors blocked ACh- and nicotine-induced catecholamine release completely, with half-maximal doses between 50 and 300 $\mu M$, depending on the inhibitors. The efficiency of MEPase inhibitors to block catecholamine secretion induced by excess potassium was less pronounced and depended on the amount of $K^+$ used to stimulate the cells. Thus, 1m$M$ CBZ-Gly-Leu-amide blocked $\sim$75% of the release elicited by 55 m$M$ $K^+$, while its inhibitory effect at 25 m$M$ or 100 m$M$ $K^+$ was reduced to less than 50%. Similarly, release induced by veratridine ($10^{-4}$ $M$) or batrachotoxin ($10^{-6}$ $M$) is only partially inhibited ($\sim$50%) by 1 m$M$ concentrations of the MEPase inhibitors. Their inhibitory action on the stimulus secretion cascade is rapid and requires preincubation of less than 2 minutes. With the exception of the irreversible inhibitor, which was the most potent investigated, the effects of oligopeptide MEPase inhibitors are readily reversible after changing the incubation media. Comparable doses of inhibitors of the other classes of proteases (Umezawa and Goyagi, 1977) did not affect at all the secretory response or showed only a strong (nonspecific?) anticholinergic effect, presumably acting like other lipophilic anesthetics known to interfere with the function of cholinergic receptors (Creveling *et al.*, 1982). The effects of MEPase inhibitors as well as inhibitors of other classes of proteases on $Ca^{2+}$-induced catecholamine release from digitonin permeabilized chromaffin cells were found to be nonspecific and rather small (less than 30%), arguing against their direct involvement in exocytotic fusion-related processes.

Localization of MEPases in chromaffin cells has been studied with high-resolution fluorescence microscopy. The fluorescent derivative of the irreversible MEPase inhibitor was discerned on the plasma membrane, inside the cytosol, and, after permeabilizing the cells, in association with intracellular granular structures. Similarly, MEPase activities were identified in association with isolated plasma membranes and chromaffin granules as well as in the postmicrosomal fraction of the soluble cell contents. Several distinct protein bands, which bound the fluorescent irreversible inhibitor of MEPase, were allocated to each of these subcellular fractions after inspection of SDS–polyacrylamide gels under UV illumination. These results clearly indicate the occurrence of more than one metalloendoprotease in bovine adrenal chromaffin cells; which of them is relevant to the secretory process remains to be proved.

No interference of MEPase inhibitors with the synexin-mediated aggregation and fusion of isolated chromaffin granules $in$ $vitro$ was detectable. On the other hand, MEPase inhibitors (1 m$M$) increased by ~50% the viscosity of pure actin solutions as well as of chromaffin granule–actin complexes (Fowler and Pollard, 1982a,b; as described in Section III), implying a metalloendoprotease involvement in the assembly of the microfilaments and their binding to the chromaffin granule membrane. These results might be relevant for the intracellular transduction of the stimulus signal and seem to be in accordance with the well-documented susceptibility of the microfilaments to proteolysis and protease activity (Applegate and Reisler, 1983).

Experiments with intact cells showed no interference by MEPase inhibitors of $K^+$ or veratridine-induced membrane depolarization as detected by optical methods (Friedman $et$ $al.$, 1985a), suggesting that these compounds do not interfere with the ionic conductances of either $K^+$ or $Na^+$ channels, respectively. While no effects of MEPase inhibitors were detectable on the influx of $^{45}Ca^{2+}$, the efflux was significantly increased, both under resting conditions and upon stimulation of the cells with ACh, potassium, or veratridine (Lelkes $et$ $al.$, 1984). While these results still await concomitant measurements of the free intracellular calcium concentration, we can speculate that the accelerated $Ca^{2+}$-efflux might cause substantial reduction in free intracellular calcium content with subsequent suppression of all those events that require elevated intracellular calcium to induce catecholamine release.

The simplest interpretation of these data is that MEPase inhibitors might indeed be acting on metalloendoproteases. Other sites of interaction, however, can be considered for polypeptide MEPase inhibitors which show an order of potency similar to that for interaction with authentic metalloendoprotease. One of the candidates which might be affected either directly or indirectly by MEPase inhibitors appears to be protein kinase C. Phosphorylation of proteins, located on the cytoplasmic face of the plasma membrane, is largely inhibited by MEPase inhibitors *in vitro*. This effect might be due to a direct inhibition of an endogenous protein kinase C or indirectly by the activation of a membrane-bound phosphatase. In any case, these results provide for the first time direct evidence for a possible link between phosphorylation, calcium channels, metalloendoproteases, and the secretory process. While there is no evidence for a direct role in membrane fusion, as originally assumed, the existing data suggest their involvement in other cellular processes related to the transduction of the stimulus signal.

## VI. ENERGETICS OF EXOCYTOSIS

The problem of how energy is involved in the process of exocytosis is perhaps the least understood of any of the problems discussed in this review. It is clear that some source of energy is necessary. A less direct reason is that secretion from chromaffin cells is highly temperature dependent. Yet, many processes, some discussed in this review, are temperature dependent without obvious involvement of classical sources of energy, such as ATP. On the other hand, protein kinase activity as well as phosphorylation of specific lipids by definition need ATP. Yet, it is also clear that at present neither of these processes are unambiguously implicated in exocytosis.

In studies of secretion from intact cells, there is substantial evidence of need for sources of metabolic energy. For example, metabolic inhibitors such as FCCP, rotenone, NaCN, Na azide, and 2-deoxyglucose block epinephrine secretion from acutely dissociated bovine chromaffin cells (Pollard *et al.*, 1984). Indeed, similar drugs inhibit catecholamine secretion from the perfused intact adrenal gland (summarized in Viveros, 1975). As iterated above, however, so many cell functions depend upon ATP that it is unclear whether these requirements for energy metabolism are directly related to secretion or to simply the maintenance of the living state.

A variety of proposals for how energy utilization might be related to exocytosis have been advanced. Some of these have been evaluated to some extent. Among the earliest theories was the concept that muscle proteins, such as actin and myosin, might be involved either in granule movement or in the fusion process itself. The arguments for a role for myosin have been summarized by Pollard *et al.* (1978); they are not very compelling. The specific involvement of actin (see Section IV of this review), however, is still under active study.

Another approach has focused on chemiosmotic properties of the chromaffin granules themselves and the possible relevance of these properties to exocytotic release. Incubation of chromaffin granules isolated in sucrose with MgATP and chloride induces osmotic lysis (Oka *et al.*, 1965). The mechanism involves electrogenic transport of protons driven by a membrane ATPase activity (see discussion of granule ATPase in Section III,B). The inward movement of protons causes the granule to become acidic inside as well as electrically positive, and chloride moves into the granule, apparently through specific channels (Pazoles and Pollard, 1978). The result is an increase in the osmotic strength of the granule interior and resulting lysis of the granule (Creutz and Pollard, 1980).

The formulation of these mechanisms into a chemiosmotic hypothesis for exocytosis has been proposed by Pollard *et al.* (1978). Briefly, if such an osmotic mechanism were involved in release, one would expect secretion from intact or permeabilized cells to be inhibited by elevated osmotic strength, to be dependent upon ATP, and to be promoted by the more permeant anions. As shown by Pollard *et al.* (1984), however, these expectations are borne out only generally in intact chromaffin cells. Indeed, there are many deviations from what one would expect if chemiosmotic chromaffin granule properties *in vitro* were exactly those of granules in the secreting cell.

ATP seems definitely involved. This is particularly evident in studies of high-voltage permeabilized cells (Baker and Knight, 1978) and digitonin permeabilized cells (Dunn and Holz, 1983; Wilson and Kirshner, 1983). Holz *et al.* (1983), however, have questioned the significance of the $H^+$ electrochemical gradient promoted by the granule membrane ATPase in this process. Elevation of osmotic strength does indeed block secretion (Pollard *et al.*, 1984; Hampton and Holz, 1983) in intact cells, but the mechanism may be more complicated than hitherto supposed (see Section V,A for further discussion). The conclusion at this point, then, is that the chemiosmotic hypothesis as presently formulated does not explain in quantitative detail the properties of secreting chromaffin cells. It is also equally evident that there is no alternative explanation presently available for how exocytosis is powered.

Finally, there is one profoundly disquieting aspect of trying to model secretion mechanisms of chromaffin cells from properties of chromaffin granules *in vitro*. That is the fact that the osmotic properties of isolated chromaffin granules appear to be quite different from the osmotic properties of chromaffin granules within the intact cells. For example, chromaffin granules in high-voltage permeabilized (Baker and Knight, 1978) and digitonin permeabilized (Wilson and Kirshner, 1983; Dunn and Holz, 1983) cells do not seem to undergo the ATP-Cl-induced osmotic lysis described above for isolated granules. Furthermore, the osmotic fragility curve for granules within intact cells is shifted toward much lower osmotic strength than granules isolated in sucrose or other media (Hampton and Holz, 1983; compare Creutz and Pollard, 1980; Hiram *et al.*, 1982). The reasons for these deviations are not known, but their existence does make difficult the parallel reasoning that implicity accompanies studies on isolated granules. Understanding the basis of these differences is likely to be fundamental to our eventual understanding of how exocytosis occurs and how energy is utilized in the process.

## VII. CONCLUSIONS

As is apparent from perusal of this review, enormous amounts of information are available on the ultrastructure and biochemistry of secretion from chromaffin cells. Yet, each of the sections of this review is dominated by profound, unsolved problems. Our new information on the ultrastructure of the chromaffin granule itself is an example of such an unsolved problem. The granule, as shown by new fast-freezing technology, contains an intragranular membrane-limited vesicle. This vesicle may be part of a mechanism for maintaining heterogeneous vesicle constituents in separate compartments. What is in this vesicle? Another observation that generates new problems is that the zones of contact between plasma membrane and granule membrane prior to fission seem to be punctate, not extensive. What is forming these contact points? Of what are they composed?

Of course, little is known about the basic mechanisms for assembly of secretory granules, even in the most well-characterized tissues. However, synthesis of the low-molecular-weight catecholamines and their insertion into the granule are understood well enough that our main concerns now include questions of physical and temporal integration. How are the several synthetic, translocating, and energetic functions physically arranged on or around the granule? Are there molecular relationships between the biosynthetic enzymes, or are they separate enzymes that have come together in a biosynthetic sequence by statistical coincidence? Is the catecholamine transporter on the granule membrane a useful general example of such a site in nervous tissue? Are there separate transporters for efflux? Is the uptake system studied in mature granules the same as that in nascent granules? Is the role of ATP in granules just that of a salt or pH buffer? How is the storage complex within the granule formed and what is it made of?

The cellular integration of organelle movement, dislocation, and secretion may indeed by controlled by cytoskeletal elements such as actin and tubulin. Yet, the cytoskeleton is composed of many other proteins, themselves also regulated by other proteins. It is clear from both biochemical and ultrastructural criteria that interactions between granules and the "cytoskeleton" occur. How these interactions are regulated and integrated with the secretory response are big problems for the future.

Finally, summarizing the problems involved in our analysis of membrane contact and fusion would take an essay nearly as long as the space devoted to the subject. Is calcium concentration or calcium flux across the membrane the critical signal for initiation of secretion? Is calcium indeed the critical signal? If calcium is the signal, does it work alone or does it activate yet another factor? Do granule aggregation and fusion events adequately model the events occurring in the cell during secretion?

The problem of how the secretion process is energized remains. This was the shortest section of all because the subject has remained a great mystery. We truly have no idea of how energy is coupled to secretion. It is true that biological energy rests in structure as well as in the capacity to break energy-rich bonds, and that the chromaffin granule seems to have an enormous amount of osmotic energy tied up in the core structure. Might this be a repository of potential energy for the process? What is the evidence that metabolic energy is needed for anything other than "housekeeping" chores associated with maintenance of a secretion-prone state? The answers to these questions will, we hope, be available in the not too distant future.

ACKNOWLEDGMENTS

We thank Mrs. Joan Mok and Mrs. Sandy Cohen for help in typing the manuscript of this review.

## REFERENCES

Abbs, M. T., and Phillips, J. H. (1980). Organization of the proteins of the chromaffin granule membrane. *Biochim. Biophys. Acta.* **595,** 200–221.

Abdel-Latif, A. A., Akhtar, R. A., and Hawthorne, J. N. (1977). Acetylcholine increases the breakdown of triphosphoinositide of rabbit iris muscle prelabelled with [$^{32}$P]phosphate. *Biochem. J.* **162,** 61–73.

Abou-Donia, M. M., and Viveros, O. H. (1981). Tetrahydrobiopterin increases in adrenal medulla and cortex: A factor in the regulation of tyrosine hydroxylase. *Proc. Natl. Acad. Sci. U.S.A.* **78,** 2703–2706.

Adnan, N. A., and Hawthorne, J. N. (1981). Phosphatidylinositol labelling in response to activation of muscarinic receptors in bovine adrenal medulla. *J. Neurochem.* **36,** 1858–1860.

Akhtar, R. A., and Abdel-Latif, A. A. (1980). Requirement for calcium ions in acetylcholine-stimulated phosphodiesterase cleavage of phosphatidylinositol 4,5-biphosphate in rabbit iris smooth muscle. *Biochem. J.* **192,** 783–791.

Ames, M. M., Lerner, P., and Lovenberg, W. (1978). Tyrosine hydroxylase: Activation by protein phosphorylation and end-product inhibition. *J. Biol. Chem.* **253,** 27–31.

Amy, C. M., and Kirshner, N. (1981). Phosphorylation of adrenal medulla cell proteins in conjunction with stimulation of catecholamine secretion. *J. Neurochem.* **36,** 847–854.

Applegate, D., and Reisler, E. (1983). Protease-sensitive regions in myosin subfragment 1. *Proc. Natl. Acad. Sci. U.S.A.* **80,** 7109–7112.

Apps, D. K. (1982). Proton translocating ATPase of chromaffin granule membranes. *Fed. Proc.* **41,** 2775–2780.

Apps, D. K., and Schatz, G. (1979). An adenosine triphosphatase isolated from chromaffin granule membranes is closely similar to $F_1$-adenosine triphosphatase of mitochondria. *Eur. J. Biochem.* **100,** 411–419.

Apps, D. K., Pride, J. G., and Phillips, J. H. (1980). Both the transmembrane pH gradient and the membrane potential are important in the accumulation of a means by resealed chromaffin granule ghosts. *FEBS Lett.* **111,** 386–390.

Argueros, L., and Daniels, A. J. (1981). Manganese as agonist and antagonist of calcium ions: Dual effect upon catecholamine release from adrenal medulla. *Life Sci.* **28,** 1535–1540.

Ashkenazi, R., Finberg, J. P. M., and Youdim, M. B. H. (1983). Behavioral response to combined treatment with selective inhibitors of MAO-A and B and the selective inhibitor of 5-HT uptake. *Br. J. Pharmacol.* **79,** 765–771.

Aunis, D., and Perrin, D. (1984). Chromaffin granule membranes–F-actin interaction and spectrin-like protein of subcellular granules: A possible relationship. *J. Neurochem.* **42,** 1558–1569.

Aunis, D., Miras-Portugal, M. T., and Mandel, P. (1973). Bovine adrenal medullary dopamine β-hydroxylase: Purification by affinity chromatography, kinetic studies and presence of essential histidyl residues. *Biochim. Biophys. Acta* **327,** 331–327.

Aunis, D., Miras-Portugal, M. T., and Mandel, P. (1974). Bovine adrenal medullary dopamine β-hydroxylase: Studies on structure. *Biochim. Biophys. Acta* **365,** 273–295.

Aunis, D., Guerold, B., Bader, M. F., and Ciesielski-Treska, J. (1980a). Immunocytochemical and biochemical demonstration of contractile proteins in chromaffin cells in culture. *Neuroscience* **5,** 2261–2277.

Aunis, D., Hesketh, J. E., and Devilliers, G. (1980b). Immunohistochemical and immunocytochemical localization of myosin, chromogranin A, and dopamine $\beta$-hydroxylase in nerve cells in culture and in adrenal glands. *J. Neurocytol.* **9**, 255–274.

Axelrod, J. (1962). Purification and properties of phenylethanolamine *N*-methyltransferase. *J. Biol. Chem.* **237**, 1657–1660.

Azzi, A., Chance, B., Radda, G. K., and Lee, C. P. (1969). A fluorescence probe of energy-dependent structure changes in fragmented membranes. *Proc. Natl. Acad. Sci. U.S.A.* **62**, 612–619.

Bader, M. F., and Aunis, D. (1983). The 97-kd $\alpha$-actinin-like protein in chromaffin granule membranes from adrenal medulla: Evidence for localization on the cytoplasmic surface and for binding to actin filaments. *Neuroscience* **8**, 165–181.

Bader, M. F., Ciesielski-Treska, J., Thierse, D., Hesketh, J. E., and Aunis, D. (1981). Immunocytochemical study of microtubules in chromaffin cells in culture and evidence that tubulin is not an integral protein of the chromaffin granule membrane. *J. Neurochem.* **37**, 917–933.

Baetge, E. E., Moon, H. M., Kaplan, B. B., Park, D. H., Reis, D. J., and Joh, T. H. (1983). Identification of clones containing DNA complementary to phenylethanolamine *N*-methyltransferase mRNA. *Neurochem. Int.* **5**, 611–617.

Baker, P. F., and Knight, D. E. (1978). Calcium-dependent exocytosis in bovine adrenal medullary cells with leaky plasma membranes. *Nature (London)* **276**, 620–622.

Baker, P. F., and Knight, D. E. (1981). Calcium control of exocytosis and endocytosis in bovine adrenal medullary cells. *Philos. Trans. R. Soc. London Ser. B* **296**, 83–103.

Baker, P. F., and Knight, D. E. (1984). Calcium control of exocytosis in bovine adrenal medullary cells. *TINS* **7**(4), 120–126.

Baker, P. F., Knight, D. E., and Niggli, V. (1982). Protein phosphorylation accompanies calcium-dependent exocytosis in "leaky" bovine adrenal medullary cells. *J. Physiol. (London)* **332**, 118P.

Bakhle, Y., and Youdim, M. B. H. (1979). The metabolism of 5-hydroxytryptamine and phenylethylamine in perfused rat lung and *in vitro*. *Br. J. Pharmacol.* **65**, 147–154.

Banerjee, D. K., Ornberg, R. L., Youdim, M. B. H., Heldman, E., and Pollard, H. B. (1985). Endothelial cells from bovine adrenal medulla develop capillary-like growth patterns in culture. *Proc. Natl. Acad. Sci. U.S.A.* **82**, 4702–4706.

Bashford, C. L., Radda, G. K., and Ritchie, G. A. (1975a). Energy-linked function of the chromaffin granule. *FEBS Lett.* **50**, 21–24.

Bashford, C. L., Radda, G. K., and Ritchie, G. A. (1975b). The effect of uncouplers on catecholamine incorporation by vesicles of chromaffin granules. *Biochem. J.* **148**, 153–155.

Bashford, C. L., Casey, R. P., Radda, G. K., and Ritchie, G. A. (1976). Energy coupling in adrenal chromaffin granules. *Neuroscience* **1**, 399–412.

Baydoun, E. A.-H., and Northcote, D. H. (1981). The extraction from maize (*Zea mays*) root cells of membrane-bound protein with $Ca^{2+}$-dependent ATPase activity and its possible role in membrane fusion *in vitro*. *Biochem. J.* **193**, 781–792.

Baxter, D. A., Johnston, D., and Strittmatter, W. J. (1983). Protease inhibitors implicate metalloendoprotease in synaptic transmission at the mammalian neuromuscular junction. *Proc. Natl. Acad. Sci. U.S.A.* **80**, 4174–4178.

Bear, E. L., and Friend, D. S. (1982). Modifications of anionic lipid domains preceding membrane fusion in guinea pig sperm. *J. Cell Biol.* **92**, 604–615.

Belpaire, F., and Laduron, P. M. (1968). Tissue fractionation and catecholamines. *Biochem. Pharmacol.* **17**, 411–421.

Bennett, J. (1983). Regulation of photosynthesis by reversible phosphorylation of the light-harvesting chlorophyll a/b protein. *Biochem. J.* **212**, 1–13.

Bental, M. (1983). The interaction of chromaffin granules and chromaffin granule ghosts with natural and model membranes. M.Sc. thesis, Feinberg Graduate School at the Weizmann Institute of Science, Rehovoth, Israel.

Bental, M., Lelkes, P. I., Scholma, J., Hoekstra, D., and Wilschut, J. (1984). $Ca^{++}$ independent, protein-mediated fusion of chromaffin granule ghosts with liposomes. *Biochim. Biophys. Acta* **774**, 296–300.

Bernier-Valentin, F., Aunis, D., and Rousset, B. (1983). Evidence for tubulin-binding sites on cellular membranes: Plasma membranes, mitochondrial membranes, and secretory granule membranes. *J. Cell Biol.* **97**, 209–216.

Berridge, M. J. (1983). Rapid accumulation of inositol trisphosphate reveals that agonists hydrolyse polyphosphoinositides instead of phosphatidylinositol. *Biochem. J.* **212**, 849, 858.

Berridge, M. J., Downes, C. P., and Hanley, M. R. (1982). Lithium amplifies agonist-dependent phosphatidylinositol responses in brain and salivary glands. *Biochem. J.* **206**, 587–595.

Berridge, M. J., Dawson, R. M. C., Downes, C. P., Heslop, J. P., and Irvine, R. F. (1983). Changes in the levels of inositol phosphates after agonist-dependent hydrolysis of membrane phosphoinositides. *Biochem. J.* **212**, 473–482.

Bilah, M. M., and Lapetina, E. G. (1982). Rapid decrease of phosphatidylinositol 4,5-bisphosphate in thrombin-stimulated platelets. *J. Biol. Chem.* **257**, 12705–12708.

Bjerrum, O. J., Helle, K. B., and Bock, E. (1979). Immunochemically identical hydrophilic and amphiphilic forms of the bovine adrenomedullary dopamine β-hydroxylase. *Biochem. J.* **181**, 231–237.

Blakeborough, P., Louis, C. F., and Turner, A. J. (1981). The structure and organization of dopamine β-hydroxylase in the chromaffin granule membrane. *Biochim. Biophys. Acta* **669**, 33–38.

Bohn, M. C. (1983). Role of glucocorticoids in expression and development of phenylethanolamine N-methyltransferase (PNMT) in cells derived from neural crest: A review. *Psychoneuroendocrinology* **8**, 381–390.

Braun, G., Lelkes, P. I., and Nir, S. (1985). Effect of cholesterol on $Ca^{2+}$-induced aggregation and fusion of sonicated phosphatidylserine/cholesterol vesicles. *Biochim. Biophys. Acta* **812**, 688–694.

Breemen, C. V., Aaronson, P., and Lontzenhiser, R. (1979). Sodium–calcium interactions in mammalian smooth muscle. *Pharmacol. Rev.* **30**(2), 167–208.

Bregestonski, P. D., Miledi, R., and Parker, I. (1980). Blocking of frog endplate channels by the organic calcium agonist B600. *Proc. R. Soc. London Ser. B* **211**, 15–24.

Brocklehurst, J. R., Freedman, R. B., Hancock, D. J., and Radda, G. K. (1970). Membrane studies with polarity-dependent and excimer-forming fluorescent probes. *Biochem. J.* **116**, 721–723.

Brooks, J. C., and Treml, S. (1983). Catecholamine secretion by chemically skinned cultured chromaffin cells. *J. Neurochem.* **40**, 468–473.

Brooks, J. C., Treml, S., and Brooks, M. (1984). Thiophosphorylation prevents catecholamine secretion by chemically skinned chromaffin cells. *Life Sci.* **35**, 569–574.

Buckley, J. T., Lefebvre, Y. A., and Hawthorne, J. N. (1971). Identification of an actively phosphorylated component of adrenal medulla chromaffin granules. *Biochim. Biophys. Acta* **239**, 517–519.

Burgess, G. M., Godfrey, P. P., McKinney, J. S., Berridge, M. J., Irvine, R. F., and

Putney, J. W. (1984). The second messenger linking receptor activation to internal Ca$^{++}$ release in liver. *Nature (London)* **309**, 63–66.

Burgoyne, R. D., and Geisow, M. J. (1981). Specific binding of $^{125}$I-calmodulin to and protein phosphorylation in adrenal chromaffin granule membranes. *FEBS Lett.* **131**, 127–131.

Burgoyne, R. D., and Geisow, M. J. (1982a). Effect of Ca$^{2+}$, calmodulin and trifluoperazine on protein phosphorylation in adrenal chromaffin granule membranes. *Biochem. Soc. Trans.* **10**, 267–268.

Burgoyne, R. D., and Geisow, M. J. (1982b). Phosphoproteins of the adrenal chromaffin granule membrane. *J. Neurochem.* **39**, 1387–1396.

Burridge, K., and Phillips, J. H. (1975). Association of actin and myosin with secretory granule membranes. *Nature (London)* **254**, 526–529.

Carlsson, A., Hillarp, N.-A., and Waldeck, B. (1963). Analysis of the Mg$^{++}$-ATP-dependent storage mechanism in the amine granules of the adrenal medulla. *Acta Physiol. Scand.* **59** (Suppl. 215), 1–38.

Casey, R. P., Njus, D., Radda, G. K., and Sehr, P. A. (1977). Adenosine triphosphate-evoked catecholamine release in chromaffin granules. *Biochemistry* **16**, 972–977.

Castagna, M., Takai, Y., Kaibuchi, K., Sano, K., Kikkawa, U., and Nishizuka, Y. (1982). Direct activation of Ca$^{2+}$-activated, phospholipid-dependent protein kinase by tumor-promoting phorbol esters. *J. Biol. Chem.* **257**, 7847–7851.

Chandler, D., and Heuser, J. E. (1980). Arrest of membrane fusion events in mast cells by quick freezing. *J. Cell Biol.* **86**, 666–674.

Chang, Ta-C. L., and Sweeley, C. C. (1963). Characterization of lipids from canine adrenal glands. *Biochemistry* **2**, 592–604.

Ciaranello, R. D. (1977). Regulation of phenylethanolamine *N*-methyltransferase synthesis and degradation. *Mod. Pharmacol. Toxicol.* **10**, 497–525.

Ciaranello, R. D. (1978). Regulation of phenylethanolamine *N*-methyltransferase synthesis and degradation. *Mol. Pharmacol.* **14**, 478–489.

Ciaranello, R. D., Jackobowitz, D., and Axelrod, J. (1973). Effect of dexamethasone on phenylethanolamine *N*-methyltransferase in chromaffin tissue of the neonatal rat. *J. Neurochem.* **20**, 799–805.

Ciaranello, R. D., Wong, D. L., and Berenbeim, D. M. (1978). Regulation of phenylethanolamine *N*-methyltransferase in rat adrenal glands. II. Control of PNMT thermal stability by an endogenous stabilizing factor. *Mol. Pharmacol.* **14**, 490–501.

Cidon, S., and Nelson, N. (1983). A novel ATPase in the chromaffin granule membrane. *J. Biol. Chem.* **258**, 2892–2898.

Cohen, F. S., Zimmerberg, J., and Finkelstein, A. (1980). Fusion of phospholipid vesicles with planar phospholipid bilayer membranes. II. Incorporation of a vesicular membrane marker into planar membrane. *J. Gen. Physiol.* **75**, 251–270.

Cohen, F. S., Akabas, M. H., Zimmerberg, J., and Finkelstein, A. (1984). Parameters affecting the fusion of unilamellar phospholipid vesicles with planar bilayer membranes. *J. Cell. Biol.* **98**, L054–1062.

Cohen, P. (1982). The role of protein phosphorylation in neural and hormonal control of cellular activity. *Nature (London)* **296**, 613–620.

Connett, R. J., and Kirshner, N. (1970). Purification and properties of bovine phenylethanolamine *N*-methyltransferase. *J. Biol. Chem.* **245**, 329–334.

Corcoran, J. J., and Kirshner, N. (1983a). Inhibition of calcium uptake, sodium uptake, and catecholamine secretion by methoxyverapamil (D600) in primary cultures of adrenal medulla cells. *J. Neurochem.* **40** (4), 1106–1109.

Corcoran, J. J., and Kirshner, N. (1983b). Effect of manganese and other divalent cations on calcium uptake and catecholamine secretion by primary cultures of bovine adrenal medulla cells. *Cell Calcium* **4**, 127–137.

Corcoran, J. J., Wilson, S. P., and Kirshner, N. (1984). Flux of catecholamines through chromaffin vesicles in cultured bovine adrenal medullary cells. *J. Biol. Chem.* **259**, 6208–6214.

Couch, C. B., and Strittmatter, W. J. (1983). Rat myoblast fusion requires metalloendoprotease activity. *Cell* **32**, 257–265.

Couch, C. B., and Strittmatter, W. J. (1984). Specific blockers of myoblast fusion inhibit a soluble and not the membrane-associated metalloendoprotease in myoblasts. *J. Biol. Chem.* **259**, 5396–5399.

Coupland, R. E. (1965). Electron microscopic observations on the structure of the rat adrenal medulla. The ultrastructure and organization of chromaffin cell in the normal adrenal medulla. *J. Anat.* **99**, 231–254.

Coupland, R. E., Pyper, A. S., and Hopwood, D. (1964). A method for differentiating between noradrenaline- and adrenaline-storing cells in the light and electron microscope. *Nature (London)* **20**, 1240–1242.

Craig, S. W., and Pollard, T. D. (1982). Actin-binding proteins. *TIBS,* **March,** 88–92.

Craine, J. E., Daniels, G. H., and Kaufman, S. (1973). Dopamine $\beta$-hydroxylase: The subunit structure and anion activation of the bovine adrenal enzyme. *J. Biol. Chem.* **248**, 7838–7844.

Creba, J. A., Downes, C. P., Hawkins, P. T., Brewster, G., Michell, R. H., and Kirk, C. J. (1983). Rapid breakdown of phosphatidylinositol 4-phosphate and phosphatidylinositol 4,5-bisphosphate in rat hepatocytes stimulated by vasopressin and other $Ca^{++}$-mobilizing hormones. *Biochem. J.* **212**, 733–747.

Creutz, C. D. (1977). Isolation, characterization and localization of bovine adrenal medullary myosin. *Cell Tissue Res.* **178**, 17–38.

Cruetz, C. E. (1981a). Secretory vesicle–cytosol interactions in exocytosis: Isolation by $Ca^{2+}$-dependent affinity chromatography of proteins that bind to the chromaffin granule membrane. *Biochem. Biophys. Res. Commun.* **103**, 1395–1400.

Creutz, C. E. (1981b). Cis-unsaturated fatty acids induce the fusion of chromaffin granules aggregated by synexin. *J. Cell Biol.* **91**, 247–256.

Creutz, C. E., and Harrison, J. R. (1984). Clathrin light chains and secretory vesicle binding proteins are distinct. *Nature (London)* **308**, 208–210.

Creutz, C. E., and Pollard, H. B. (1981). A cell-free model for protein–lipid interactions in exoxytosis. *Biophys. J.* **37**, 119–120.

Creutz, C. E., and Sterner, D. C. (1983). Calcium dependence of the binding of synexin to isolated chromaffin granules. *Biochem. Biophys. Res. Commun.* **114**, 355–364.

Creutz, C. E., Pazoles, C. J., and Pollard, H. B. (1978). Identification and purification of an adrenal medullary protein (synexin) that causes calcium-dependent aggregation of isolated chromaffin granules. *J. Biol. Chem.* **253**, 2858–2866.

Creutz, C. E., Pazoles, C. J., and Pollard, H. B. (1979). Self-association of synexin in the presence of calcium: Correlation with synexin-induced membrane fusion and examination of the structure of synexin aggregates. *J. Biol. Chem.* **254**, 553–558.

Creutz, C. E., Scott, J. E., Pazoles, C. J., and Pollard, H. B. (1982). Further characterization of the aggregation and fusion of chromaffin granules by synexin as a model for compound exoycytosis. *J. Cell Biochem.* **18**, 87–97.

Creutz, C. E., Dowling, L. G., Sando, J. J., Villar-Palasi, C., Whipple, J. H., and Zaks, W. J. (1983). Characterization of the chromobindins: Soluble proteins that bind to the chromaffin granule membrane in the presence of $Ca^{2+}$. *J. Biol. Chem.* **258,** 14664–14674.

Creveling, C. R., McNeal, E., Daly, J. W., and Brown, G. B. (1983). Depolarization of brain vesicle preparations and binding of batrachotoxins: Blockage by local anesthetics. *Mol. Pharmacol.* **23,** 350–358.

Cullis, P. R., deKruiff, B., Hope, M. J., Verkleij, A. J., Nayar, R., Farren, S. B., Tilcock, C., Madden, T. D., and Bally, M. B. (1983). Structural properties of lipids and their functional roles in biological membranes in membrane fluidity in biology. *In* "Concepts of Membrane Structure" (R. C. Alaia, ed.), Vol. 1, pp. 39–81. Academic Press, New York.

Dabrow, M., Zaremba, S., and Hogue-Angeletti, R. A. (1980). Specificity of synexin-induced chromaffin granule aggregation. *Biochem. Biophys. Res. Commun.* **96,** 1164–1171.

Daniels, A. J., Williams, R. J. P., and Wright, P. E. (1978). The character of the stored molecules in chromaffin granules of the adrenal medulla: A nuclear magnetic resonance study. *Neuroscience* **3,** 573–585.

Da Prada, M., Orsit, R., and Pletscher, A. (1975). Discrimination of monoamine uptake by membranes of adrenal chromaffin granules. *Br. J. Pharmacol.* **53,** 257–265.

Davis, B., and Lazarus, N. R. (1976). An *in vitro* system for studying insulin release caused by secretory granules–plasma membrane interaction: Definition of the system. *J. Physiol. (London)* **256,** 709–729.

Dawson, R. M. C., and Clarke, N. (1972). D-Myoinositol 1 : 2-cyclic phosphate 2-phosphohydrolase. *Biochem. J.* **127,** 113–118.

Dawson, A. P., and Irvine, R. F. (1984). Inositol (1,4,5) trisphosphate-promoted $Ca^{++}$ release from microsomal fractions of rat liver. *Biochem. Biophys. Res. Commun.* **120,** 858–864.

De Robertis, E., and Vaz Ferreira, A. (1957). Electron microscopic study of the excretion of catechol-containing droplets in the adrenal medulla. *Exp. Cell Res.* **12,** 568–574.

Derome, G., Tseng, R., Mercier, P., Lemaire, I., and Lemaire, S. (1981). Possible muscarinic regulation of catecholamine secretion mediated by cyclic GMP in isolated bovine adrenal chromaffin cells. *Biochem. Pharmacol.* **30,** 855–860.

Donnelly, C. H., Richelson, E., and Murphy, D. L. (1976). Properties of monoamine oxidase in mouse neuroblastoma NIE-115 cells. *Biochem. Pharmacol.* **25,** 1639–1643.

Douglas, W. W. (1975). Secretomotor control of adrenal medullary secretion: Synaptic membrane and ionic events in stimulus-secretion coupling. *Handb. Physiol. Sect. 7, Endocrinol.* **55,** 367–388.

Dowd, D. J., Edwards, C., Englert, D., Mazurkiewicz, J. E., and Ye, H. Z. (1983). Immunofluorescent evidence for exocytosis and internalization of secretory granule membrane in isolated chromaffin cells. *Neuroscience* **10,** 1025–1033.

Downes, C. P., and Michell, R. H. (1982). Phosphatidylinositol 4-phosphate and phosphatidylinositol 4,5-biphosphate: Lipids in search of a function. *Cell Calcium* **3,** 467–502.

Drummond, A. H., Bushfield, M., and MacPhee, C. H. (1984). Thyrotropin-releasing hormone-stimulated [$^3$H]inositol metabolism in $GH_3$ pituitary tumor cells. Studies with lithium. *Mol. Pharmacol.* **25,** 201–208.

Duncan, C. J. (1983). Role of calcium in triggering the release of transmitters at the neuromuscular junction. *Cell Calcium* **4,** 171–193.

Dunn, L. A., and Holz, R. W. (1983). Catecholamine secretion from digitonin-treated adrenal medullary chromaffin cells. *J. Biol. Chem.* **258**, 4989–4993.

Duong, L. T., and Fleming, P. J. (1983). The asymmetric orientation of cytochrome $b_{561}$ in bovine chromaffin granule membranes. *Arch. Biochem. Biophys.* **228**, 332–341.

Durell, J., Garland, J. T., and Friedel, R. O. (1969). Acetylcholine action: Biochemical aspects. *Science* **165**, 862–866.

Duzgunes, N., and Papahadjopoulos, D. (1983). Ionotropic effects on phospholipid membranes: Calcium/magnesium specificity in binding, fluidity and fusion. *In* "Membrane Fluidity in Biology" (R. C. Aloia, ed.), Vol. 1. Academic Press, New York.

Duzgunes, N., Wilschut, J., Fraley, R., and Papahadjopoulos, D. (1981a). Studies on the mechanism of membrane fusion. Role of head-group composition in calcium- and magnesium-induced fusion of mixed phospholipid vesicles. *Biochim. Biophys. Acta* **642**, 182–195.

Duzgunes, N., Nir, S., Wilschut, J., Bentz, J., Newton, C., Portis, A., and Papahadjopoulos, D. (1981b). Calcium- and magnesium-induced fusion of mixed phosphatidylserine/phosphatidylcholine vesicles: Effect of ion binding. *J. Membr. Biol.* **59**, 115–125.

Eckerdt, R., Dahl, G., and Gratzl, M. (1981). Membrane fusion of secretory vesicles and liposomes. Two different types of fusion. *Biochim. Biophys. Acta* **646**, 10–22.

Eytan, G. D., and Almary, T. (1983). Melittin-induced fusion of acidic liposomes. *FEBS Lett.* **156**, 29–32.

Farquhar, M. G. (1981). Membrane recycling in secretory cells: Implications for traffic of products and specialized membranes within the golgi complex. *Methods Cell Biol.* **23**, 400–427.

Fenwick, E. M., Fajdiga, P. B., Howe, N. B. S., and Livett, B. G. (1978). Functional and morphological characterization of isolated bovine adrenal medullary cells. *J. Cell Biol.* **76**, 12–30.

Fenwick, E. M., Marty, A., and Neher, E. (1982). Sodium and calcium channels in bovine chromaffin cells. *J. Physiol.* (London) **331**, 599–635.

Fety, R., and Renaud, B. (1983). Time course study of changes in the activity of the catecholamine synthesizing enzymes in the rat medulla oblongata after intraventricular injection of 6-hydroxydopamine. *Brain Res.* **272**, 277–282.

Finberg, J. P. M., and Youdim, M. B. H. (1983). Monoamide oxidases. In: *Handb. Neurochem.* **4**, 293–315.

Fisher, S. K., Holz, R. W., and Agranoff, B. W. (1981). Muscarinic receptors in chromaffin cell cultures mediate enhanced phospholipid labeling but not catecholamine secretion. *J. Neurochem.* **37**, 491–497.

Fischer-Colbrie, R., Schachinger, M., Zangerle, R., and Winkler, H. (1982). Dopamine $\beta$-hydroxylase and other glycoproteins from the soluble content and the membranes of adrenal medulla chromaffin granules. *J. Neurochem.* **38**, 725–732.

Flatmark, T. (1982). The dopamine $\beta$-hydroxylating system of bovine adrenal chromaffin granules. *In* "From Cyclotrons to Cytochromes: Essays in Molecular Biology and Chemistry" (N. O. Kaplan and A. Robinson, eds.), pp. 431–444. Academic Press, New York.

Fleming, P. J., and Saxena, A. (1982). Reconstitution of the membrane-bound form of dopamine $\beta$-hydroxylase. *Biophys. J.* **37**, 99–100.

Fowler, V. M., and Pollard, H. B. (1982a). Chromaffin granule membrane–F-actin interaction are calcium sensitive. *Nature (London)* **295**, 336–339.

Fowler, V. M., and Pollard, H. B. (1982b). *In vitro* reconstitution of chromaffin granule–

cytoskeleton interactions: Ionic factors influencing the association of F-actin with purified chromaffin granule membranes. *J. Cell Biochem.* **18,** 295–311.

Fowler, C. J., and Tipton, K. F. (1982). Deamination of 5-hydroxytryptamine by both forms of monoamine oxidase in the rat brain. *J. Neurochem.* **38,** 733–738.

Frederick, J. M., Hollyfield, J. G., and Strittmatter, W. J. (1983). Metalloendoprotease required for exocytosis of glycine by retinal neurons in xenopus. *J. Cell Biol.* **97,** 171A (Abstr. No. 645).

Friedman, J. E., Lelkes, P. I., Rosenheck, K., and Oplatka, A. (1980). The possible implication of membrane-associated actin in stimulus-secretion coupling in adrenal chromaffin cells. *Biochem. Biophys. Res. Commun.* **96,** 1717–1723.

Friedman, J. E., Lavie, E., Lelkes, P. I., Rosenheck, K., Schneeweiss, F., and Schneider, A. S. (1985a). Membrane potential catecholamine secretion by bovine adrenal chromaffin cells: Use of tetraphenylphosphonium distribution and carbocyanine dye fluorescence. J. Neurochem. **44,** 1391–1402.

Friedman, J. E., Lelkes, P. I., Rosenheck, K., and Oplatka, A. (1985b). Control of stimulus–secretion coupling in adrenal medullary chromaffin cells by microfilament specific macromolecules. Submitted.

Frye, R. A., and Holz, R. W. (1983). Phospholipase $A_2$ inhibitors block catecholamine secretion and calcium uptake in cultured bovine adrenal medullary cells. *Mol. Pharmacol.* **23,** 547–550.

Frye, R. A., and Holz, R. W. (1984). The relationship between arachidomic acid release and catecholamine secretion from cultured bovine adrenal chromaffin cells. *J. Neurochem.* **43,** 146–150.

Fuller, G. M., Brinkley, B. R., and Boughter, J. M. (1975). Immunofluorescence of mitotic spindles using monospecific antibody against bovine brain tubulin. *Science* **187,** 948–951.

Gabay, S., and Valcourt, A. J. (1968). Studies of monoamine oxidase. *Biochim. Biophys. Acta* **159,** 440–450.

Gabizon, R., Yetinson, T., and Schuldiner, S. (1982). Photoinactivation and identification of the biogenic amine transporter in chromaffin granules from bovine adrenal medulla. *J. Biol. Chem.* **257,** 15145–15152.

Gad, A. E. (1983). Cationic polypeptide-induced fusion of acid liposomes. *Biochim. Biophys. Acta* **728,** 377–382.

Garcia, L. A., Schenkmann, S., Araujo, P. S., and Chaimovich, H. (1983). Fusion of small unilamellar vesicles induced by bovine serum albumin fragments. *Braz. J. Med. Biol. Res.* **16,** 89–96.

Garrick, N., and Murphy, D. L. (1982). Differences in selectivity toward norepinephrine compared to serotonin. *Biochem. Pharmacol.* **31,** 4061–4067.

Geffen, L. B. (1981). Dopamine β-hydroxylase antibodies as probes of noradrenergic neurons. *Proc. Aust. Physiol. Pharmacol. Soc.* **12,** 1–9.

Godfrey, P. P., and Putney, J. W. (1984). Receptor-mediated metabolism of the phosphoinositides and phosphatidic acid in rat lacrimal acinar cells. *Biochem. J.* **218,** 187–195.

Goldstein, J. L., Anderson, R. G., and Brown, M. S. (1979). Coated pits, coated vesicles and receptor-mediated endocytosis. *Nature (London)* **279,** 679.

Goridis, C., and Neff, N. H. (1971a). Monoamine oxidase in sympathetic nerve: A transmitter specific enzyme type. *Br. J. Pharmacol.* **43,** 814–820.

Goridis, C., and Neff, N. H. (1971b). Evidence for a specific monoamine oxidase associated with sympathetic nerve. *Neuropharmacology* **10,** 557–564.

Gratzl, M., Schudt, C., Eckerdt, R., and Dahl, G. (1980a). Fusion of isolated biological membranes. *Membr. Struct. Funct.* **3**, 59–92.

Gratzl, M., Eckerdt, R., and Dahl, G. (1980b). The role of $Ca^{2+}$ as a trigger for membrane fusion. *In* "Biochemistry and Biophysics of the Pancreatic B - Cell" (W. J. Malaisse and I.-B. Taeljedal, eds.), pp. 144–149. Thieme, Stuttgart.

Grynszpan-Winograd, O. (1971). Morphological aspects of exocytosis in the adrenal medulla. *Philos. Trans. R. Soc. London Ser. B* **261**, 291–292.

Hadjiconstantinou, M., Cohen, J., and Neff, N. H. (1983). Epinephrine: A potential neurotransmitter in retina. *J. Neurochem.* **41**, 1440–1444.

Hampton, R. Y., and Holz, R. W. (1983). Effects of changes in osmolarity on the stability and function of cultured chromaffin cells and the possible role of osmotic forces in exocytosis. *J. Cell Biol.* **96**, 1082–1088.

Harish, O. E., Levy, R., Rosenheck, K., and Oplatka, A. (1984). Possible involvement of actin and myosin in $Ca^{2+}$ transport through the plasma membrane of chromaffin cells. *Biochem. Biophys. Res. Commun.* **119**, 652–656.

Hartshorne, D. J., and Siemankowski, R. F. (1981). Regulation of smooth muscle actomyosin. *Annu. Rev. Physiol.* **43**, 519–530.

Hasegawa-Sasaki, H., and Sasaki, T. (1983). Phytochemagglutinin induces rapid degradation of phosphatidylinositol 4,5-biphosphate and transient accumulation of phosphatidic acid and diacylglycerol in a human cell line, CCRF-CEM. *Biochim. Biophys. Acta* **754**, 305–314.

Hawkins, M., and Breakefield, X. O. (1978). Monoamine oxidase A and B in cultured cells. *J. Neurochem.* **30**, 1391–1397.

Hawthorne, J. N., and Swilen, A. F. (1982). Phosphatidylinositol metabolism in the adrenal medulla. *Cell Calcium* **3**, 351–358.

Haycock, J. W., Bennett, W. F., George, R. J., and Waymire, J. C. (1982a). Multiple-site phosphorylation of tyrosine hydroxylase: Differential regulation by 8-bromo-cAMP and acetylcholine. *J. Biol. Chem.* **257**, 13699–13703.

Haycock, J. W., Meligeni, J. A., Bennett, W. F., and Waymire, J. C. (1982b). Phosphorylation and activation of tyrosine hydroxylase mediate the acetylcholine-induced increase in catecholamine biosynthesis in adrenal chromaffin cells. *J. Biol. Chem.* **257**, 12641–12648.

Heldman, E., Levine, M. A., Morita, K., and Pollard, H. B. (1984). Potassium and nicotine-stimulated catecholamine release from cultured chromaffin cells are mediated by two different modes of calcium flux. *Soc. Neurosci. Annu. Meet., 14th.*

Helle, K. B., and Serck-Hanssen, G. (1981). Different forms of dopamine $\beta$-hydroxylase in vesicles. *In* "Chemical Neurotransmission 75 Years" (L. Stjarne, P. Hedquist, H. Lagercrantz, and A. Wennmalm, eds.), pp. 85–90. Academic Press, New York.

Helle, K. B., Flatmark, T., Serck-Hanssen, G., and Lonning, S. (1971). An improved method for the large-scale isolation of chromaffin granules from bovine adrenal medulla. *Biochim. Biophys. Acta* **226**, 1–8.

Helle, K. B., Serck-Hanssen, G., and Bock, E. (1978). Complexes of chromogranin A and dopamine $\beta$-hydroxylase among the chromogranins of the bovine adrenal medulla. *Biochim. Biophys. Acta* **533**, 396–407.

Helle, K. B., Pihl, K. E., and Serck-Hanssen, G. (1982). Hydrophilic and amphiphilic forms of dopamine $\beta$-hydroxylase in early and mature stages of the bovine adrenomedullary granules. *Adv. Biosci.* **36**, 217–224.

Hersey, R. M., and Distefano (1979). Control of phenylethanolamine N-methyltransferase by glucocorticoids in cultured bovine adrenal medullary cells. *J. Pharmacol. Exp. Ther.* **209**, 147–152.

Hesketh, J. E., Aunis, D., Mandel, P., and Devilliers, G. (1978). Biochemical and morphological studies of bovine adrenal medullary myosin. *Biol. Cell.* **33**, 199–208.

Hesketh, J. E., Ciesielski-Treska, J., and Aunis, D. (1981). A phase-contrast and immunofluorescence study of adrenal medullary chromaffin cells in culture: Neurite formation, actin and chromaffin granule distribution. *Cell Tissue Res.* **218**, 331–343.

Hillarp, N. A. (1959). Further observations on the state of the catecholamines stored in the adrenal medullary granules. *Acta Physiol. Scand.* **47**, 271–279.

Hiram, Y., Nir, A., and Zinder, O. (1982). Tensile strength of the chromaffin granule membrane. *Biophys. J.* **39**, 65–69.

Hiram, Y., Nir, A., Greenberg, A., and Zinder, O. (1984). Temperature effects in the stimulus-secretion process from isolated chromaffin cells. *Biophys. J.* **45**, 651–658.

Hoekstra, D. (1982). Role of lipid phase separations on membrane hydration in phospholipid vesicle fusion. *Biochemistry* **21**, 2833–2840.

Hoeldtke, R., and Kaufman, S. (1977). Bovine adrenal tyrosine hydroxylase: Purification and properties. *J. Biol. Chem.* **252**, 3160–3169.

Hoffman, P. G., Zinder, O., Nikodijevik, O., and Pollard, H. B. (1976). ATP-stimulated transmitter release and cAMP synthesis in isolated chromaffin granules. *J. Supramol. Struct.* **4**, 151–184.

Hogue-Angeletti, R., Nolan, J., and Caspar, S. (1983). Chromaffin granule dopamine $\beta$-monooxygenase: Membrane and soluble forms. *Fed. Proc., Fed. Am. Soc. Exp. Biol.* **42**, 2023.

Hokfelt, T., Fuxe, K., Goldstein, M., and Johansson, O. (1974). Immunohistochemical evidence for the existence of adrenaline neurons in the rat brain. *Brain Res.* **66**, 235–251.

Hokin, M., and Hokin, L. (1953). Effects of acetylcholine on phospholipids in the pancreas. *J. Biol. Chem.* **209**, 549–558.

Hokin, M. R., Benfey, B. G., and Hokin, L. E. (1958). Phospholipids and adrenaline secretion in guinea pig adrenal medulla. *J. Biol. Chem.* **233**, 814–817.

Holz, R. N. (1978). Evidence that catecholamine transport into chromaffin vesicles is coupled to vesicle membrane potential. *Proc. Natl. Acad. Sci. U.S.A.* **75**, 5190–5194.

Holz, R. N. (1979). Measurement of membrane potential of chromaffin granules by the accumulation of triphenylmethylphosphonium cation. *J. Biol. Chem.* **254**, 6703–6709.

Holz, R. W., Senter, R. A., and Frye, R. A. (1982). Relationship between $Ca^{2+}$ uptake and catecholamine secretion in primary dissociated cultures of adrenal medulla. *J. Neurochem.* **39**, 635–646.

Holz, R. W., Senter, R. A., and Sharp, R. R. (1983). Evidence that the $H^+$-electrochemical gradient across membranes of chromaffin granules is not involved in exocytosis. *J. Biol. Chem.* **258**, 7506–7513.

Holzbauer, M., Bull, M., Youdim, M. B. H., and Wooding, F. B. P. (1973). Subcellular distribution of steroids in the adrenal gland. *Nature (London)* **242**, 117–118.

Hong, K., Duzgunes, N., and Papahadjopoulos, D. (1981). Role of synexin in membrane fusion. Enhancement of calcium-dependent fusion of phospholipid vesicles. *J. Biol. Chem.* **256**, 3641–3644.

Hong, K., Duzgunes, N., and Papahadjopoulos, D. (1982). Modulation of membrane fusion by calcium binding proteins. *Biophys. J.* **37**, 297–305.

Hortnagl, H., Winkler, H., and Lochs, H. (1972). Membrane proteins of chromaffin granules: Isolation and partial characterization of two proteins. *Biochem. J.* **129**, 187–192.

Hotchkiss, A., Pollard, H. B., Scott, J. and Axelrod, J. (1981). Release of arachidonic acid from adrenal chromaffin cell cultures during secretion of epinephrine. *Fed. Proc., Fed. Am. Soc. Exp. Biol.* **40**, 256.

Houseay, M. D., and Tipton, K. F. (1974). A kinetic evaluation of monoamine oxidase activity in rat liver mitochondrial outer membrane. *Biochem. J.* **139**, 649–652.

Hunt, T. (1983). Phosphorylation and the control of protein synthesis. *Philos. Trans. R. Soc. London Ser. B* **302**, 127–134.

Ingebretsen, O. C., and Flatmark, T. (1979). Active and passive transport of dopamine in chromaffin granule ghosts isolated from bovine adrenal medulla. *J. Biol. Chem.* **254**, 3833–3839.

Irvine, R. R. (1982). The enzymology of stimulated inositol lipid turnover. *Cell Calcium* **3**, 295–309.

Irvine, R. F., Letcher, A. J., and Dawson, R. M. (1984). Phosphatidylinositol 4,5-bisphosphate phosphodiesterase and phosphomonoesterase activities of rat brain. *Biochem. J.* **218**, 177–185.

Ito, S. (1983). Time course of release of catecholamine and other granular contents from perifused adrenal chromaffin cells of guinea pig. *J. Physiol. (London)* **341**, 153–167.

Jarrott, B., and Iversen, L. L. (1971). Noradrenaline metabolizing enzymes in normal and sympathetically denervated vas deferens. *J. Neurochem.* **18**, 1–16.

Jockusch. B. M., Burger, M. M., DaPrada, M., Richards, J. G., Chaponnier, C., and Gabbiani, G. (1977). α-actinin attached to membranes of secretory vesicles. *Nature (London)* **270**, 628–629.

Joh, T., and Goldstein, M. (1973). Isolation and characterization of multiple forms of phenylethanolamine $N$-methyltransferase. *Mol. Pharmacol.* **9**, 117–129.

Joh, T. H., and Reis, D. J. (1975). Different forms of tyrosine hydroxylase in central dopaminergic and noradrenergic neurons and sympathetic ganglia. *Brain Res.* **85**, 146–151.

Joh, T. H., Kapit, R., and Goldstein, M. (1969). A kinetic study of particulate bovine adrenal tyrosine hydroxylase. *Biochim. Biophys. Acta* **171**, 378–380.

Joh, T. H., Park, D. H., and Reis, D. J. (1978). Direct phosphorylation of brain tyrosine hydroxylase by cyclic AMP-dependent protein kinases: Mechanism of action. *Proc. Natl. Acad. Sci. U.S.A.* **75**, 4744–4748.

Joh, T. H., Baetge, E. E., Kaplan, B. B., Ross, M. E., Brodsky, M. J., Albert, V. R., Park, D. H., and Reis, D. J. (1981). Catecholamine synthetic enzymes probably share common gene coding sequences. *Neurosci. Abstr.* **7**, 206.

Johnson, R. G., and Scarpa, A. (1976). Internal pH of isolated chromaffin granules. *J. Biol. Chem.* **251**, 2189–2191.

Johnson, R. G., and Scarpa, A. (1979). Proton motive force and catecholamine transport in isolated chromaffin granules. *J. Biol. Chem.* **254**, 3750–3760.

Johnson, R. G., Carlson, N. J., and Scarpa, A. (1978). Delta pH and catecholamine distribution in isolated chromaffin granules. *J. Biol. Chem.* **253**, 1512–1521.

Johnson, R. G., Pfister, D., Carty, S. E., and Scarpa, A. (1979). Biological amine transport in chromaffin ghosts: Coupling to the transmembrane proton and potential gradients. *J. Biol. Chem.* **254**, 10963–10972.

Johnson, R. G., Carty, S. E., and Scarpa, A. (1981). Proton substrate stoichiometries during active transport of biogenic amines in chromaffin ghosts. *J. Biol. Chem.* **256**, 65773–5780.

Johnson, R. G., Carty, S. E., Hayflick, S., and Scarpa, A. (1982). Mechanisms of accumulation, tyramine, metaraminol and isoproterenol in isolated chromaffin granules and ghosts. *Biochem. Pharmacol.* **31**, 815–823.

Johnston, J. P. (1968). Some observations upon a new inhibitor of monoamine oxidase in brain tissue. *Biochem. Pharmacol.* **17**, 1285–1297.

Joseph, S. K., Thomas, A. P., Williams, R. J., Irvine, R. F., and Williamson, J. R. (1984). Myoinositol 1,4,5-triphosphate. A second messenger for the hormonal mobilization of intracellular $Ca^{++}$ in liver. *J. Biol. Chem.* **259**, 3077–3081.

Kao, L.-S., and Schneider, A.S. (1985). Muscarinic receptors on bovine chromaffin cells mediate a rise in cytosolic calcium that is independent of extracellular calcium. *J. Biol. Chem.* **260**, 2019–2022.

Kardo, H., Wolosewick, J. J., and Pappas, G. D. (1982). The microtrabecular lattice of the adrenal medulla revealed by polyethylene glycol embedding and stereo electron microscopy. *J. Neurosci.* **2**, 57–65.

Kaufman, S. (1963). The structure of the phenylalanine-hydroxylation cofactor. *Proc. Natl. Acad. Sci. U.S.A.* **50**, 1085–1093.

Kaufman, S. (1974). Properties of the pterin-dependent aromatic amino acid hydroxy-lases. *In* "Aromatic Amino Acids in the Brain" (CIBA Foundation), pp. 81–115. Elsevier, Amsterdam.

Kawasaki, K., Sato, S. B., and Ohnishi, S. (1983). Membrane fusion activity of reconstituted vesicles of influenza virus hemagglutinin glycoproteins. *Biochim. Biophys. Acta* **733**, 286–290.

Kearney, E. B., Saloch, J. I., Walker, W. H., Song, R. L., Kenney, W. C., Zeszoteck, E., and Singer, T. P. (1971). The covalently bound flavin of hepatic monoamine oxidase. I. Isolation and sequence of a flavin peptide and evidence for binding at the 8 position. *Eur. J. Biochem.* **24**, 321–327.

Kelner, K. and Pollard, H. B. (1985). Glucocorticoid receptors and regulation of phenyl-ethanolamine-$N$-methyl transferase activity in cultured chromaffin cells. *J. Neuroscience* **5**, 2161–2168.

Kiang, N.-L., Krusius, T., Finne, J., Margolis, R. U., and Margolis, R. K. (1982). Glyco-proteins and proteoglycans of the chromaffin granule matrix. *J. Biol. Chem.* **257**, 1651–1652.

Kidokoro, Y., and Ritchie, A. K. (1980). Chromaffin cell action potentials and their possible role in adrenalin secretion from rat adrenal medulla. *J. Physiol. (London)* **307**, 199–216.

Kilpatrick, D. L., Ledbetter, F. H., Carson, K. A., Kirshner, A. G., Slepetis, R., and Kirshner, N. (1980). Stability of bovine adrenal medulla cells in culture. *J. Neurochem.* **35**, 679–692.

Kilpatrick, D. L., Ledbetter, F. H., Carson, K. A., Kirshner, A. G., Slepetis, R., and Kirshner, N. (1980). Stability of bovine adrenal medulla cells in culture. *J. Neurochem.* **35**, 679–692.

Kirshner, N. (1957). Pathway of noradrenaline formation from dopa. *J. Biol. Chem.* **226**, 821–825.

Kirshner, N. (1962). Uptake of catecholamines by a particulate fraction of adrenal medulla. *J. Biol. Chem.* **237**, 2311–2317.

Kirshner, N., and Goodall, MdC. (1957). The formation of adrenaline from noradrenaline. *Biochim. Biophys. Acta* **24**, 658–659.

Knight, D. E., and Baker, P. F. (1983a). The phorbol ester TPA increases the affinity of exocytosis for calcium in "leaky" adrenal medullary cells. *FEBS Lett.* **160**, 98–100.

Knight, D. E., and Baker, P. F. (1983b). Stimulus-secretion coupling in isolated bovine adrenal medulla cells. *Exp. Physiol.* **68**. 23–143.

Knight, D. E., and Kestenen, N. T. (1983). Evoked transient intracellular free $Ca^{++}$ changes and secretion in isolated bovine adrenal medullary cells. *Proc. R. Soc. London Ser. B* **218**, 177–199.

Knoth, J., Handloser, K., and Njus, D. (1980). Electrogenic epinephrine transport in chromaffin granule ghosts. *Biochemistry* **19**, 2938–2942.

Knoth, J., Isaacs, J. M., and Njus, D. (1981). Amine transport in chromaffin granule ghosts. *J. Biol. Chem.* **256**, 6541–6543.

Koenigsberg, R. L., Cote, A., and Trifaro, J. M. (1982). *Neuroscience* **7**, 2277–2286.

Kondo, H., Wolosewick, J. J., and Pappas, G. D. (1982). The microtrabecular lattice of the adrenal medulla revealed by polyethylene glycol embedding and stereo electron microscopy. *J. Neurosci.* **2**, 57–65.

Konig, P., Hortnagl, H., Kostron, H., Sapinsky, H., and Winkler, H. (1976). The arrangement of dopamine $\beta$-hydroxylase and chromomembrin B in the membrane of chromaffin granules. *J. Neurochem.* **27**, 1539–1541.

Konings, F., and DePotter, W. (1981). Calcium-dependent *in vitro* interaction between bovine adrenal medullary cell membranes and chromaffin granules as a model for exocytosis. *FEBS Lett.* **126**, 103–106.

Konings, F., and DePotter, W. (1982). A role for sialic acid containing substrates in the exocytosis-like *in vitro* interaction between adrenal medullary plasma membranes and chromaffin granules. *Biochem. Biophys. Res. Commun.* **106**, 1191–1195.

Konings, F., and DePotter, W. (1983). Protein phosphorylation and the exocytosis-like interaction between isolated adrenal medullary plasma membranes and chromaffin granules. *Biochem. Biophys. Res. Commun.* **110**, 55–60.

Konings, F., Majchrowicz, B., and DePotter, W. (1982). The exocytosis-like effect of bovine adrenal medullary plasma membranes on the integrity of chromaffin granules. *Arch. Int. Pharmacodyn.* **260**, 282–283.

Kuczenski, R. T., and Mandel, A. J. (1972). Regulatory properties of soluble and particulate rat brain tyrosine hydroxylase. *J. Biol. Chem.* **247**, 3114–3122.

Kuhn, D. M., and Lovenberg, W. (1983). Hydroxylases. *Handb. Neurochem.* **4**, 133–150.

Laduron, P. M. (1975). Evidence for a localization of dopamine $\beta$-hydroxylase with the chromaffin granules. *FEBS Lett.* **52**, 132–134.

Lapetina, E. G., and Michell, R. H. (1973). Phosphatidylinositol metabolism in cells receiving extracellular stimulation. *FEBS Lett.* **31**, 1–10.

Lazarides, E., and Weber, K. (1974). Actin antibody: The specific visualization of actin filaments in nonmuscle cells. *Proc. Natl. Acad. Sci. U.S.A.* **71**, 2268–2273.

Lee, R. W. H., and Trifaro, J. M. (1981). Characterization of anti-actin antibodies and their use in immunocytochemical studies on the localization of actin in adrenal chromaffin cells in culture. *Neuroscience* **6**, 2087–2108.

Lee, R. W. H., Mashyashi, W. E., and Trifaro, J. M. (1979). Two forms of cytoplasmic actin in adrenal chromaffin cells. *Neuroscience* **4**, 843–852.

Lee, V., Shelanski, M. L., and Greene, L. A. (1977). Specific neural and adrenal medullary antigens detected by antisera to clonal PC12 pheochromocytoma cells. *Proc. Natl. Acad. Sci. U.S.A.* **74**, 5021–5025.

Lefebvre, Y. A., White, D. A., and Hawthorne, J. N. (1976). Diphosphoinositide metabolism in bovine adrenal medulla. *Can. J. Biochem.* **54**, 746–753.

Lelkes, P. I., Lavie, E., Naquira, D., Schneeweiss, F., Schneider, A. S., and Rosenheck, K. (1980). Acetylcholine-induced *in vitro* fusion between cell membrane vesicles and chromaffin granules from the bovine adrenal medulla. *FEBS Lett.* **115**, 129–133.

Lelkes, P. I., and Friedman, J. E. (1985). Interaction of French-pressed liposomes with isolated bovine adrenal chromaffin cells. I. Characterization of the cell-liposome interactions. *J. Biol. Chem.* **260**, 1796–1803.

Lelkes, P. I., Naquira, D., Friedman, J. E., Rosenheck, K., and Schneider, A. S. (1982). Plasma membrane vesicles from bovine adrenal chromaffin cells: Characterization and fusion with chromaffin granules. *Adv. Biosci.* **36**, 143–150.

Lelkes, P. I., Brocklehurst, K. W., Morita, K., and Pollard, H. B. (1984). Metalloendoproteases in bovine adrenal chromaffin cells: Their localization and involvement in stimulus–secretion coupling. *In* "Molecular Biology of Peripheral Catecholamine Storing Tissues," Colmar, France, abstract p. 104.

Lentendre, C. H., MacDonnell, P. C., and Guroff, G. (1977). The biosynthesis of phosphorylated tyrosine hydroxylase by organ cultures of rat adrenal medulla and superior cervical ganglia: A correction. *Biochem. Biophys. Res. Commun.* **76**, 615–617.

Lever, J. D. (1955) Electron microscopic observations on the normal and denervated adrenal medulla of the rat. *Endocrinology* **57**, 621–635.

Levine, M., Morita, K., and Pollard, H. B. (1985). Enhancement of norepinephrine biosynthesis by ascorbic acid in cultured bovine chromaffin cells. *J. Biol. Chem.* (in press).

Levine, M., Asher, A., Pollard, H. B., and Zinder, O. (1983). Ascorbic acid and catecholamine secretion from cultured chromaffin cells. *J. Biol. Chem.* **258** (21), 13111–13115.

Levine, R. A., Kuhn, D. M., Williams, A. C., and Lovenberg, W. (1981a). The influence of aging on biogenic amine synthesis: The role of the hydroxylase cofactor. *In* "Influence of Age on the Pharmacology of Psychoactive Drugs" (A. Raskin, D. S. Robinson, and J. Levine eds.), pp. 37–46. Elsevier, Amsterdam.

Levine, R. A., Miller, L. P., and Lovenberg, W. (1981b). Tetrahydrobiopterin in striatum: Localization in dopamine nerve terminals and role in catecholamine synthesis. *Science* **214**, 919–921.

Lichtenberg, D., Freire, E., Schmidt, C. F., Barenholz, Y., Felgner, P. L., and Thompson, T. E. (1981). Effect of surface curvature on stability, thermodynamic behavior, and osmotic activity of dipalmitolphosphatidylcholine single lamellar vesicles. *Biochemistry* **20**, 3462–3467.

Litosch, I., Lin, S.-H., and Fain, J. N. (1983). Rapid changes in hepatocyte phosphoinositides induced by vasopressin. *J. Biol. Chem.* **258**, 13727–13732.

Livett, B. G., Dean, D. M., Whelan, L. G., Udenfriend, S., and Rossier, J. (1981). Co-release of enkephalin and catecholamines from cultured adrenal chromaffin cells. *Nature (London)* **289**, 317–319.

Livett, B. G., Day, R., Elde, R. P., and Howe, P. R. C. (1982). Co-storage of enkephalins and adrenaline in the bovine adrenal medulla. *Neuroscience* **7**, 1323–1332.

Ljone, T., Skotland, T., and Flatmark T. (1976). Purification and characterization of dopamine $\beta$-hydroxylase from bovine adrenal medulla. *Eur. J. Biochem.* **61**, 525–533.

Lovenberg, W., Bruckwick, E., and Hanbauer, I. (1975). ATP, cyclic AMP, and magnesium increase the affinity of rat striatal tyrosine hydroxylase for its cofactor. *Proc. Natl. Acad. Sci. U.S.A.* **72**, 2955–2958.

Lovenberg, W., Ames, M. M., and Lerner, P. (1978). Mechanisms of short-term regulation of tyrosine hydroxylase. *In* "Psychopharmacology: A Generation of Progress" (M. A. Lipton, A. De Mascio, and K. F. Killam, eds.), pp. 247–259. Raven, New York.

Low, M. G., and Weglicki, W. B. (1983). Resolution of myocardial phospholipase C into several forms with distinct properties. *Biochem. J.* **215**, 325–334.

MacPhee, C. H., and Drummond, A. H. (1984). Thyrotropin-releasing hormone stimulates rapid breakdown of phosphatidylinositol 4,5-bisphosphate and phosphatidylinositol 4-phosphate in $GH_3$ pituitary tumor cells. *Mol. Pharmacol.* **25**, 193–200.

McHugh, E. M., McGee, R., Jr., and Fleming, P. J. (1985). Biosynthesis of multiple forms of dopamine $\beta$-hydroxylase in rat pheochromocytoma (PC 12) cells. *J. Biol. Chem.* **260**, 4409–4417.

Martin, T. F. J. (1983). Thyrotropin-releasing hormone rapidly activates the phosphodiesterase hydrolysis of polyphosphoinositides in $GH_3$ pituitary cells. *J. Biol. Chem.* **258**, 14816–14822.

Meligeni, J. A., Haycock, J. W., Bennett, W. F., and Waymire, J. C. (1982). Phosphorylation and activation of tyrosine hydroxylase mediate the cAMP-induced increase in catecholamine biosynthesis in adrenal chromaffin cells. *J. Biol. Chem.* **257**, 12632–12640.

Meyer, D. I., and Burger, M. M. (1979). The chromaffin granule surface: The presence of actin and the nature of its interaction with the membranes. *FEBS Lett.* **56**, 327–331.

Michell, R. H. (1975). Inositol phospholipids and cell surface function. *Biochim. Biophys. Acta* **415**, 81–147.

Molinoff, P. B., Brimijoin, S., Weinshilboum, R., and Axelrod, J. (1970). Neurally mediated increase in dopamine $\beta$-hydroxylase activity. *Proc. Natl. Acad. Sci. U.S.A.* **66**, 453–458.

Moore, K. E., and Phillipson, O. T. (1975). Effects of dexamethasone on phenylethanolamine *N*-methyltransferase and adrenaline in the brains and superior cervical ganglia of adult and neonatal rats. *J. Neurochem.* **25**, 289–294.

Morganroth, V. H., III, Hegstrand, L. R., Rothe, R. H., and Greengard, P. (1975). Evidence for involvement of protein kinase in the activation by adenosine $3',5$-monophosphate of brain tyrosine 3-monooxygenase. *J. Biol. Chem.* **250**, 1946–1948.

Morihara, K. (1974). Comparative specificity of microbial proteinases. *Adv. Enzymol.* **41**, 179–243.

Morris, S. J., Sudhoff, T. C., and Haynes, D. H. (1982a). Calcium-promoted resonance energy transfer between fluorescently labeled proteins during aggregation of chromaffin granule membranes. *Biochim. Biophys. Acta* **693**, 425–436.

Morris, S. J., Hughes, J. M. X., and Whittaker, V. P. (1982b). Purification and mode of action of synexin: A protein-enhancing calcium-induced membrane aggregation. *J. Neurochem.* **39**, 529–536.

Muller, T. W., and Kirshner, N. (1975). ATPase and phosphatidylinositol kinase activities of adrenal chromaffin vesicles. *J. Neurochem.* **24**, 1155–1161.

Mundy, D. I., and Strittmatter, W. J. (1983). Role of metalloendoprotease in exocytosis by adrenal chromaffin cells. *J. Cell Biol.* **97**, 171A (Abstr. No. 646).

Mundy, D. I., and Strittmatter, W. J. (1985). Requirement for metalloprotease in exocytosis: Evidence in mast cells and adrenal chromaffin cells. *Cell* **40**, 645–656.

Nayar, R., Hope, M. J., and Cullis, P. R. (1982). Phospholipids as adjuncts for calcium ion stimulated release of chromaffin granule contents: Implications of mechanisms of exocytosis. *Biochemistry* **21**, 4583–4589.

Neff, N. H., and Fueutes, J. A. (1976). The use of selective monoamine oxidase inhibitor drugs for evaluating pharmacological and physiological mechanisms. *Ciba Found. Symp. New Ser.* (39), 163–187.

Nir, S., Bentz, J., and Wilschut, J. (1980). Mass action kinetics of phosphatidylserine vesicle fusion as monitored by coalescence of internal vesicle volumes. *Biochemistry* **19**, 6030–6036.

Nir, S., Bentz, J., Milschut, J., and Duzgunes, N. (1983). Aggregation and fusion of phospholipid vesicles. *Prog. Surf. Sci.* **13**, 1–124.

Nishizuka, Y. (1984). The role of protein kinase C in cell surface signal transduction and tumour promotion. *Nature (London)* **308**, 693–698.

Njus, D., and Radda, G. K. (1979). A potassium ion diffusion potential causes adrenaline uptake in chromaffin granule ghosts. *Biochem. J.* **180**, 579–585.

Njus, D., Sehr, P. A., Radda, G. K., Ritchie, G. A., and Seeley, P. J. (1978). Phosphorus-31 nuclear magnetic resonance studies of active proton translocation in chromaffin granules. *Biochemistry* **17**, 4337–4343.

Njus, D., Knoth, J., and Zallakian, M. (1981). Proton linked transport in chromaffin granules. *Curr. Top. Bioenerg.* **11**, 107–147.

Odenwald, W. F., and Morris, S. J. (1983). Identification of a second synexin-like adrenal medullary and liver protein that enhances calcium-induced membrane aggregation. *Biochem. Biophys. Res. Commun.* **112**, 147–154.

Ogawa, M., and Inouye, A. (1979). Responses of the transmembrane potential coupled to the ATP-evoked catecholamine release in isolated chromaffin granules. *Jpn. J. Physiol.* **29**, 309–325.

Ohsako, S., and Deguchi, T. (1983). Phosphatidic acid mimicks the muscarinic action of acetylcholine in cultured bovine chromaffin cells. *FEBS Lett.* **152**, 62–66.

Oka, M., Ohuchi, T., Yoshida, H., and Imaizumi, R. (1965). Effect of adenosine triphosphate and magnesium on the release of catecholamines from adrenal medullary granules. *Biochim. Biophys. Acta* **97**, 170–171.

Oka, M., Isosaki, M., and Watanabe, J. (1982). Calcium flux and catecholamine release in isolated bovine adrenal medullary cells: Effects of nicotinic and muscarinic stimulation. *Adv. Biosci.* **36**, 29–36.

O'Malley, K. L., Mauron, A., Raese, J., Barcas, J. D., and Larry, K. (1983). Genes for catecholamine biosynthesis: Cloning by expression and identification of the cDNA for rat dopamine β-hydroxylase. *Proc. Natl. Acad. Sci. U.S.A.* **80**, 2161–2165.

Orchard, J. L., Davis, J. S., Larson, R. E., and Farese, R. V. (1984). Effects of carbachol and pancreozymin (cholecystokinin-octapeptide) on polyphosphoinositide metabolism in the rat pancreas *in vitro*. *Biochem. J.* **217**, 281–287.

Ornberg, R. L., and Reese, T. S. (1981). Beginnings of exocytosis in *Limulus* amebocytes. *J. Cell Biol.* **90**, 40–54.

Osborn, M., Franke, W. W., and Weber, K. (1977). Visualization of a system of filaments 7–10 nm thick in cultured cells of an epitheliod line (PtK 2) by immunofluorescence microscopy. *Proc. Natl. Acad. Sci. U.S.A.* **74**, 2490–2494.

Osborne, N. N., and Nesselhut, T. (1983). Adrenaline: Occurrence in the bovine retina. *Neurosci. Lett.* 3933–3936.

Padbury, J. F., Lam, R. W., Hobel, C. J., and Fisher, D. A. (1983). Identification and partial purification of phenylethanolamine *N*-methyltransferase in the developing ovine lung. *Pediatr. Res.* **17**, 362–367.

Palade, G. E., and Bruns, R. R. (1968). Structural modulations of plasmalemmal vesicles. *J. Cell Biol.* **37**, 633–648.

Papahadjopoulos, D. (1978). Calcium induced phase changes and fusion in natural and model membranes. *In* "Membrane Fusion" (G. Poste and G. L. Nicholson, eds.), pp. 756–780. North Holland Publ., Amsterdam.

Park, D. H., Baetge, E. E., Kaplan, B. B., Albert, V. R., Reis, D. J., and Joh, T. H. (1982). Different forms of adrenal phenylethanolamine *N*-methyltransferase: Species specific post-translational modification. *J. Neurochem.* **38**, 410–414.

Pastan, I., and Willingham, M. C. (1983). Receptor-mediated endocytosis: Coated pits, receptosomes, and the Golgi. *TIBS* **8**, 250–254.

Patzak, A., Bock, G., Fischer-Colbrie, R., Schaunstein, K., Schmidt, W., Lingg, G., and Winkler, H. (1984). Exocytotic exposure and retrieval of membrane antigens of chromaffin granules: Quantitative evaluation of immunofluorescence on the surface of chromaffin cells. *J. Cell Biol.* **98**, 1817–1824.

Pazoles, C. J., and Pollard, H. B. (1978). Evidence for stimulation of anion transport in ATP-evoked transmitter release from isolated secretory vesicles. *J. Biol. Chem.* **253**, 3962–3969.

Pazoles, C. J., Clagget, C. E., Creutz, C. E., Pollard, H. B., and Weinbach, E. C. (1980). Identification and subcellular localization of catalase activity in bovine adrenal medulla and cortex. *Arch. Biochem. Biophys.* **200**, 434–443.

Pendleton, R. G., Gessner, G., and Sawyer, J. (1978). Studies on the distribution of phenylethanolamine *N*-methyltransferase and epinephrine in the rat. *Res. Commun. Chem. Pathol. Pharmacol.* **21**, 315–325.

Phillips, J. H. (1973). Phosphatidylinositol kinase. A component of the chromaffin-granule membrane. *Biochem. J.* **136**, 579–587.

Phillips, J. H. (1974a). Transport of catecholamines by resealed chromaffin granule "ghosts." *Biochem. J.* **144**, 311–318.

Phillips, J. H. (1974b). Steady-state kinetics of catecholamine transport in chromaffin granule ghosts. *Biochem. J.* **144**, 319–325.

Phillips, J. H., and Allison, Y. P. (1978). Proton translocation by the bovine chromaffin granule membrane. *Biochem. J.* **170**, 661–672.

Phillips, J. H., and Slater, A. (1975). Actin in the adrenal medulla. *FEBS Lett.* **56**, 327–331.

Phillips, J. H., Allison, Y. P., and Morris, S. J. (1977). The distribution of calcium, magnesium, copper and iron in the bovine adrenal medulla. *Neuroscience* **2**, 147–152.

Phillips, J. H., Burridge, K., Wilson, S. P., and Kirshner, N. (1983). Visualization of the exocytosis/endocytosis secretory cycle in culture adrenal chromaffin cells. *J. Cell Biol.* **97**, 1906–1917.

Pohorecky, L. A., and Wurtman, R. J. (1968). Induction of epinephrine-forming enzyme by glucocorticoids: Steroid hydroxylation and induction effect. *Nature (London)* **219**, 392–394.

Poisner, A. M., and Cooke, P. (1975). Microtubules in the adrenal medulla. *Ann. N.Y. Acad. Sci.* **253**, 653–669.

Pollard, H. B., and Scott, J. H. (1982). Synhibin: A new calcium-dependent membrane-binding protein that inhibits synexin-induced chromaffin granule aggregation and fusion. *FEBS Lett.* **150**, 201–206.

Pollard, H. B., Zinder, O., and Hoffman, P. G. (1976a). *In* "Data Book on Cell Biology" (P. L. Altman and D. D. Katz, eds.), pp. 359–362. Fed. Am. Soc. Exp. Biol., Washington, D.C.

Pollard, H. B., Zinder, O., Hoffman, P. G., and Nikodijevik, O. (1976b). Regulation of the transmembrane potential of isolated chromaffin granules by ATP, ATP analogs, and external pH. *J. Biol. Chem.* **251**, 4544–4550.

Pollard, H. B., Pazoles, C. J., Creutz, G. E., and Zinder, O. (1978). The chromaffin granule and possible mechanisms of exocytosis. *Int. Rev. Cytol.* **58**, 159–197.

Pollard, H. B., Shindo, H., Creutz, C. E., Pazoles, C. J., and Cohen, J. S. (1979). Internal pH, $^{31}$P- and state of ATP in adrenergic chromaffin granules determined by nuclear magnetic resonance spectroscopy. *J. Biol. Chem.* **254**, 1170–1177.

Pollard, H. B., Creutz, C. E., Fowler, V. M., Scott, J. H., and Pazoles, C. J. (1982). Calcium-dependent regulation of chromaffin granule movement, membrane contact, and fusion during exocytosis. *Cold Spring Harbor Symp. Quant. Biol.* **46**, 819–833.

Pollard, H. B., Scott, J. H., and Creutz, C. E. (1983). Inhibition of synexin activity and exocytosis from chromaffin cells by phenothiazine drugs. *Biochem. Biophys. Res. Commun.* **113**, 908–915.

Pollard, H. B., Pazoles, C. J., Creutz, C. E., Scott, J. H., Zinder, O., and Hotchkiss, A. (1984). An osmotic mechanism for exocytosis from dissociated chromaffin cells. *J. Biol. Chem.* **259**, 1114–1121.

Prentki, M., Biden, T. J., Janjic, D., Irvine, R. F., Berridge, M. J., and Wollheim, C. D. (1984). Rapid mobilization of $Ca^{++}$ from rat insulinoma microsomes by inositol 1,4,5-trisphosphate. *Nature (London)* **309**, 562–564.

Putney, J. W., Weiss, S. J., Van De Walle, C. M., and Haddas, R. A. (1980). Is phosphatidic acid a calcium ionophore under neurohumoral control? *Nature (London)* **284**, 345–347.

Putney, J. W., Burgess, G. M., Halenda, S. P., McKinney, J. S., and Rubin, R. P. (1983). Effects of secretagogues on [$^{32}$P]phosphatidylinositol 4,5-bisphosphate metabolism in the exocrine pancreas. *Biochem. J.* **212**, 483–488.

Ramu, A., Pazoles, C. J., Creutz, C. E., and Pollard, H. B. (1981). Catecholamine transport by isolated chromaffin granules. *J. Biol. Chem.* **256**, 1229–1234.

Ramu, A., Levine, M., and Pollard, H. B. (1983). Chemical evidence that catecholamines are transported across the chromaffin granule membrane as noncationic species. *Proc. Natl. Acad. Sci. U.S.A.* **80**, 2107–2111.

Rand, R. P. A. (1981). Interacting phospholipid bilayers: Measured forces and induced structural changes. *Annu. Rev. Biophys. Bioeng.* **10**, 277–314.

Rand, R. P., Reese, T. S., and Miller, R. G. (1981). Phospholipid bilayer deformations associated with interbilayer contact and fusion. *Nature (London)* **293**, 237–238.

Rasnick, D., and Powers, J. C. (1978). Active site directed irreversible inhibition of thermolysin. *Biochemistry* **17**, 4363–4369.

Rebecchi, M. J., and Gershengorn, M. C. (1983). Thyroliberin stimulates rapid hydrolysis of phosphatidylinositol 4,5-bisphosphate by a phosphodiesterase in rat mammotropic pituitary cells. *Biochem. J.* **216**, 287–294.

Reichardt, L. F., and Kelley, R. B. (1983). A molecular description of nerve terminal function. *Annu. Rev. Biochem.* **52**, 871–926.

Rendu, F., Marche, P., MacLouf, J., Girard, A., and Levy-Tolendano, S. (1983). Triphosphoinositide breakdown and dense body release as the earliest events in thrombininduced activation of human platelets. *Biochem. Biophys. Res. Commun.* **116**, 513–519.

Rose, K. M., Stetler, D. A., and Jacob, S. T. (1983). Phosphorylation of RNA polymerase: Specific association of protein kinase NII with RNA polymerase I. *Philos. Trans. R. Soc. London Ser. B* **302**, 135–142.

Saavedra, J. M. (1980). Brain and pineal adrenaline: Its level, synthesis and possible function in stress. *Dev. Neurosci.* **8**, 37–45.

Saavedra, J. M., Palkovits, M., Brownstein, M. J., and Axelrod, J. (1974). Localization of phenylethanolamine N-methyltransferase in the rat brain nuclei. *Nature (London)* **248**, 695–696.

Sabban, E. L., Hadman, M., and Goldstein, M. (1984). Effect of the ionophore monesin of post-translational processing of dopamine β-hydroxylase. *Fed. Proc., Fed. Am. Soc. Exp. Biol.* **43**, 2004.

Salach, J. I., Singer, T. P., Yasunobu, K. T., Minamura, N., and Youdim, M. B. H. (1976). Cysteinyl flavin in monoamine oxidase from the central nervous system. *Ciba Found. Symp. New Ser.* (39), 49–60.

Salama, G., Johnson, R. G., and Scarpa, A. (1980). Spectrophotometry measurements of transmembrane potential and pH gradients in chromaffin granules. *J. Gen. Physiol.* **75**, 109–140.

Saxena, A., and Fleming, P. J. (1983). Isolation and reconstitution of the membranebound form of dopamine β-hydroxylase. *J. Biol. Chem.* **258**, 4147–4152.

Scherman, D., Jamdon, P., and Henry, J. P. (1983). Characterization of the monoamine carrier of chromaffin granule membrane by binding of [2-$^3$H]dihydrotetrabenazine. *Proc. Natl. Acad. Sci. U.S.A.* **80**, 584–588.

Scherman, D., and Henry, J.-P. (1981). pH-dependence of the ATP-driven uptake of noradrenaline by bovine chromaffin granule ghosts. *Eur. J. Biochem.* **116**, 535–539.

Schliwa, M. (1984). Mechanisms of intracellular organelle transport. *In* "Cell and Muscle Motility" (J. W. Shay, ed.), Vol. 5, pp. 1–406. Plenum, New York.

Schmidt, W., Patzak, A., Ling, G., and Winkler, H. (1983). Membrane events in adrenal chromaffin cells during exocytosis: A freeze-etching analysis after rapid cryofixation. *Eur. J. Cell Biol.* **32**, 31–37.

Schneider, A. S., Cline, H. T., Rosenheck, K., and Sonenberg, M. (1981). Stimulus-secretion coupling in isolated adrenal chromaffin cells: Calcium channel activation and possible role of cytoskeletal elements. *J. Neurochem.* **37**, 567–575.

Sen, R., and Sharp, R. R. (1981). High molecular weight catecholamine-ATP aggregates are absent from the chromaffin granule aqueous phase. *Biochem. J.* **195**, 329–332.

Sen, R., Sharp, R. R., Domino, L. E., and Domino, E. F. (1979). Composition of the aqueous phase of chromaffin granules. *Biochim. Biophys. Acta* **587**, 75–78.

Shukla, S. D. (1982). Phosphatidylinositol-specific phospholipase C. *Life Sci.* **30**, 1323–1335.

Silver, M. A., and Jacobowitz, D. M. (1979). Specific uptake and retrograde flow of antibody to dopamine β-hydroxylase by central nervous system noradrenergic neurons *in vivo*. *Brain Res.* **167**, 62–75.

Skotland, T., and Ljones, T. (1979). Dopamine β-monooxygenase: Structure, mechanism and properties of the enzyme-bound copper. *Inorg. Perspect. Biol. Med.* **2**, 151–180.

Slater, E. P., Zaremba, S., and Hogue-Angeletti, R. A. (1981). Purification of membrane-bound dopamine β-hydroxylase from chromaffin granules: Relation to soluble dopamine β-hydroxylase. *Arch. Biochem. Biophys.* **211**, 288–296.

Slotkin, T. A. (1973). Hypothetical model of catecholamine uptake into adrenal medullary storage vesicles. *Life Sci.* **13**, 675–678.

Slotkin, T. A., and Kirshner, N. (1971). Uptake, storage, and distribution of amines in bovine adrenal medullary vesicles. *Mol. Pharmacol.* **7**, 581–592.

Smith, A. D., and Winkler, H. (1972). Fundamental mechanism in the release of catecholamines. *Handb. Exp. Pharmacol.* **33**, 538–617.

Smith, J. E., and Reese, T. S. (1980). Use of aldehyde fixatives to determine the rate of synaptic transmitter release. *J. Exp. Biol.* **89**, 19–29.

Smith, U., Smith, D. S., Winkler, H., and Ryan, J. W. (1973). Exocytosis in the adrenal medulla demonstrated by freeze-etching. *Science* **179**, 79–82.

Streb, H., Irvine, R. F., Berridge, M. J., and Schulz, I. (1984). Release of Ca$^{++}$ from a nonmitochondrial intracellular store in pancreatic acinar cells by inositol 1,4,5-trisphosphate. *Nature (London)* **306**, 67–69.

Struck, D. K., Hoekstra, D., and Pagano, R. E. (1981). Use of resonance energy transfer to monitor membrane fusion. *Biochemistry* **20**, 4093–4099.

Sudhof, T. C., Walker, J. H., and Obrocki, J. (1982). Calelectrin self-aggregates and promotes membrane aggregation in the presence of calcium. *EMBO J.* **1**, 1167–1170.

Sudhof, T. C., Ebbecke, M., Walker, J. H., Fritsche, U., and Bonstead, C. (1984). Isolation of mammalian calelectrins: A new class of ubiquitous Ca$^{2+}$-regulation proteins. *Biochemistry* **23**, 1103–1109.

Suematsu, E., Hirata, M., Hashimoto, T., and Kuriyama, H. (1984). Inositol 1,4,5-trisphosphate releases Ca$^{++}$ from intracellular store sites in skinned single cells of porcine coronary artery. *Biochem. Biophys. Res. Commun.* **120**, 481–485.

Sussman, K., Pollard, H. B., Leitner, J. W., Nesher, R., Adler, J., and Cerasi, E. (1983). Differential control of insulin secretion and somatostatin receptor recruitment in isolated pancreatic islets. *Biochem. J.* **214**, 225–230.

Tada, M., and Katz, A. M. (1982). Phosphorylation of the sarcoplasmic reticulum. *Annu. Rev. Physiol.* **44**, 401–424.

Takai, Y., Kishimoto, A., Iwasa, Y., Kawahara, Y., Mori, T., and Nishizuka, Y. (1979). Calcium-dependent activation of a multifunctional protein kinase by membrane phospholipids. *J. Biol. Chem.* **254**, 3692–3695.

Taugner, G. (1971). The membrane of catecholamine storage vesicles from adrenal medulla: Catecholamine fluxes and ATPase activity. *Nauyn-Schmiedebergs Arch. Exp. Pathol. Pharmakol.* **270**, 392–402.

Taugner, G. (1972). The membrane of catecholamine storage vesicles of adrenal medulla: Uptake and release of noradrenaline in relation to the pH. *Nauyn-Schmiedebergs Arch. Exp. Pathol. Pharmakol.* **274**, 299–314.

Tessel, R. E., and Burgess, S. K. (1980). Changes in the release and content of endogenous epinephrine, norepinephrine and dopamine induced by KCl, veratridine and amphetamine within rat hypothalamus *in vivo. Dev. Neurosci.* **8**, 53–58.

Theonen, H., Mueller, R. A., and Axelrod, J. (1970). Neuronally dependent induction of phenylethanolamine $N$-methyltransferase by 6-hydroxydopamine. *Biochem. Pharmacol.* **19**, 669–673.

Tipton, K. F., Spires, P. C., and Youdim, M. B. H. (1975). Beef adrenal monoamine oxidase. *Biochem. Pharmacol.* **21**, 2197–2205.

Tischler, A. S., Perlman, R. L., Nunnemacher, G., Morse, G. M., DeLellis, R. A., Wolfe, H. J., and Sheard, B. E. (1982). Long-term effects of dexamethasone and nerve growth factor on adrenal medullary cells cultured from young rats. *Cell Tissue Res.* **225**, 525–542.

Treiman, M., Weber, W., and Gratzl M. (1983). 3',5'-Cyclic adenosine monophosphate- and $Ca^{2+}$-calmodulin-dependent endogenous protein phosphorylation activity in membranes of the bovine chromaffin secretory vesicles: Identification of two phosphorylated components as tyrosine hydroxylase and protein kinase regulatory subunit type II. *J. Neurochem.* **40**, 661–669.

Trifaro, J. M. (1977). Common mechanisms of hormone secretion. *Annu. Rev. Pharmacol. Toxicol.* **17**, 27–47.

Trifaro, J. M. (1969a). Phospholipid metabolism and adrenal medullary activity. I. The effect of acetylcholine on tissue uptake and incorporation of orthophosphate-$^{32}$P into nucleotides and phospholipids of bovine adrenal medulla. *Mol. Pharmacol.* **5**, 382–392.

Trifaro, J. M. (1969b). The effect of $Ca^{++}$ omission on the secretion of catecholamines and the incorporation of orthophosphate-$^{32}$P into nucleotides and phospholipids of bovine adrenal medulla during acetylcholine stimulation. *Mol. Pharmacol.* **5**, 424–427.

Trifaro, J. M., and Dworkind, J. (1975). Phosphorylation of the membrane components of chromaffin granules: Synthesis of diphosphatidylinositol and presence of phosphatidylinositol kinase in granule membranes. *Can. J. Physiol. Pharmacol.* **53**, 479–492.

Trifaro, J. M., and Lee, R. W. H. (1980). Morphological characteristics and stimulus-secretion coupling in bovine adrenal chromaffin cell cultures. *Neuroscience* **5**, 1533–1546.

Trifaro, J. M., and Ulpian, C. (1976). Isolation and characterization of myosin from the adrenal medulla. *Neuroscience* **1**, 483–488.

Trifaro, J. M., Collier, B., Lastowecka, A., and Stern, D. (1972). Inhibition by colchicine and vinblastine of acetylcholine induced catecholamine release from the adrenal gland: An anticholinergic action, not an effect upon microtubules. *Mol. Pharmacol.* **8**, 264–267.

Trifaro, J. M., Ulpian, C., and Preiksaitis, H. (1978). Anti-myosin stains chromaffin cells. *Experientia* **34**, 1568–1571.

Tycho, B., and Maxfield, F. R. (1982). Rapid acidification of endocytic vesicles containing $\alpha_2$-macroglobulin. *Cell* **28**, 643–651.

Udenfriend, S., and Kilpatrick D. L. (1983). Biochemistry of the enkephalins and enkephalin-containing peptides. *Arch. Biochem. Biophys.* **221**, 309–323.

Umezawa, H., and Aoyagi, T. (1977). Activities of proteinase inhibitors of microbial origin. *In* "Proteinases in Mammalian Cells and Tissues" (A. J. Barrett, ed.), pp. 637–662. North-Holland Publ., Amsterdam.

Ungar, A., and Phillips, J. H. (1983). Regulation of the adrenal medulla. *Physiol. Rev.* **63**, (3), 787–843.

Unsicker, K., Rieffert, B., and Ziegler, W. (1980). Effects of cell culture conditions, nerve growth factor, dexamethasone and cyclic AMP on adrenal chromaffin cells *in vitro*. *In* "Histochemistry and Cell Biology of Autonomic Neurons" (O. Eranko *et al.*, eds.), pp. 51–59. Raven, New York.

Uster, P. S., and Deamer, D. W. (1981). Fusion competence of phosphatidylserine-containing liposomes quantitatively measured by a fluorescence resonance energy transfer assay. *Arch. Biochem. Biophys.* **209**, 385–395.

Van der Gugten, J. N., Palkovits, M., Wijnen, H. L. J. M., and Versteeg, D. H. G. (1976). Regional distribution of adrenaline in rat brain. *Brain Res.* **107**, 171–175.

Van Orden, L. S., Burke, J. P., Redick, J. A., Rybarczyk, K. E., Van Orden, D. E., Baker, H. A., and Hartman, B. K. (1977). Immunocytochemical evidence for particulate localization of phenylethanolamine *N*-methyltransferase in adrenal medulla. *Neuropharmacology* **16**, 129–133.

Verkleij, A. J. (1984). Lipidic intramembranous particles. *Biochim. Biophys. Acta* **779**, 43–63.

Viveros, O. H. (1975). Mechanism of secretion of catecholamines from adrenal medullary. *Handb. Physiol. Endocrinol.* pp. 389–426.

Viveros, O. H., Arqueros, L., Connett, R. J., and Kirshner, N. (1969). Mechanism of secretion from the adrenal medulla. *Mol. Pharmacol.* **5**, 69–82.

Viveros, O. H., Diliberto, E. J., Hazum, E., and Chang, K. J. (1979). Opiate-like materials in the adrenal medulla: evidence for storage and secretion with catecholamines. *Mol. Pharm.* **16**, 1101–1108.

Von Euler, U. S., and Lishajko, F. (1969). Effects of some metabolic co-factors and inhibitors on transmitter release and uptake in isolated adrenergic nerve granules. *Acta Physiol. Scand.* **77**, 298–307.

Vulliet, P. R., Langan, T. A., and Weiner, N. (1980). Tyrosine hydroxylase: A substrate of cyclic AMP-dependent protein kinase. *Proc. Natl. Acad. Sci. U.S.A.* **77**, 92–96.

Wada, A., Yanagihara, N., Izumi, F., Salcurai, S., and Kobayashi, H. (1983a). Trifluoperazine inhibits $^{45}Ca$ uptake and catecholamine secretion and synthesis in adrenal medullary cells. *J. Neurochem.* **40**, 481–486.

Wada, A., Sakurai, S., Kobayashi, H., Yanagihara, N., and Izumi, F. (1983b). Suppression by phospholipase $A_2$ inhibitors of secretion of catecholamines from isolated adrenal medullary cells by suppression of cellular calcium uptake. *Biochem. Pharmacol.* **32**, 1175–1178.

Walker, J. H. (1982). Isolation from cholinergic synapses of a protein that binds to membranes in a calcium-dependent manner. *J. Neurochem.* **39**, 815–823.

Walker, W. H., Kearney, E. B., Seng, R. L., and Singer, T. P. (1971). The covalently bound flavin of hepatic monoamine oxidase. II. Identification and properties of cysteinyl riboflavin. *Eur. J. Biochem.* **24**, 328–331.

Wallace, E. F., Krantz, M. J., and Lovenberg, W. (1973). Dopamine $\beta$-hydroxylase, a tetrameric glycoprotein. *Proc. Natl. Acad. Sci. U.S.A.* **70**, 2253–2255.

Wasserman, G., and Tramezzini, J. H. (1963). Separate distribution of adrenoline- and noradrenaline-secreting cells in the adrenal of snakes. *Gen. Comp. Endocrinol.* **3**, 480–481.

Waymire, J. C., Waymire, K. G., Boehme, R., Noritake, D., and Wardell, J. (1977).

Regulation of tyrosine hydroxylase by cyclic 3',5'-adenosine monophosphate in cultured neuroblastoma and cultured dissociated bovine adrenal chromaffin cells. *Mod. Pharmacol. Toxicol.* **10**, 327–363.

Waymire, J. C., Bennett, W. F., Boehme, R., Hankins, L., Gilmer-Waymire, K., and Haycock, J. W. (1983). Bovine adrenal chromaffin cells: High yield purification and viability in suspension culture. *J. Neurosci. Methods* **7**, 329–351.

West, G. B., Shepherd, D. M., and Hunter, R. B. (1951). Adrenaline and noradrenaline concentrations in adrenal glands at different ages and in some diseases. *Lancet* **261**, 966–969.

Whitaker, M. J., and Baker, P. F. (1983). Calcium-dependent exocytosis in an *in vitro* secretory granule plasma membrane preparation from sea urchin eggs and the effects of some inhibitors of cytoskeletal function. *Proc. R. Soc. London Ser. B* **216**, 397–413.

White, J., Kielian, M., and Helenius, A. (1983). Membrane fusion proteins of enveloped animal viruses. *Q. Rev. Biophys.* **16**, 151–195.

Wilkins, J. A., and Lin, S. (1981). Association of actin with chromaffin granule membranes and the effect of cytochalasin B on the polarity of actin filament elongation. *Biochim. Biophys. Acta* **642**, 55–66.

Wilschut, J., Duzgunes, N., Fraley, R., and Papahadjopoulos, D. (1980). Studies on the mechanism of membrane fusion: Kinetics of calcium ion induced fusion of phosphatidylserine vesicles. *Biochemistry* **19**, 6011–6021.

Wilschut, J., Duzgunes, N., and Papahadjopoulos, D. (1981). Calcium/magnesium specificity in membrane fusion: Kinetics of aggregation and fusion of phosphatidylserine vesicles and the role of bilayer curvature. *Biochemistry* **20**, 3126–3133.

Wilson, S. P., and Kirshner, N. (1983). Calcium-evoked secretion from digitonin-permeabilized adrenal medullary chromaffin cells. *J. Biol. Chem.* **258**, 4994–5000.

Wilson, S. P., and Viveros, O. H. (1981). Primary culture of adrenal chromaffin cells in a chemically defined medium. *Exp. Cell. Res.* **133**, 159–169.

Wilson, S. P., Chang, K.-J., and Viveros, O. H. (1982). Proportional secretion of opioid peptides and catecholamines from adrenal chromaffin cells in culture. *J. Neurosci.* **2**, 1150–1165.

Winkler, H. (1976). The composition of adrenal chromaffin granules: An assessment of controversial results. *Neuroscience* **1**, 65–80.

Winkler, H. (1977). The biogenesis of adrenal chromaffin granules. *Neuroscience* **2**, 657–683.

Winkler, H. (1982). The proteins of catecholamine-storing organelles. *Scand. J. Immunol. Suppl.* **9**, 75–96.

Winkler and Carmichael (1982). The chromaffin granule. *In* "The Secretory Granule" (A. Poisner and J. M. Trifaro, eds.). Elsevier, North Holland.

Winkler, H., and Westhead, E. W. (1980). The molecular organization of adrenal chromaffin granules. *Neuroscience* **5**, 1803–1823.

Wood, J. G., Seeling, L. L., Benjamin, C. P. (1971). Cytochemistry of epinephrine and norepinephrine adrenomedullary cells. *Histochemie* **28**, 183–197.

Wurtman, R. J., and Axelrod, J. (1965). Adrenaline synthesis: Control by the pituitary gland and adrenal glucocorticoids. *Science* **150**, 1464–1465.

Wurtman, R. J., and Axelrod, J. (1966). Control of enzymatic synthesis of adrenaline in the adrenal medulla by adrenal cortical steroids. *J. Biol. Chem.* **241**, 2301–2305.

Wurtman, R. J., Hefti, F., and Melamed, E. (1980). Precursor control of neurotransmitter synthesis. *Pharmacol. Rev.* **32**, 315–335.

Yamauchi, T., and Fujisawa, H. (1979). *In vitro* phosphorylation of bovine adrenal tyrosine hydroxylase by adenosine 3':5'-monophosphate-dependent protein kinase. *J. Biol. Chem.* **254,** 503–507.

Yamauchi, T., Nakata, H., and Fujisawa, H. (1981). A new activator protein that activates tryptophan 5-monooxygenase and tyrosine 3-monooxygenase in the presence of $Ca^{2+}$, calmodulin-dependent protein kinase. *J. Biol. Chem.* **256,** 5404–5409.

Youdim, M. B. H., and Finberg, J. P. M. (1982). Monoamine oxidase inhibitor antidepressants. *In* "Psychopharmacology" (D. G. Grahame-Smith, A Hippius, and H. Winoker, eds.), pp. 38–57. Excerpta Medica, Amsterdam.

Youdim, M. B. H., and Finberg, J. P. M. (1984) Monoamine oxidase inhibitor antidepressants. *In* "Psychopharmacology" (D. G. Grahame-Smith, A. Hippius, and H. Winoker, eds.). Excerpta Medica, Amsterdam. (In press).

Youdim, M. B. H., and Holzbauer, M. (1976). Physiological aspects of oxidative deamination of monoamines. *Ciba Found. Symp. New Ser.* (39), 105–131.

Youdim, M. B. H., Banerjee, D. K., and Pollard, H. B. (1984). Isolated chromaffin cells from adrenal medulla contain primarily monoamine oxidase B. *Science* **224,** 619–621.

Youdim, M. B. H., Banerjee, D. K., and Pollard, H. B. (1985a). Monoamine metabolism and monoamine oxidase (MAO) activity in isolated cultured chromaffin cells. *J. Pharm. Pharmacol.* (In press).

Youdim, M. B. H., Finberg, J. P. M., and Tipton, K. F. (1985b). Monoamine oxidases. *Handb. Exp. Pharmacol.* (In press).

Youdim, M. B. H., Heldman, E., Banerjee, D. K., and Ornberg, R. L. (1985c). Discrete catecholamine metabolism and release in isolated adrenal medullary chromaffin and endothelial cells: Comparison with PC12 cells. *Proc. Int. Union Physiol., Jerusalem.*

Zaremba, S., and Hogue-Angeletti, R. A. (1981). Transmembrane nature of chromaffin granule dopamine $\beta$-hydroxylase. *J. Biol. Chem.* **256,** 12310–12315.

Zinder, O., Hoffman, P. G., Bonner W. M., and Pollard, H. B. Comparison of chemical properties of purified plasma membranes and secretory vesicle membranes from the bovine adrenal medulla. *Cell Tiss. Res.* **188,** 153–170.

Zimmerberg, J., Cohen, F. S., and Finkelstein, A. (1980). Micromolar $Ca^{2+}$ stimulates fusion of lipid vesicles with planar bilayers containing a calcium-binding protein. *Science* **210,** 906–908.

# Compartmentation of Second Messenger Action: Immunocytochemical and Biochemical Evidence

JEFFREY F. HARPER,\*,† MARI K. HADDOX,†
ROY A. JOHANSON,\* ROCHELLE M. HANLEY,\*
AND ALTON L. STEINER\*,†

*Departments of Internal Medicine\* and Pharmacology†
University of Texas Medical School at Houston
Houston, Texas*

## I. INTRODUCTION

### A. OVERVIEW

Extensive work has been reported by a number of investigators approaching the problems of compartmentalized second messenger action. They have produced a body of evidence strongly suggesting that compartmentalization plays a vital role in cellular regulation, including the following:

1. Immunocytochemical localization of second messengers and the proteins controlled by cAMP, cGMP, and $Ca^{2+}$ often show distinct subcellular patterns best explained by compartmentation.

2. Cyclic AMP-dependent protein kinase (cA-PK) isozymes can be activated independently by hormonal stimulation of some intact cells. Additionally, regulation of soluble and particulate cA-PK appears at times to be under differential hormonal control. Under these circumstances, intracellular cyclic AMP is apparently available to only one isozyme, establishing that functional compartmentation exists.

197

3. Few cytoplasmic proteins are truly soluble *in vivo*. The aqueous cytoplasm of any cell is sparse, and occupation of cellular space by extensive cytoskeletal networks reduces the cellular space occupied by water. The cytoplasm is not a liquid through which rapid, free diffusion occurs. Less than 20% of cellular protein diffuses unhindered through the viscous cytoplasm.

4. Discrete subcellular compartments exist which are defined by limiting membrane barriers. In particular, potential mechanisms by which cyclic AMP affects nuclear events have been explored and will be reviewed in this article.

## B. Description of Second Messenger Systems

This review probes evidence that second messenger system compartmentation occurs and how it may be regulated. We do not attempt to review comprehensively the molecular details of second messenger action except as they relate directly to compartmentation. Since an understanding of second messenger action is, however, necessary for understanding its compartmentation, a brief summary of current knowledge, with reference to relevant reviews, is provided here.

### 1. *Cyclic AMP*

Cyclic AMP serves as the second messenger for numerous hormones, including many catecholamines, prostaglandins, and peptide hormones. Cyclic AMP is synthesized intracellularly from ATP by the membrane-associated enzyme complex adenylate cyclase. Hormone binding to a receptor signals the catalytic unit of adenylate cyclase to increase cyclic AMP synthesis rate via an intermediate protein $G_s$ (Gilman, 1984; Schramm and Selinger, 1984).

The only known mechanism by which cyclic AMP regulates eukaryotic cellular function is through activation of cyclic AMP-dependent protein kinases (cA-PKs), of which two general isozymic types exist (Corbin *et al.*, 1975; for review see Doskeland and Ogreid, 1981). The holoenzyme is a tetramer consisting of two catalytic and two regulatory subunits. Kinase activity is regulated by cyclic AMP binding to two sites on each of the regulatory (R) subunits of the cA-PK holoenzyme. Binding of R subunits to the catalytic (C) subunits inhibits activity; cyclic AMP bound to R promotes dissociation of the R from C subunits, freeing and thereby activating the catalytic units. Activated cA-PK C subunits catalytically phosphorylate diverse proteins. Both activation and inhibition of enzymatic functions of the substrate proteins are effected through phosphorylation. The two cA-PK isozymes differ only in the R subunits; the C subunits of each isozyme are essentially identical, and so the *in vitro* substrate specificity of each isozyme is identical. No function for free cyclic AMP-bound R subunits in eukaryotes has been demonstrated *in vivo,* although an analogous cyclic AMP binding protein (catabolite activator protein, CAP) regulates transcription in prokaryotes when cyclic AMP is bound (Ullmann and Danchin, 1983).

Cyclic AMP action is terminated via two pathways. Cyclic AMP is hydrolyzed to 5'-AMP by several cyclic nucleotide phosphodiesterase isozymes (Beavo *et al.,* 1982); 5'-AMP cannot activate cA-PK. Cyclic AMP can also be removed by efflux from the cell (Barber and Butcher, 1983); extracellular cyclic AMP cannot reach intracellular cA-PK. Enzyme activities regulated by covalent phosphorylation are counterregulated by protein phosphatase-catalyzed dephosphorylation. Four classes of protein phosphatase account for the cA-PK terminating phosphatase activities found in eukaryotic cells (Ingebritsen and Cohen, 1983). Various factors regulate these phosphatases. Of particular importance in the context of this review is the finding that an inhibitor of phosphatase 1 activity (Inhibitor 1; $I_1$) inhibits only when it is itself phosphorylated, and it is only phosphorylated by cA-PK (Ingebritsen *et al.,* 1983).

## 2. *Calcium Ion*

Many hormonal interactions at receptors other than those coupled to adenylate cyclase regulate $Ca^{2+}$ entry into cells. The molecular details of how this is accomplished are not clear, but may involve the regulated turnover of polyphosphorylated phosphatidylinositols to liberate inositol 1,4,5-trisphosphate. The inositol trisphosphate so produced acts as a second messenger to stimulate $Ca^{2+}$ release from intracellular pools (Nishizuka, 1984).

Intracellular actions of $Ca^{2+}$ are mediated via $Ca^{2+}$ binding proteins, including calmodulin, protein kinase C, and troponin C. $Ca^{2+}$-bound calmodulin is able to bind to and thus activate a variety of enzymes, including several protein kinases, one cyclic nucleotide phosphodiesterase, and neuronal adenylate cyclase (Moore and Dedman, 1982). Protein kinase C generally phosphorylates cellular proteins distinct from those phosphorylated by cA-PK and calmodulin-regulated protein kinases (Nishizuka, 1984; Nestler and Greengard, 1983). It requires $Ca^{2+}$ and phosphatidylserine and is activated by diacyl glycerol produced by hormone-activated cleavage of inositol trisphosphate from phosphatidylinositol 4,5-bisphosphate. Diacyl glycerol reduces the protein kinase C requirement for $Ca^{2+}$ such that enzyme activation can occur at physiological $Ca^{2+}$ concentrations.

These second messenger systems each interact in numerous ways. Implications of these interactions on compartmentation of hormonal actions will be explored in Section II,C,2.


## II. Compartmentation of Second Messengers


### A. Potential for Second Messenger Compartmentation


#### 1. *"Nonsoluble" Cytoplasm*

Although ~60% of the cellular protein is found in the supernatant fraction after cell disruption and centrifugation, studies employing diverse experimental techniques make it clear that in the intact cell few proteins are totally soluble. The cytosol, i.e., the soluble fraction yielded by the centrifugation of disrupted cells, probably bears little resemblance to the aqueous cytoplasm, which along with the cytomatrix constitutes the total cytoplasm of the living cell (for a more complete review of the data supporting this conclusion and of the controversies regarding it, see Clegg, 1984). Four unique experimental lines of evidence leading to this conclusion can be summarized as follows:

1. In intact *Euglena* subjected to centrifugal force, the contents of the living cell are stratified and can be dissected and analyzed. The soluble phase which rises above the particulate layers contains very little protein. Enzyme activities conventionally found in the *Euglena* cell extract cytosol are not detectable in the intact cell aqueous cytoplasm. The majority of the protein in the intact *Euglena* is associated with intracellular structures (Kempner and Miller, 1968a,b).

2. The diffusion characteristics of exogenous and endogenous proteins into and out of the cytoplasm of *Xenopus* oocytes can be determined after they are injected with a gelatin reference phase. Using this technique, it has been concluded that over 80% of the cellular protein exists, at least in part, in a nondiffusive form (Paine, 1984).

3. High-voltage electron microscopy of whole cell mounts has revealed a pervasive filament network in the cytoplasm named the microtrabecular lattice. The spaces between the trabeculae are devoid of proteins and are water-rich (Porter *et al.*, 1983).

4. Electron spin resonance measurements of the viscosity of the wa-

ter in cytoplasm have led to the conclusion that the aqueous component of cytoplasm is extremely dilute in macromolecule content (Mastro and Keith, 1984).

These studies and others like them have led to the conclusion that the aqueous cytoplasm does not contain a concentrated solution of enzymes, as inferred from the cell fractionation studies. It appears that very few "cytosolic" enzymes, i.e., those found in the supernatant after cell extract centrifugation, are actually totally free in solution inside the cell. Rather, it is envisioned that there exists a dynamic equilibrium between the soluble state and a bound state in association with cytomatrical structures. Compartmentation and order are achieved without physical barriers by the selective affinity of proteins for each other (Masters, 1984).

## 2. *Regulated Accumulation of Proteins in Nucleus*

The movement of proteins between nucleus and cytoplasm was first detected by Goldstein (1958) during his studies of nuclear transplantation from radiolabeled to nonradiolabeled *Amoeba proteus*. The possibility that this movement might form the basis of a regulatory mechanism was suggested in the next decade by the nuclear transplantation experiments of Gurdon (1968). He examined the functional consequences of placing somatic cell nuclei isolated from *Xenopus* into cytoplasmic environments different from those from which they had been taken. These studies led to the conclusion that both the condensation state of the chromosomes and the primary nuclear events of gene transcription and DNA replication are controlled by the cell cytoplasm. The nucleocytoplasmic exchange of information appeared to be mediated by the migration of proteins between the cytoplasm and the nucleus.

In 1970, Gurdon reported that histones extracted from the nucleus would, upon injection into the *Xenopus* oocyte cytoplasm, reenter the nucleus and concentrate there at a level 150 times that in the cytoplasm, while similarly injected bovine albumin simply diffused throughout the cell and did not preferentially associate with any subcellular compartment. This initiated a continuing series of experiments by many investigators into the identity of mechanisms that govern selective distribution of proteins between the nucleus and cytoplasm (for reviews, see DeRobertis, 1983; Bonner, 1978). A major conclusion to be drawn from these studies is that proteins isolated from the nucleus will return and concentrate there upon microinjection into the cytoplasm, while proteins of cytoplasmic origin will remain in the cytoplasm. A third class of proteins, those distributing evenly between the nucleus and the cytoplasm, has also been identified.

The nuclear membrane does not appear to be the primary mechanism governing partition of proteins between the nucleus and cytoplasm. The nuclear membrane does constitute a diffusion barrier to the entry of microinjected foreign proteins or dextran molecules into the nucleus. The rate of nuclear entry of these molecules correlates with the limiting size of the nuclear membrane pores (5–9 nm) such that bovine albumin (65,000 Da) enters very slowly and IgG (165,000 Da) is almost completely excluded. Size of the protein does not constitute a critical factor for distribution of cellular proteins that are extracted and reinjected. Within the cell there exist small cytoplasmic proteins, e.g., 36,000-Da HCa, that do not enter the nucleus at all upon microinjection (Dabauvalle and Franke, 1984), and large nuclear proteins, e.g., 148,000-Da RN1 (Feldherr *et al.*, 1983) and 165,000-Da nucleoplasmin (Dingwall *et al.*, 1982), that enter the nucleus so rapidly after microinjection into the cytoplasm that a process of mediated transport has been proposed. Moreover, damage to the nuclear envelope so that it is no longer a permeability barrier does not hamper exclusion of proteins of cytoplasmic origin from the nucleus, and proteins of nuclear origin are still retained within the nucleoplasm (Feldherr and Pomerantz, 1978). Presumably, protein–protein and protein–nucleic acid interactions of sufficiently high affinity function to concentrate the true nuclear proteins within the nucleus against the concentration gradient of the cytoplasm in the intact cell.

The signal allowing a protein to enter the nucleus and concentrate there appears to lie within the molecular structure of the protein itself. Only one fragment of nucleoplasmin cleaved into two parts retains the ability to enter and concentrate within the nucleus (Dingwall *et al.*, 1982). The data suggest that the signal for nuclear association of nucleoplasmin is contained in a small segment near the C-terminus. Another protein, simian virus large T antigen, is found predominantly in the nucleus of infected cells. A mutant strain of the virus has been isolated in which the large T does not enter and concentrate in the nucleus, but rather remains in the cytoplasm. The mutation that accomplishes the loss of nuclear association of this molecule was recently found to be a simple change, a single amino acid substitution of Lys-128 to Asn (Scheidtmann *et al.*, 1984).

What then can be proposed for the type of proteins discussed in this review—molecules that are typically cytoplasmic but that on occasion, such as after hormone stimulation, appear to exist as a subfraction in association with the nucleus? A precedent for an alteration in the intracellular localization of protein can be found in mechanisms governing cell differentiation during embryonic development. Proteins of cytoplasmic origin during one stage of embryogenesis become nuclear associated as the organism proceeds into the next stage of development.

At least three possible mechanisms can be suggested for modification of a cytoplasmic protein to the form required to become a nuclear protein:

1. The appearance within the cytoplasm of another component that binds the cytoplasmic protein and confers upon this complex the properties required for nuclear association;

2. A posttranslational modification of the protein that confers the "signal property" of nuclear entry and accumulation; and

3. The development within the nucleus of binding sites specific for the normally cytoplasmic protein.

An example of the first mechanism is represented by snRNA binding proteins during early development in *Xenopus*. These proteins are found in the cytoplasm during the earliest stages of development, but enter the nucleus at the late blastula stage (Zeller *et al.*, 1983). While in the cytoplasm the proteins are devoid of RNA, but the nuclear entry coincides with the synthesis and cytoplasmic appearance of UsnRNA.

A difference in posttranslational modification state may regulate the intracellular distribution of large T antigen. Although the majority of large T is located in the nucleus, a small fraction is found associated with the plasma membrane. The membrane-associated large T is acylated, whereas the nuclear-associated protein is not, and the nuclear-associated protein is much more highly phosphorylated than the membrane-associated protein (Klockman and Deppert, 1983; Lanford and Butel, 1980).

## B. Evidence for Functional Second Messenger Compartmentation

### 1. *Methods*

*a. Biochemical.* No one method provides conclusive proof for the existence of intracellular second messenger system compartmentation, because no method is without potential artifacts. Selective hormonal activation of intracellular enzymes implies that second messenger compartments may exist. In analysis of such phenomena, activation during tissue homogenization must be excluded. Changes in the activation state of cA-PK are discussed elsewhere in this review. Another technique, biochemical fractionation, allows one to determine compartmentation within organelles of any substance. Two known artifacts must be avoided—loss of substances from organelles and adsorption of substances to organelles. A number of techniques have been devised to overcome these limitations (nuclear isolation in nonaqueous solutions, for instance), but it remains impossible to prove that what is obtained in the test tube was part of that compartment *in vivo*. It is also impossible to isolate intact cytosolic "compartments" defined *in situ* by kinetic or cytoskeletal constraints, although studies of selective enzyme activation may point to the conclusion that such compartments exist.

  *b. Immunocytochemical.* Immunocytochemical techniques can provide information to substantiate or even go beyond that achievable with biochemical tools. Cells are analyzed individually with immunocytochemistry, so heterogenous tissues may be used. Further, since cells can be frozen or fixed *in situ* prior to manipulation, one need not worry about artifactual shifts of location (if fixation has been proper). Moreover, specifically altered second messengers within a small cellular area can be detected immunocytochemically where biochemical methods yield ambiguous results. Biochemical techniques are too insensitive to measure localized, discrete changes within whole cells, although biochemical methods applied to an isolated organelle fraction can reveal the change detected on intact cells immunochemically.

  Immunocytochemical techniques are subject to problems distinct from those of biochemical techniques. Lack of immunocytochemical detection conveys no information. Such a lack may be artifactual, reflecting interference by steric hindrance, protein denaturation, or excessive fixation. Only with fully efficient fixation (which is difficult to prove) can one be certain that apparent *in vivo* locations of antigens are valid. We hope that use of amorphous ice sublimation from unfixed frozen tissue pieces prior to embedding and sectioning will overcome this limitation (Section III,B).

  Other potential problems are readily overcome. Polyclonal antisera taken from animals contain antibodies to multiple antigens (everything to which the animal has competently made a response). Recognition of antigens other than the one of interest in immunocytochemical localization studies is a potential problem that requires careful controls. Use of affinity-purified antisera can overcome many of these problems, but only if absolutely pure antigen is used as the affinity matrix (lest antisera raised to and purified by trace contaminants lead to spurious results). One could also use antigen purified by completely different processes for immunization and purification, respectively. Monoclonal antibodies, of course, are free of problems caused by multiple antibodies, but display other limitations. Relatively small, not necessarily unique segments of molecules are recognized by antibodies.

Thus, several distinct antigens may be recognized by one antibody. Neither use of monoclonal antibodies nor affinity purification of polyclonal antisera overcome such inherent cross-reactivity. Indeed, the situation is potentially worse with monoclonal antibodies. All molecules of a monoclonal antibody cross-react with proteins that share epitopes, but different antibodies in a polyclonal antiserum likely react differently to proteins distinct from the immunizing antigen. The group average response of the polyclonal antiserum should be greater toward the immunizing antigen than toward any cross-reacting antigen. The perfect antibody does not exist. The hazard always exists that immunocytochemical detection with any one antibody may localize merely cross-reactive antigens. Use of multiple antisera, each recognizing cellular antigens with distinct cross-reactivities, helps guard against this possibility.

Problems of interpretation exist. Apparent changes in immunocytochemical localization of a component might be explainable in several ways. For instance, increased localization of nuclear cA-PK in glucagon-treated rat liver (Koide et al., 1981) might be caused by an increased amount of cA-PK in nuclei (because of enhanced delivery to nuclei, transport through nuclear pores, or retention within nuclei), but there need not be physically more cA-PK within nuclei to see increased localization. There might be increased cA-PK concentrations within subnuclear sites due to shifts within the nucleus. Increased local concentration would make detection easier, due to coalescence of diffuse staining. Alternatively, increased staining might reflect an increased ability to detect existing cA-PK without intracellular shift. Antigenicity could be altered by conformational change or covalent modification upon activation. It is also possible that altered association with binding sites exists such that either cA-PK is less sterically hindered to antibody access or more cA-PK is retained on the section during preparation and staining.

Even more questions can be raised regarding localization studies of cyclic AMP. We have found (Harper and Steiner, unpublished) that only certain antisera recognize nuclear cyclic AMP in ACTH-stimulated rat adrenal cortex. All of these antisera recognize cytoplasmic cyclic AMP, and all recognize isoproterenol-stimulated nuclear cyclic AMP in rat parotid. Lack of recognition of adrenal nuclear cyclic AMP has not been explained. We do know that recognition of adrenal nuclear cyclic AMP is achieved only with those antisera that recognize 8-bromo-cyclic AMP. Whether the adrenal contains unique nuclear cyclic AMP binding proteins, whether cyclic AMP is bound by cA-PK in a unique way in the adrenal, or even whether it is uniquely bound cyclic

AMP that is detected is unknown. We do know that cA-PK-bound cyclic AMP can be detected by anticyclic AMP sera *in vitro* (Harper and Steiner, unpublished). We believe that during immunochemical staining the unbound cyclic AMP is washed away from the tissue slices, leaving only bound cyclic AMP to be detected (Ortez *et al.*, 1980).

c. *Power of Combined Approach.* There are many valid uses of immunocytochemical techniques. With proper control of staining, one can be sure that antigen exists (within the limits of antibody specificity stated above). This is especially valuable with heterogenous tissues, and it pinpoints where within cells antigen exists. Immunocytochemical techniques further can be used to determine the effects of hormonal stimulation on intracellular localization patterns. Examples of such hormonally induced changes in localization for second messenger system components are provided in Sections II,B,2,a and II,B,4,b. Biochemical techniques are necessary to analyze for mechanisms underlying changes in staining pattern. As stated above, however, biochemical techniques alone cannot prove the site of antigen localization. Concomitant use of biochemical and immunocytochemical techniques surmounts the potential problems of using just one technique. The two methods differ in limitations, and each allows one to gather data not obtainable by the other. Further, where the results obtained by the two techniques overlap and agree, one has enhanced confidence that the results are correct.

## 2. Cyclic Nucleotides and Protein Kinase

a. *Immunocytochemical Evidence. i. Cyclic nucleotides.* The diversity of mechanisms controlled by cAMP in mediating hormone action in different tissues grew with the sensitivity of methods for cyclic AMP developed during the late 1960s (Steiner *et al.*, 1969; Gilman, 1970). This research established cAMP as a universal second messenger for $\beta$-adrenergic agents and many polypeptide hormones. Experiments were based on criteria of Sutherland and co-workers (Robison *et al.*, 1971) to establish the identity of a second messenger of hormonal action. Hormone action via cyclic AMP should be substantiated by (1) hormone activation of adenylate cyclase from homogenates of the tissue, (2) hormone-induced accumulation of cAMP in an appropriate dose-dependent manner in incubated tissue, (3) potentiation by a cyclic-AMP phosphodiesterase inhibitor, and (4) hormone action mimicked by exogenous cAMP or its dibutyryl analog. Cellular compartmentation did not enter into the then existent theories.

It was generally believed that the cellular actions of these messengers took place in the cytoplasm which was assumed to be a uniform soluble environment. The messenger, particularly cAMP, was believed to function in the soluble environment by activating soluble enzyme systems responsive to the second messenger. The predominant approach to the biochemical elucidation of cAMP action was to homogenize tissues and determine the effect of cAMP on soluble enzymes from the homogenate. Such studies helped to identify enzymes regulated by cAMP. Moreover, the enzymes controlling cAMP concentration were recognized through studies on regulation of adenylate cyclase and cyclic nucleotide phosphodiesterases. After the discovery of cAMP-dependent protein kinases by Walsh *et al.* (1968) and subsequent recognition by Corbin *et al.* (1975) that two isozymes of cA-PK exist in most mammalian tissues, a general principle evolved that all actions of cAMP are accomplished by phosphorylation of specific substrates in cell by cAMP-dependent protein kinases (Kuo and Greengard, 1969). The discovery of a specific cGMP-dependent protein kinase with significant homology to the type II cA-PK led to the concept that the mechanism of cGMP action must somehow parallel that of cAMP, although the addition of exogenous cGMP to tissue preparations usually produced only the action of cAMP, making interpretation difficult.

To understand how cyclic nucleotides act and how regulation is accomplished, we hypothesized that the second messengers acted at specific sites in cells and within certain cells in heterogeneous tissues. In this hypothesis, the action of cyclic nucleotides was assumed to be compartmentalized within the cell, and we believed that an experimental approach based on this hypothesis would yield evidence of compartmentation. We therefore developed during the early 1970s an immunocytochemical approach to investigate the actions of cyclic nucleotides. Given the uncertainty concerning function of cGMP in the cell, we expected that this immunocytochemical approach might provide clues to such functions of cGMP.

We had developed antisera to cAMP in 1968 (Steiner *et al.,* 1969). Initially we were frustrated by the difficulty of measuring cAMP in tissue extracts utilizing enzyme cycling techniques. We could measure only a few samples per week and encountered many obstacles with these tedious procedures. We reasoned that the cyclic phosphate of cAMP and the charge groups on the purine nucleus could be important antigenic determinants that would help distinguish cAMP from other adenine nucleotides. We followed the procedures of Falbriard *et al.* (1967) and added a succinyl group at the ribose $2'-O$ position of cAMP. We then coupled the $2'-O$-succinyl-cAMP to a protein (human serum albumin or keyhole limpet hemocyanin), immunized rabbits, and elicited antisera to the cyclic nucleotide. We made an iodinated derivative of cAMP, succinyl-cAMP [125]I-labeled tyrosine methyl ester, and developed a radioimmunoassay for cAMP that was sensitive and very specific. We could measure cAMP in small amounts of tissue extract, and unlike investigators using earlier methods, we could do so without purification of the cAMP. We found that some cAMP antisera could distinguish cAMP from ATP by six orders of magnitude. This discrimination helped explain our ability to measure cAMP in tissue extracts without purification. We subsequently utilized a similar approach to make antiserum to cGMP (Steiner *et al.*, 1972).

Three laboratories initially collaborated in utilizing antibodies to cAMP to provide clues to the role(s) of cAMP in biological systems: Bloom, Hoffer, and Battenberg at the National Institutes of Health, Parker and Wedner of Washington University, St. Louis, and Steiner at the Albany Medical College. We originally decided to investigate which cell types within tissues respond to hormones with changes in cyclic AMP content and hence presumably cAMP action. The first studies were performed on cryostat cut frozen sections in which cAMP was localized in parotid sections from rats previously injected with isoproterenol or saline (Wedner *et al.*, 1972). Isoproterenol-stimulated fluorescence was observed in the basal portion of the acinar cells and the basket cells directly beneath them; ductile cells did not fluoresce. This study showed that the stimulated increase in cAMP was localized predominantly to the acinar cell, the target cell for isoproterenol in salivary gland. We were encouraged by these results because for the first time it was possible to determine which cells in a heterogenous tissue respond with cAMP accumulation.

Immunocytochemical studies were also performed on sections of rat cerebellum after decapitation (Bloom *et al.*, 1972). Increased fluorescence was visualized within 150 seconds of decapitation in Purkinje cells and in the granular layer, indicating a role for cAMP in these cells in this heterogeneous tissue. Interestingly, the glial cells did not fluoresce significantly. In a subsequent study, Siggins *et al.* (1973) applied 10–100 $\mu M$ norepinephrine to the exposed rat cerebellar cortex. Again the number of Purkinje cells stained increased significantly. With electrical stimulation to the locus ceruleus in the rat, the number of Purkinje cells staining for cAMP increased from 15 to 75%. No increase was seen in cerebellum from sham-operated animals or in animals pretreated with 6-hydroxydopamine. On the basis of these findings, cAMP was proposed to be the second messenger for the inhibitory pathway from the locus cereleus to the cerebellar Purkinje cells.

The utility of this immunocytochemical procedure was amplified further in studies with rat peritoneal mast cells. In these cells the stimulant, histamine releasing agent 48/80, causes degranulation of the mast cells. This action is accompanied by a decreased intracellular cAMP that can be detected biochemically within 15 seconds, with return to control levels by 30 minutes. Immunocytochemically detected cyclic AMP decreased markedly within 2 minutes after mast cell stimulation by 48/80. Fluorescent staining returned to baseline at 30 minutes. These immunocytochemical results paralleled the biochemical determination of cAMP concentration within the rat peritoneal mast cell and showed that it was also possible to detect decreased intracellular cAMP by the immunocytochemical procedure (Steiner et al., 1976).

Immunocytochemistry also allowed improved resolution of cyclic nucleotide localization within cells. Studies with human peripheral lymphocytes (Wedner et al., 1975) illustrated the utility of the immunocytochemical approach in single cell preparations because they showed that different stimuli to cAMP production in these cells caused cAMP to be localized in different areas of the cell. Phytohemagglutinin (PHA), prostaglandin $E_1$ (PGE$_1$), and isoproterenol induce prompt additive increases in intracellular cAMP measured biochemically when incubated with lymphocytes (Smith et al., 1971). In cells incubated with PHA, a patchy immunofluorescence pattern for cyclic AMP was visualized along the external plasma membrane with no fluorescence in the nucleus; after PGE$_1$, all the fluorescence was found in the cytoplasm; with isoproterenol, staining was dispersed throughout the cell, including the nucleus. These patterns appeared within 2 minutes of incubation with the stimulant, persisted through 30 minutes of incubation, and remained characteristic for each of the three agents. The authors concluded that the patterns visualized by cAMP immunocytochemistry were indicative of in vivo hormone-dependent cAMP action.

A good example of how cellular compartmentation undetectable by classical biochemical means can be studied immunocytochemically was provided in experiments done in collaboration with Pryzwansky (Pryzwansky et al., 1981). We labeled directly cyclic nucleotide antisera with different fluorescent conjugates: anti-cAMP with fluorescein isothiocyanate and anti-cGMP with rhodamine. These chromophores emit fluorescence at different wavelengths and cause either red or green color, respectively, to be detected by fluorescence microscopy. Also directly labeled were antibodies to granular products of polymorphonuclear leukocytes that are important in the process of phagocytosis. A phagosome is formed within seconds of exposure of the leukocytes to zymosan particles; it is eventually internalized. Differential fixation and permeabilization techniques were used to observe either exclusively external cyclic nucleotide (cell fixation by 2% paraformaldehyde) or cyclic nucleotide throughout the cell (permeabilization by cold acetone and methanol after paraformaldehyde fixation). We found that within 30 seconds there was increased detection of cAMP in the forming phagosome at the plasma membrane of zymosan particle-activated leukocytes (detected in fixed nonpermeabilized cells). Cytoplasmic pools of cAMP and cGMP were also visualized after fixation and permeabilization. Both plasma membrane and cytoplasmic pools of cAMP could be detected in the leukocytes, concentrated at the site of phagocytosis. Neither intracellular nor extracellular cGMP appeared to be involved in the forming phagosome. An antiserum to the regulatory subunit of type I cA-PK ($R^I$) was also tested. $R^I$ was detected in the phagosome; we speculated that this was the binding protein for localized cAMP in the area of the phagosome and that phosphorylation events catalyzed by associated C units were involved in the initial events of phagocytosis. This work illustrates the utility of immunocytochemical technology when applied to a biological system with extremely localized activation of cyclic AMP action. No alteration of total cellular cyclic AMP concentration can be detected under these conditions by biochemical analysis.

We have used the immunocytochemical approach to localize cGMP in a number of biological systems. Initial work was done with dog thyroid tissue in which we showed marked differences in the localization of cAMP and cGMP (Fallon *et al.*, 1974). cGMP was localized to the plasma membrane border of thyroid follicular cells that were in contact with thyroglobulin, while cAMP was visualized diffusely in cytoplasm. Stimulation of dog thyroid slices by TSH and acetylcholine, agents known to increase the concentration of cAMP and cGMP, respectively, in dog thyroid, showed increased fluorescence for the appropriate cyclic nucleotide in cytoplasm of follicular cells by 5 minutes. No change was observed in fluorescence intensity for the unaffected cyclic nucleotide. Absorption control sera, passed through the appropriate cyclic nucleotide affinity resin, showed no fluorescence in either control or hormone-stimulated thyroid tissue. These studies indicated that cyclic nucleotide immunocytochemistry could detect differences in cAMP and cGMP localization within individual cells and pointed out a potential role for cGMP and its specific protein kinase in membrane-directed events within the thyroid. The method, moreover, has shown that cGMP and cAMP are localized to different parts of the cell in many tissues. One of the most dramatically different localization patterns is found in rat liver, where we showed that cAMP is sinusoidally localized, while cGMP is found predominantly within nuclei (Fig. 1).

Koide *et al.* (1978) determined the localization of cGMP in regenerat-

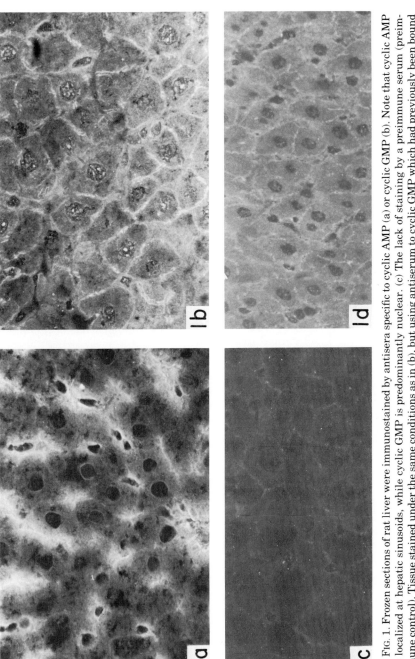

FIG. 1. Frozen sections of rat liver were immunostained by antisera specific to cyclic AMP (a) or cyclic GMP (b). Note that cyclic AMP is localized at hepatic sinusoids, while cyclic GMP is predominantly nuclear. (c) The lack of staining by a preimmune serum (preimmune control). Tissue stained under the same conditions as in (b), but using antiserum to cyclic GMP which had previously been bound by cyclic GMP in solution, is shown in (d) (absorption control). Originally published by Ong et al. (1975) and reprinted with permission.

ing rat liver after partial hepatectomy and correlated the immunocyto-chemical results with the measurement of guanylate cyclase activity in plasma membrane preparations and in isolated nuclei. Even though there was no change in total cGMP concentration in liver after hepa-tectomy as measured by radioimmunoassay, we found distinct changes in cGMP localization by the immunocytochemical technique. Within 8 hours after partial hepatectomy, the plasma membranes showed in-creased fluorescence, which peaked at 18 hours, while the nuclear membrane and nucleoli displayed increased cGMP fluorescence begin-ning at 12 hours and continuing until 24 hours postsurgery. Particu-late guanylate cyclase activity started to increase at the same time that enhanced cGMP staining was found at the plasma membrane (8 hours). Isolated nuclei showed biochemically increased guanylate cy-clase activity beginning at 12 hours, again correlating well with the immunocytochemical results. This study showed that the increased synthesis of cGMP was compartmentalized in the regenerating hepato-cyte to plasma membrane and nucleus at different times following partial hepatectomy. These changes were detected immunocytochemi-cally, even though the total tissue content of cGMP and total guany-late cyclase activity did not change, and they provided important clues for appropriate biochemical investigation.

The nuclear localization for cGMP has been a consistent finding. Cyclic GMP is found in nuclei from rat liver, intestine, testis (Ong et al., 1975), and adrenal cortex (Whitley *et al.*, 1975). The nuclear sites of cGMP localization have included nuclear membrane, nucleolus, and a fine reticular pattern. A particularly interesting localization for cGMP was along meiotic chromosomes in primary spermatocytes (Spruill and Steiner, 1976). We investigated the chromosomal localization for cGMP further with studies on the giant polytene chromosome from salivary glands of *Drosophila melanogaster* (Spruill *et al.*, 1978). The giant chromosomes were removed from salivary gland and fixed with 2% paraformaldehyde. Identical chromosomal preparations were visu-alized by phase and fluorescence microscopy. Distinct specific chromo-somal banding patterns were seen for cGMP, and they correlated with certain chromosomal puff areas. Cyclic GMP immunofluorescence was dramatically increased at locus 93D within 30 minutes after heat shock to the salivary gland *in vivo*. Heat induces puffing and RNA polymerase activity in these giant chromosomes at known sites, in-cluding 93D (Jamrich *et al.*, 1977). These results suggested that cyclic GMP was involved in at least some of the active chromosomal regions. Cyclic AMP was not detected on these giant chromosomes.

Despite our findings over the past 10 years that cGMP is localized by immunocytochemistry to nuclear elements, we have been unable to determine the binding proteins for this cyclic nucleotide or to discover the role cGMP plays in nuclear events. We have found that the cGMP protein kinase localizes at the nucleolus in parallel with cGMP in a number of biological systems, indicating that cGMP might act through its protein kinase at a number of nuclear sites. The limited quantity of tissue available from isolated nuclei has hindered our attempts to determine whether cGMP or its binding protein associate with specific nuclear acceptor proteins, DNA, or proteins of the nuclear matrix.

*ii. Protein kinases.* For the past few years, we have continued to develop these immunocytochemical techniques. We have focused on the effectors of second messenger action, e.g., cyclic nucleotide-regulated protein kinases, a specific cA-PK substrate $I_1$ (Inhibitor 1 of phosphatase type 1), and calmodulin. The procedures involved in the preparation of the cA-PK immunogens and the generation of specific antibodies, performed in collaboration with Beavo and colleagues at the University of Washington, are reviewed in detail by Kapoor and Steiner (1982). Generation of antisera to subunits of the cAMP kinases has also been reported by Fleisher *et al.* (1976), Hofmann *et al.* (1977), Uno *et al.* (1977), and Schwoch *et al.* (1980). The regulatory subunits of the cAMP-dependent protein kinases, the reconstituted cAMP holoenzymes, and the cGMP-dependent protein kinase proved to be good immunogens. The native catalytic subunit of cA-PK has proved to be a poor antigen, but a rabbit antiserum was nevertheless produced (Steiner *et al.*, 1978). Schwoch *et al.* (1980) and Murtaugh *et al.* (1982) improved titer by using catalytic subunit modified by treatment with glutaraldehyde prior to conjugation with keyhole limpet hemocyanin. This procedure led to the production of high-affinity antisera. We have used an affinity-purified anti-C (glutaraldehyde conjugated) serum for immunocytochemistry (Murtaugh *et al.*, 1982).

We have detected altered localization of protein kinases in a variety of tissues after hormonal stimulation. For example, within 5 minutes after glucagon administration to rats *in vivo*, increased C and $R^I$ immunofluorescence was found in both hepatocyte cytoplasm and in nucleus. $R^{II}$ localization also increased in nuclei, but this change was not detected until 15 minutes after glucagon administration (Koide *et al.*, 1981).

We have seen nuclear localization for C, $R^I$, $R^{II}$, and cG kinase in diverse tissues with or without hormonal stimulation of cAMP or cGMP accumulation in the tissue. Several experimental models of hormonal activation of target cell hyperplasia in normally very slowly dividing (or $G_0$ state) cells have been studied, including estrogen-stimulated uterus (Flandroy *et al.*, 1983), liver regeneration (Steiner *et al.* 1978), and isoproterenol-stimulated parotid (Harper and Steiner, unpublished). ACTH (corticotropin) -stimulated hypertrophy has also been investigated (Harper *et al.*, 1981). We have used these systems to investigate the function of cyclic AMP, cyclic GMP, and $Ca^{2+}$-calmodulin in mediation of hormonal signals stimulating cellular growth. Amazingly similar results have been found by immunocytochemical techniques with each tissue, even though the activating hormones are of distinctly different classes: peptide, steroid, or catecholamine. In most cases, increased cyclic AMP and cA-PK immunofluorescence are found in nuclei relatively quickly (within 30 minutes). In each case, increased $R^I$ localization occurs before any change can be detected in $R^{II}$, which is not localized to nuclei until after several hours. C localization is generally concurrent in time and location with the sum of $R^I$ and $R^{II}$. Cyclic GMP and cG-PK increase at the same time increased nuclear calmodulin immunofluorescence is observed, which is later than increases for $R^I$ and concurrent with or later than $R^{II}$. An example of these changes is shown in Fig. 2, where calmodulin is localized in rat adrenal cortex. Adrenals were removed from rats following dexamethasone suppression of endogenous ACTH secretion (panel A) or 11 hours after injection of repository ACTH to dexamethasone-treated rats (panel B). Nuclear, predominantly nucleolar calmodulin is seen only in the ACTH-stimulated adrenal.

Studies of estradiol-stimulated uterine growth showed similarity with other tissues we have studied. Within 12 hours after injection of 17$\beta$-estradiol into immature rats, sharply increased staining for cGMP, cG-PK, and calmodulin was observed within the nucleoli of only those uterine cell types which are under estrogen-regulated growth control. By 20–24 hours after estradiol injection, a more dispersed, reticular distribution of the nuclear fluorescence was observed. cAMP fluorescence changed only in cytoplasm, in contrast to the general pattern seen with isoproterenol or ACTH in their respective target tissues.

Browne *et al.* (1980) utilized antibodies for cA-PK and tubulin in studies of mitosis in kangaroo rat (PTK) cells. $R^{II}$ and cG-PK were localized to the mitotic spindle during different stages of mitosis, although $R^I$ and C were not detected there. In another study, Browne *et al.* (1982) localized $R^{II}$ to microtubules in interphase cells. These results suggest a role for $R^{II}$ in the regulation of microtubular function. These findings are consistent with the observation (Theurkauf and Vallee, 1982) that $R^{II}$ is intimately associated with the rat brain microtubule-associated protein MAP-2. Means and co-workers localized calmodulin

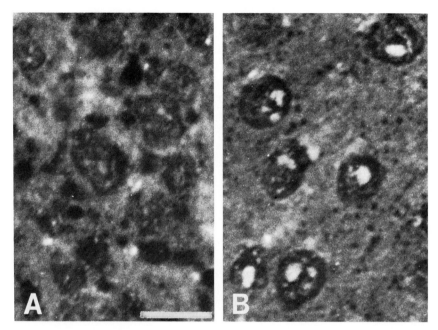

FIG. 2. Hormonal stimulation of many tissues alters the immunocytochemical localization of important regulatory molecules. This figure demonstrates the effect ACTH has on calmodulin localization in rat adrenal cortex. (A) Calmodulin localization in adrenal cortex taken from a rat that had been injected with dexamethasone for the previous 21 hours (to suppress endogenous ACTH secretion). Contrast that to (B) in which calmodulin is localized in adrenal from a rat injected with dexamethasone and for the final 11 hours with repository ACTH in gelatin. The exogenous ACTH produces marked localization of calmodulin in nucleoli. The calibration bar indicates 10 μm. Originally published by Harper and Steiner (1983).

to microtubules immunocytochemically (Marcum *et al.*, 1978); we have confirmed their results (unpublished). We speculate that cyclic nucleotide protein kinases act in concert with other intracellular messengers such as calcium to regulate the activity of microtubules.

Localization of other enzymes important in the potential regulation of cyclic GMP action has been performed by Ariano (1983). She showed immunocytochemically that cyclic GMP, soluble guanylate cyclase, and cG-PK are localized to the same discrete intracellular areas of rat rostral caudate–putamen complex cells, as is phosphodiesterase localized histochemically. The medium-spiny neurons contained most of the localized cyclic GMP system components. Electron microscope immunocytochemistry revealed discrete localization of all of the components of cyclic GMP metabolism confined to the postsynaptic region of asymmetrical (but not symmetrical) terminal boutons. She suggested that since the cyclic GMP components were localized together at the synaptic region, cyclic GMP is functionally important in neuronal communication.

b. *Biochemical Evidence.* i. *Compartmentation of cyclic AMP-dependent protein kinase actions.* Hormones activate adenylate cyclase through interaction with membrane-bound receptors. The ultimate response any particular cell makes to an individual hormone depends both on the presence of appropriate receptors on that cell membrane and on intracellular reactions developing subsequent to the hormone–receptor interaction. Consequences of the hormone–receptor interaction will determine cellular responses to any hormone. In some cases, the particular interactions can lead to compartmentalized cA-PK activation; apparently in that case, cyclic AMP synthesis stimulated by one hormone can produce different intracellular consequences than that stimulated by another. Thus, different hormones, each acting through cyclic AMP, produce different intracellular biochemical effects. Several investigators have found that hormonal stimulation of a cell can produce selective cyclic AMP-dependent protein kinase activation.

Byus *et al.* (1978) showed that activation of human peripheral lymphocytes by 10 $\mu M$ concanavalin A leads to mitogenesis and activation of only type I cA-PK. No mitogenesis is observed after stimulation by either 100 $\mu M$ concanavalin A or 0.1 m$M$ dibutyryl-cyclic AMP, conditions under which both cA-PK isozymes are activated. The observed selective mitogenic response to agents which all raise intracellular cyclic AMP was theorized to be regulated by selective stimulant-dependent cA-PK type I activation.

Similar results on selective cA-PK$^I$ activation were obtained in rat liver. Schwoch (1978) and Byus *et al.* (1979) found that graded doses of glucagon or dibutyryl cyclic AMP produce graded effects on cA-PK activation such that low doses selectively activate type I cA-PK in isolated hepatocytes, while higher doses activate both isozymes. Maximal glycogenolysis was achieved at drug doses that selectively activate type I kinase, indicating that type I kinase is sufficient for regulation of glycogenolysis; no further activation (nor inhibition) developed upon stimulation of type II kinase at higher glucagon doses.

The observations that type I cA-PK could be activated selectively in liver or lymphocytes may indicate merely that type I isozyme is more sensitive to activation by cyclic AMP than is type II in most tissues. Thus, slight elevations of cyclic AMP could affect type I selectively without any need to invoke distinct pools of cA-PK. Results by Livesey *et al.* (1982) counter this argument with their finding that $PGE_2$ selectively activates cA-PK type II, but that parathyroid hormone (PTH) activates both isozymes in osteoblast-rich cells derived from newborn rat calvaria.

Several factors must be considered when interpreting the data from these experiments. Only cytosolic soluble cA-PK was analyzed. Any cA-PK associated with membranes was removed by centrifugation prior to application of the supernatant containing cA-PK activity to the isozyme separation columns. Further, the possibility that multiple cell types account for selective cA-PK activation was not eliminated in any of the studies cited above.

The problems of isozyme sensitivity to cyclic AMP and of cell type homogeneity were addressed by Ng *et al.* (1983) and Livesey *et al.* (1984) with experiments using T 47D human breast carcinoma cells. $PGE_2$-stimulated cyclic AMP accumulation activates equally each cA-PK isozyme in this cell line. Calcitonin, on the other hand, activates type II isozyme fully in intact cells without any effect on type I cA-PK. Measurement of activation *in vitro* shows that type II isozyme is activated by cyclic AMP at a $K_a$ 60% higher than is type I. Thus, selective activation of type II isozyme in cultured T 47D cells by calcitonin is not due merely to intrinsic isozyme sensitivity to cyclic AMP. Rather, intracellular compartmentation of the cyclic AMP generated by calcitonin stimulation must be different from that following stimulation with $PGE_2$.

None of these studies addressed the possibility that subcellular cA-PK shifts from particulate to soluble fractions (or vice versa) may have accounted for at least some of the observed selective effects of activation. One series of experiments has shown that differential effects of hormone actions may be accounted for by such a phenomenon without selective cA-PK isozyme activation. Hayes and Brunton have shown that isoproterenol activates both membrane-associated and cytosolic cA-PK in rat heart, while $PGE_1$ stimulates only cytosolic cA-PK (Hayes *et al.*, 1979). Although both isoproterenol and $PGE_1$ stimulate cyclic AMP accumulation and activate cA-PK, only isoproterenol increases $dP/dt$ and activates glycolytic enzymes known to be regulated by a cA-PK cascade. These effects apparently are not due to any inhibitory potential of $PGE_1$, since $PGE_1$ does not alter the ability of isoproterenol to produce any of these effects. The lack of $PGE_1$ effect on glycolytic enzymes correlates with the lack of ability to activate particulate cA-PK.

The possibility that multiple cell types account for the disparate cA-PK activation has subsequently been addressed and rejected in independent laboratories by Hayes *et al.* (1982) and by Buxton and Brunton (1983). Both groups have isolated cardiomyocytes for primary culture; Hayes *et al.* report that they obtain 85% pure rat myocytes, and Buxton and Brunton obtain >92% pure rabbit myocytes. In each preparation, the differences between $PGE_1$ and isoproterenol originally seen in perfused rat heart are maintained. Buxton and Brunton (1983) showed that $PGE_1$, which triples cyclic AMP accumulation and doubles cA-PK activation, does not affect glycolytic enzyme activities. Isoproterenol, however, at either 10 n$M$ (which produces similar cyclic AMP and cA-PK increase as $PGE_1$) or at 1 $\mu M$ (maximally effective), produces the same activation of glycolytic enzymes seen in perfused heart. Again, $PGE_1$ neither activates nor inhibits the ability of isoproterenol (1 $\mu M$) to act. As in the intact heart, the apparent basis for these divergent actions is that only isoproterenol increases particulate cA-PK activity, while both agonists activate the soluble enzyme. Although the total cellular cA-PK concentration was elevated to the same extent with both stimulants, only isproterenol produced a decline in the particulate cA-PK holoenzyme from 47 to 31% of total, with a half-life of less than 1 minute. This reduction of holoenzyme reflects the release of free active C. Pharmacological probes of $Ca^{2+}$ flux suggest that the lack of $PGE_1$ effect is not due to calcium movement across the plasma membrane stimulated by either isoproterenol or $PGE_1$. Hayes *et al.* (1982) have also shown that differential effects of isoproterenol and $PGE_1$ are maintained using primary rat cardiomyocyte cultures. Isoproterenol was found to stimulate $^{32}P$ incorporation into at least 16 proteins of [$^{32}P$]$P_i$-treated cardiomyocytes, while $PGE_1$ did not affect the phosphorylation state of any protein relative to control.

    *ii. cA-PK actions in nuclei.* The nucleus is one of the more obvious and clearly definable examples of compartmentalization in the eukaryotic cell. A number of investigators have obtained results by biochemical methods which show that the second messenger cAMP, through its interaction with its intermediary proteins the cA-PKs, stimulates or regulates several cellular activities localized within the nuclear compartment. These results provide a rationale for the increased levels of cA-PK subunits observed immunocytochemically in nuclei in response to hormonal stimuli or during different stages of the cell cycle.

    The cA-PK in the nucleus can catalyze phosphorylation of nuclear proteins. It has, however, been difficult to identify specific nuclear proteins directly regulated *in vivo* by phosphorylation by cA-PK, since there are 18 different protein kinases in nuclei (for review, see Mitchell and Kleinsmith, 1983). It is probable that the cA-PKs activate other nuclear protein kinases by phosphorylation. Nevertheless, some progress has been made identifying the nuclear proteins which are phosphorylated by cA-PK. It has been shown that dibutyryl-cAMP differentially stimulates the *in vivo* phosphorylation of a number of acidic proteins in rat liver nuclei (Johnson and Allfrey, 1972). Histones H-1, H-2A, H-2B, and H-3 are all substrates for phosphorylation by cA-PK *in vitro*, but H-1 is the only histone known to be phosphorylated by cA-PK *in vivo* (Laks *et al.*, 1981; Harrison *et al.*, 1982). Walton *et al.* (1982) observed similarly stimulated phosphorylation of HMG-14 *in vitro*, but evidence on whether this occurs *in vivo* is lacking.

Rosenfeld and co-workers (Murdoch *et al.*, 1983; Rosenfeld *et al.*, 1983) have identified a chromosome-associated 23,000-Da basic protein in GH-4 rat pituitary cells that is phosphorylated in response to hormonal stimuli without measurable time lag. They have referred to this protein as the basic regulated phosphoprotein, or BRP. It is found exclusively in the nucleus at a concentration equal to about 1% of histone H-1 concentration. Cyclic AMP, apparently through cAMP-dependent protein kinase, and thyrotropin-releasing hormone, through a mechanism that is not yet clear, stimulate the phosphorylation of BRP by as much as 12-fold. Phosphorylation of BRP is associated with a transient increase in the transcription rate of as much as 20% of the actively transcribed genes.

Cyclic AMP stimulates increased synthesis of a number of specific enzymes. Experiments using cDNA probes generally show that accumulation of mRNA coding for specific proteins increases in parallel with the increased synthesis rates of these proteins. Induction of mRNA for the A subunit of lactate dehydrogenase (mRNA$^{\text{LDH}}$) in C6 rat glioma cells has been described by Jungmann and associates (Jungmann *et al.*, 1983a,b). Synthesis of mRNA$^{\text{LDH}}$ was quantified following stimulation by dibutyryl cAMP or isoproterenol. The specific mRNA concentration began to rise 90 minutes after stimulation; it peaked at 4 hours, with ~threefold greater mRNA$^{\text{LDH}}$ than control cells. The half-life of the basal mRNA$^{\text{LDH}}$ was 45 minutes; in contrast, stimulated cells exhibited two populations of mRNA$^{\text{LDH}}$ with $t_{1/2}$ of 50 minutes and 150 minutes, respectively (Jungmann *et al.*, 1983b). These data suggest that cyclic AMP may both increase the rate of LDH mRNA transcription and act to alter the turnover mechanism for the mRNA in the cytoplasm.

Cyclic AMP also increases phosphoenolpyruvate carboxykinase (PEP-CK) in rat liver. Administration of dibutyryl-cAMP to fasted-refed rats causes an eight- to ninefold increase in the functional content of mRNA coding for hepatic phosphoenolpyruvate carboxykinase in cell free protein-synthesizing systems (Iynedjian and Hanson, 1977). PEP-CK mRNA, as measured by hybridization using a cDNA probe, increased eightfold in 1 hour (Cimbala *et al.*, 1982). The administration of dibutyryl-cAMP to starved, glucose-refed rats caused a sevenfold increase in the transcription rate of the *PEP-CK* gene, as measured in isolated hepatic nuclei (Lamers *et al.*, 1982), without significant changes in the mRNA degradation rate (Beale *et al.*, 1982). Thus, it may be concluded that increased *PEP-CK* synthesis induced by cAMP reflects an increased rate of gene transcription.

A 620 base-pair (bp) 5' fragment containing 547 bp of the 5' flanking sequence of the *PEP-CK* gene has been obtained (Wynshaw-Boris *et al.*, 1984). It was ligated into the pBR327-based vector, pOPF, at the 5' end of a thymidine kinase gene which lacked its viral promotor. Dibutyryl-cyclic AMP-inducible thymidine kinase was obtained upon transfer of this chimera into thymidine kinase-deficient rat hepatoma cells. These results show that at least one cyclic AMP-regulated DNA region is contained within the 5' flanking region of the *PEP-CK* gene, although whether cA-PK or another cyclic AMP binding protein acts directly at this region is unknown. Also unknown is whether catalytic kinase activity, cyclic AMP binding R unit, or both contribute to this regulation.

Dibutyryl cAMP injected into adrenalectomized rats (Noguchi *et al.*, 1982) causes an increase *in vitro* translatable tyrosine aminotransferase mRNA (mRNA$^{TAT}$). The mRNA$^{TAT}$ activity peaks at 1 hour and returns to baseline after 2.5 hours. The increase in the rate of synthesis of tyrosine aminotransferase is proportional to the increase in the mRNA$^{TAT}$. Repeated injections of dibutyryl cAMP at 0, 1, 2.5, and 4 hours produce a rise and fall in translatable mRNA$^{TAT}$ identical to that observed after a single injection of dibutyryl-cAMP; i.e., the mRNA$^{TAT}$ response becomes densensitized to further effects of dibutyryl-cAMP. The synthesis rate of tyrosine aminotransferase protein, however, becomes greater at 5 hours with multiple dibutyryl-cAMP injections that after a single dose, suggesting that the dibutyryl-cAMP may stimulate the synthesis of a protein which specifically facilitates the translation of mRNA$^{TAT}$. Boney *et al.* (1983) utilized protein-loaded red blood cell ghosts to microinject cultured rat H35 hepatoma cells with the catalytic subunit of cAMP-dependent protein kinase, the kinase inhibitor protein, or the regulatory subunit of cAMP-dependent protein kinase. The catalytic subunit produced a two- to threefold increase in TAT synthesis. The protein kinase inhibitor protein blocked 8-bromo-cAMP-induced synthesis of the enzyme. Microinjection of the pure regulatory subunit of the kinase inhibited induction by 8-bromo-cAMP of increased aminotransferase concentrations. These results provide direct evidence that cAMP-dependent protein kinase is important in mediating the effect of cAMP on the synthesis of tyrosine aminotransferase.

At least three mechanisms may be proposed to explain how cAMP regulates gene transcription. As discussed, cA-PK phosphorylates a number of nuclear proteins, with the potential for concomitant changes in activity. Additionally, R subunits of cA-PK may bind to and regulate the activity of other proteins, or they may bind to chromatin in regulatory regions and directly regulate transcription of specific genes.

Cyclic AMP, by facilitating the association of R with other proteins, may regulate enzymatic or other activities in the cell beyond that of the catalytic subunit of the kinase. Jurgensen (1984) reported such a protein to which the cAMP-$R^{II}$ complex binds. He found that cAMP-$R^{II}$ will bind to and inhibit the activity of $Mg^{2+}$-ATP-dependent protein phosphatase. Net accumulation of phosphorylated proteins in the presence of cAMP could thus be enhanced. Interactions of $R^{II}$ with calcium-calmodulin (Hathaway et al., 1981) and calcineurin (Klee et al., 1983) suggest a close interaction between cAMP and $Ca^{2+}$. Sarkar et al. (1984) have identified a 75,000-Da protein that appears to associate with bovine brain $R^{II}$; a function for this protein has not yet been identified. These results show that there may be enzymatic or other activities independent of phosphorylation which cAMP affects via the regulatory subunits of the cAMP-dependent protein kinases.

No regulatory interaction of the R subunit of cA-PK with the promoter region of mammalian genes, in a manner analogous to the *Escherichia coli* catabolite gene activator protein (CAP), has been reported. The CAP protein contains a domain to the carboxy side of the cAMP binding domain which has been shown to interact with DNA, and this site shows homology with other DNA binding proteins (Ullmann and Danchin, 1983). In contrast, the regulatory subunits of the cAMP-dependent protein kinases contain two domains that bind cAMP and a third domain on the amino-terminal side of the cAMP binding domains. This third domain shows no recognizable homology with the DNA binding regions of the CAP protein and other DNA binding proteins (Weber et al., 1982). Thus, it does not seem that $R^I$ or $R^{II}$ might bind to DNA in a manner similar to that shown by CAP. However, direct binding by a nonhomologous site on R units is nevertheless possible. It is also possible that R (or variants of R) could interact with proteins tightly associated with specific sites on the DNA and thereby regulate transcription.

Hormones might regulate nuclear cA-PK either by activation of cA-PK preexistent in nuclei or by translocation of activated cytoplasmic cA-PK. Several groups have reported that cA-PK, either as holoenzyme or separate subunits, is translocated to nuclei and retained within them upon hormonal stimulation. Jungmann and co-workers have provided the best examples of such translocation. They showed that treatment of neonatal porcine ovarian tissue with 0.1 $\mu M$ 8-*p*-chlorophenylthio-cAMP for 15 minutes produced a large specific increase of cAMP-PK activity in nuclei (Spielvogel *et al.*, 1977) defined as such because the increased nuclear protein kinase activity could be inhibited with either the specific protein kinase inhibitor of Walsh *et al.* (1971) or antiserum to cAMP-PK. There was no detectable translocation of nuclear protein kinases other than cA-PK. Several controls proved that the nonspecific adsorption effect described by Keely *et al.* (1975) could not account for these observations. Nuclei could be washed with 0.14 $M$ NaCl without removal of the cAMP-PK activity and could be isolated with nonaqueous solvents (which should prevent cytoplasmic exchange during isolation), maintaining the specific cAMP-PK activity differences (Spielvogel *et al.*, 1977). Additional work from Jungmann and associates shows that this is not an isolated phenomenon. Similar evidence for translocation has been found following treatment of WI-38 fibroblast cells with 8-chlorophenylthio-cAMP (Jungmann *et al.*, 1976) and of C-6 glioma cells with isoproterenol (Jungmann *et al.*, 1980). The data with C-6 cells are particularly interesting. In this cultured cell isoproterenol produces a rapid and specific translocation of type I cAMP-PK without an effect upon the type II isozyme.

Translocation of cA-PK also has been found during liver regeneration (Laks *et al.*, 1981). Nuclear type I kinase concentration increased fivefold and nuclear type II by threefold at 16 hours after partial hepatic resection. This apparent translocation of cA-PK into nuclei is inhibited by prior treatment of rats with cholchicine, suggesting involvement of microtubules in the processes which produce increased nuclear cA-PK.

In summary, regulated effects of cA-PK in nuclei indicate that cAMP is compartmentalized there for a specific function(s). Data are being collected that should soon illuminate such phenomena. Perhaps both cA-PK-directed effects and separate regulation by R units control gene regulation.

*iii. Nuclear actions of cGMP.* The possibility that cGMP may be important in controlling nuclear function has not been investigated as extensively as that of cAMP. Nevertheless, some intriguing observations have been made. Our studies of cyclic nucleotide association with the polytene chromosomes of *Drosophila* (Spruill *et al.*, 1978) have shown that cGMP, but not cAMP, is preferentially localized at genetically active sites of polytene chromosomes. The association of cGMP with active chromosomal loci suggests that it may be involved in controlling RNA synthesis.

Arfmann *et al.* (1981) have studied phosphorylation of the high-mobility group proteins (HMG-1, 2, 14, and 17) in CHO cells. In studies on phosphorylation in metaphase and in interphase, they found a threefold increase in the phosphorylation of HMG-1, HMG-2, and HMG-14 (and also histone H-1), and a 50% decrease in HMG-17. The degree of phosphorylation of HMG-14 and HMG-17 in cultured cells (mouse Ehrlich ascites, L1210 and P388 leukemia, HT-29 human colon carcinoma cells, and CHO cells) is substantially greater during log-phase growth than in the plateau phase (Saffer and Glazer, 1982). Phosphorylated HMG-14 and HMG-17 were found to be preferentially associated with micrococcal nuclease-sensitive regions of the chromatin, implying that they are localized in actively transcribed sequences of the chromatin (Saffer, 1982).

*In vitro* experiments (Walton *et al.*, 1982) have shown that HMG-14 contains a major high-affinity substrate site for the cAMP- and cGMP-dependent protein kinases, and that it is preferentially phosphorylated by the cGMP-dependent protein kinase. Both HMG-14 and HMG-17 contain additional minor substrate sites for the cGMP-dependent protein kinase. It has not been established whether these phosphorylations occur *in vivo*. Zeilig *et al.* (1981) have shown that histone H-1 is preferentially phosphorylated *in vitro* by cGMP-dependent protein kinase. The preferential localization of cGMP to actively transcribed regions of the chromatin and the preferential phosphorylation of proteins associated with actively transcribed regions of DNA by cGMP-dependent protein kinase combine to suggest an *in vivo* role for cGMP in regulating gene transcription. Additionally, the possibility that cGMP might control nuclear activity through other intermediary proteins cannot be overlooked.

### 3. Calcium-Regulated Components

*a. Introduction.* Electrical and hormonal stimuli may produce nearly instantaneous increases in free cytosolic $Ca^{2+}$ from a resting concentration of $\sim 0.1 \ \mu M$ to a maximum of $10 \ \mu M$. Upon termination of the activation signal, $Ca^{2+}$ is rapidly and efficiently removed from the cytosolic compartment primarily by the high-affinity, high-capacity calcium pump within the plasma membrane. Cytosolic calcium is also efficiently taken up into the mitochondria and, in the myocyte, into a highly differentiated compartment, the sarcoplasmic reticulum. Thus, the intracellular free $Ca^{2+}$ concentration can be raised and lowered quickly, fulfilling properties of a good second messenger.

The most significant physiologic consequences of a rise in cytosolic free $Ca^{2+}$ are initiation of muscle contraction, the breakdown of glycogen, and secretion. These physiologic end points result from a series of biochemical reactions which, in mammalian cells, involve the calcium binding proteins, calmodulin, troponin C, and protein kinase C. These proteins bind $Ca^{2+}$ with an affinity constant approximately midway between resting and stimulated intracellular free $Ca^{2+}$. Binding of $Ca^{2+}$ to calmodulin or troponin C produces conformational changes that cause a hydrophobic domain to emerge. This so-called "hydrophobic pocket" enables the calcium binding proteins to bind to and activate enzymes that then perform specific cellular functions (for a review, see Moore and Dedman, 1982). In the instance of skeletal muscle thin filament, tropinin I is tightly bound to actin and inhibits actomyosin ATPase, the enzyme responsible for muscle contraction. An increase in cytosolic calcium causes tighter coupling of troponin C to troponin I such that actomyosin ATPase becomes active and the muscle contracts (for review, see Potter and Johnson, 1982). Contraction represents but one example of a localized $Ca^{2+}$-mediated event compartmentalized through enhanced affinity of a calcium binding protein (TnC) for a specific cellular structure (myofibrils).

Calmodulin is the predominant calcium binding protein in smooth muscle and in all vertebrate nonmuscle tissues examined thus far (for review, see Means and Dedman, 1980). Proteins known to be activated by calmodulin include cyclic nucleotide phosphodiesterase, myosin light-chain kinase, phosphorylase kinase, type 2b phosphatase (calcineurin), $Ca^{2+}$-ATPase, glycogen synthase kinase 4, synapsin I kinase, and (plant) NAD kinase. It is apparent from this list that calcium and calmodulin, like the cyclic nucleotides, regulate to a major degree phosphorylation conditions in cellular metabolism.

   *b. Example of Compartmentalized Calmodulin-Regulated System: Glycogen.* Glycogen metabolism consists of a highly ordered set of biochemical events tightly regulated through phosphorylation and dephosphorylation in response to hormonal stimuli. Localization of enzymes within this "soluble" non-membrane-bound compartment provides an example of compartmentalized localization of $Ca^{2+}$-regulated enzymes. As early as 1970, Meyer *et al.* reflected upon the observations of others that many of the enzymes of hepatic glycogen metabolism could be sedimented with the glycogen. They then proceeded to show biochemically that phosphorylase, phosphorylase kinase, and phosphorylase phosphatase are all strongly bound to the glycogen pellet of skeletal muscle (Meyer et al., 1970). Engel (1961) had localized glycogen to the I band of skeletal muscle, while Sigel and Pette (1969) had cytochemically localized phosphorylase at the same region. These observations were collected by Meyer et al. (1970) to produce the hypothesis that glycogen particles constitute a defined matrix of the cytosol on which the enzymes of its metabolism act.

If this hypothesis is correct, one should be able to localize to the glycogen fraction, both biochemically and histochemically, other enzymes of glycogen metabolism, including calmodulin (as a subunit of phosphorylase kinase and as a potential additional regulator), the calmodulin-dependent glycogen synthase kinase 4 (GSK4), GSK3, GSK5 (casein kinase II), the catalytic subunit of cyclic AMP-dependent protein kinase, protein phosphatase 1, protein phosphatase 2b, and protein phosphatase inhibitors 1 and 2. Purification to homogeneity of the enzymes of glycogen metabolism usually begins from solution high in concentrations of EDTA, generating "cytosolic" enzymes. In vivo, however, they are probably tightly associated with glycogen particles. Cohen (1980) showed that in rabbit skeletal muscle homogenized in 1 m$M$ CaCl$_2$, 60–70% of glycogen synthase, phosphorylase, and phosphorylase kinase remain bound to the myofibrillar fraction (i.e., bound to the glycogen-containing fraction).

A simple technique to dissolve glycogen using $\alpha$-amylase (Lillie, 1947) enabled us (Harper et al., 1980) to determine immunocytochemically that calmodulin is bound to glycogen particles in hepatocytes and skeletal muscle. The punctate glycogen-associated immunofluorescent staining of calmodulin was removed by treatment of liver slices with $\alpha$-amylase prior to staining. Livers from fasted rats also lacked punctate localized calmodulin. Calmodulin was similarly localized to plasma membranes and to nuclear elements. Nuclear and membrane-bound calmodulin remained associated in the liver of fasting rats and in liver sections treated with $\alpha$-amylase (see Fig. 3). Staining for nuclear hepatic calmodulin is also affected by partial hepatectomy, increasing in nuclei within 8 to 16 hours and decreasing in cytoplasm due to glycogen depletion (Earp, Harper, and Steiner, unpublished). Ingebritsen et al. (1983) showed with the $\alpha$-amylase technique that 50% of protein phosphatase 1 (which contributes 90% of phosphorylase phosphatase activity) was bound to glycogen in skeletal muscle extract and 10% was bound in liver extracts.

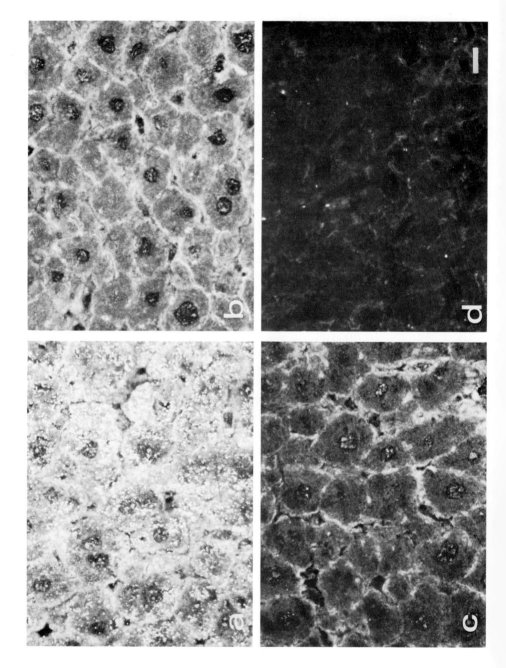

## 4. Phosphatases

*a. Biochemical.* A central concept in our current understanding of hormone action is that phosphorylation regulates key enzymes in all metabolic (and probably all neuronal) pathways. The phosphorylation state of these enzymes represents a dynamic balance between kinases and phosphatases, both hormonally sensitive. The kinases, both cyclic AMP-dependent and $Ca^{2+}$-regulated protein kinases, have been examined in great detail. Our understanding of the dephosphorylation mechanisms has lagged significantly, one of the major reasons being the lack of a unifying scheme for classifying phosphatases. Previously, protein phosphatases have been classified according to substrates, e.g., phosphorylase phosphatase, glycogen synthase phosphatase, histone phosphatase. We now recognize that these designations include multiple phosphatases acting on each of these substrates. Sorting through the pre-1983 literature on phosphatases is thus confusing at best.

In 1983, Cohen and associates proposed a generalized classification (Ingebritsen and Cohen, 1983) of the phosphoprotein phosphatases based on two criteria. Type 1 phosphatase dephosphorylates the $\beta$ subunit of phosphorylase kinase, while type 2 phosphatases prefer the $\alpha$ subunit. Type 1 phosphatase is subject to inhibition by two low-molecular-weight thermostable proteins, termed Inhibitor 1 and Inhibitor 2. Type 2 phosphatases are not sensitive to these inhibitors. Critical examination of purified phosphatases from skeletal muscle and tissue extracts utilizing all known phosphoprotein substrates has not identified any other cytosolic protein phosphatases. Types 1 and 2a show broad substrate specificity, and the specificity of type 2c is intermediate.

As noted, evidence for compartmentation of phosphatases is difficult to evaluate among laboratories because the previous classifications were imprecise. Nevertheless, such evidence has been found. Dopere and Stalmans (1982) analyzed fractions of rat liver obtained by differential centrifugation for phosphatase activity using phosphorylase *b* as

---

FIG. 3. Digestion of starch in tissue sections by $\alpha$-amylase demonstrates that calmodulin is glycogen associated. Rat liver sections were immunostained for calmodulin under several conditions. Normally fed rat liver was sectioned (a, b, and d). The section was pretreated with $\alpha$-amylase prior to immunostaining (b). Fasted rat liver was sectioned (c). Immunostaining of the liver sections shown in (a–c) was then performed. The nonspecific (control) staining is shown in (d). Note the white dots localized in (a), which are removed either by prior fasting of the rat (c) or by treating the fed rat liver section with $\alpha$-amylase (b). These white dots indicate glycogen-associated calmodulin. The calibration bar indicates $10\mu m$. Originally published by Harper *et al.* (1980), and used with permission.

substrate. They found that a higher proportion of phosphorylase phosphatase activity was associated with the nuclear fraction than in mitochondrial/lysosomal or cytosolic fractions. They did not differentiate this activity into type 1 or type 2 phosphatases according to Cohen's criteria. Nahas *et al.* (1984) attempted subcellular localization of human polymorphonuclear leukocyte phosphatases, again using substrate-dependent definitions for glycogen synthase phosphatase, phosphorylase phosphatase, and histone phosphatase. Both synthase phosphatase and phosphorylase phosphatase activity were found to be associated with the microsomal fraction, while the majority of histone phosphatase activity (75–85%) was found in the cytosol. Since multiple phosphatases act on each of these substrates, it is difficult to extrapolate these results to determine the localization of each biochemically distinct phosphatase.

Recently, Ingebritsen *et al.* (1983) systematically evaluated phosphatase activity in liver and skeletal muscle extracts. They subfractionated homogenates into cytosol, glycogen–protein complex, and microsomes. Using the criteria for discrimination among the phosphatases as established by Cohen, they found nearly exclusive cytosolic localization of all of the type 2 phosphatases. In contrast, at least half of skeletal muscle type 1 phosphatase was associated with the glycogen complex. In the liver, 20% of the type 1 phosphatase is located in the microsomal fraction, while only 10% is associated with the glycogen complex. One of the key enzymes of glycogen metabolism, glycogen synthase, is activated by net dephosphorylation (Lawrence *et al.*, 1983; Parker *et al.*, 1983), although the exact mechanisms have not been worked out. The biochemical colocalization of these two enzymes (type I phosphatase and glycogen synthase) in the glycogen pellet suggests *in vivo* regulatory interaction.

*b. Immunocytochemical.* Immunocytochemical localization of phosphatases and phosphatase inhibitors has also been limited. Polyclonal antibodies have been raised against bovine brain phosphatase 2b (Tallant *et al.*, 1983), rabbit skeletal muscle phosphatase 2a (Alemany *et al.*, 1984), and phosphatase Inhibitor 1 (Shenolikar and Steiner, 1984). Monoclonal antibodies have been generated against phosphatase 2b (Wang *et al.*, 1983). Using antibody to phosphatase 2b (calcineurin), Wood *et al.* (1980) demonstrated that calcineurin, like calmodulin, is localized at postsynaptic densities in brain. Using the same antiserum, Klumpp *et al.* (1983) found this molecule in the cell membrane of *Paramecium,* particularly in the cilia. Calcineurin, in contrast to its activator protein calmodulin, did not localize to the glycogen particles in *Paramecium.* This immunocytochemical localization has since been confirmed biochemically (J. Schultz, personal communication).

Immunocytochemical localization of phosphorylated Inhibitor 1 ($I_1$) has been carried out in this laboratory by Shenolikar and Steiner (1984). This protein is ubiquitously distributed in mammalian tissues and is a potentially important regulator of cAMP action because only cA-PK can phosphorylate $I_1$ (Cohen et al., 1979). Phosphorylated $I_1$ inhibits protein phosphatase 1 and thus amplifies the cAMP signal. A unique polyclonal antiserum we developed recognizes phospho-$I_1$ at least 200 times more avidly than dephospho-$I_1$. We believe this antibody probe is the most specific one developed for detecting a substrate of cAMP action within whole tissues. Shenolikar and Steiner (1984) reported immunocytochemical data on phospho-$I_1$ localization in several tissues of the rat. In rat liver, phospho-$I_1$ localization increases after 5 minutes of glucagon administration in vivo. Increased fluorescence is visualized throughout the cytoplasm and with particularly bright fluorescence in nuclei. Fluorescence returned to control patterns by 30 minutes. Previous biochemical studies (Foulkes et al., 1982; Nemenoff et al., 1983) have shown that dephosphorylation of normally phospho-$I_1$ is produced after insulin stimulation, while $\beta$-adrenergic agonists stimulate greater $I_1$ phosphorylation. In our immunocytochemical studies, insulin reduced glucagon-stimulated phospho-$I_1$ fluorescence in all cellular compartments of rat hepatocytes, including nuclei. These data illustrate the power of the immunocytochemical approach. The increased avidity of this polyclonal antiserum for phospho-$I_1$ versus dephospho-$I_1$ is particularly important, since it indicates not only where protein phosphatase 1 action is inhibited, but, more importantly, where cA-PK acts.

## C. Hypotheses on Compartmentation Mechanisms

### 1. Selective cA-PK Activation

Cardiac cA-PK responses to isoproterenol or $PGE_1$ are apparently regulated through selective activation of particulate cA-PK. The mechanism of selective activation, probably not mediated through selective cA-PK isozyme effect (Hayes et al., 1980), and the selective activation of cA-PK isozymes in T 47D cells, as described by Ng et al., are not well understood (Section II,B,2,b,i). Numerous theories can be advanced, but each must account for the observations that in liver and rat calvaria or T47D cells, cA-PK types I or II, respectively, are selectively activated by some, but not all hormones, and that in cardiomyocytes, only isoproterenol stimulates particulate cA-PK, even though both isoproterenol and $PGE_1$ elevate cyclic AMP to the same intracellular concentration.

Compartmentation of cyclic AMP effects may be achieved in several ways. No evidence exists to suggest that effectors other than cyclic AMP regulate the cA-PK activation state intracellularly (although compartmentation of catalytic unit inhibitors may help regulate the actions of activated kinase). We will therefore start with the assumption that a selective cyclic AMP action on cA-PK arises from compartmentation of cyclic AMP delivery to the kinase isozymes. The general term "delivery" can encompass the mechanisms responsible for both selective cytosolic isozyme activation (as in calvarial cells) and particulate versus soluble enzyme (as in cardiomyocytes); the actual mechanisms may be similar or quite different.

We believe that two general mechanisms could accomplish selective cyclic AMP delivery to compartmentalized cA-PK: by compartmentation of adenylate cyclase responsive to different agents and thus of cyclic AMP synthesis, or by kinetic compartmentation of cyclic AMP diffusion to cA-PK.

Compartmentalized adenylate cyclase and cAMP synthesis require that hormones which differentially activate cA-PK do so by activating selective adenylate cyclase subsets. The cyclic AMP so generated would then exist in separate compartments at the time synthesized. Some data suggest that compartmentation of adenylate cyclase and thus cyclic AMP synthesis is plausible. Any hypothesis based on cyclic AMP synthesis in selective pools requires that adenylate cyclase catalytic unit be confined to a particular membrane domain. Proof that this can happen is lacking, but it is known that the cytoskeleton regulates catalytic activity in some manner (for a review, see Zor, 1983). It is possible that cytoskeletal anchoring of adenylate cyclase to a particular membrane fraction limits its diffusion so that functional domains are maintained. It is further possible that different adenylate cyclase domains could respond to hormones selectively. Tolkovski and Levitski (1978) found that in turkey erythrocytes $\beta$-adrenergic agonists apparently activate all adenylate cyclase catalytic units, and that each receptor may interact with each catalytic unit with specific combinations brought about by lateral diffusion within the plasma membrane (collision coupling). They found that adenosine receptors are not separately mobile, however, but coupled to catalytic units such that adenosine stimulates only 60–70% of total adenylate cyclase activity. If the adenosine-coupled catalytic units exist in a defined membrane compartment, then selective effects of $\beta$-adrenergic stimulation could be achieved by cyclic AMP synthesis in localized areas. The newly synthesized cyclic AMP would then be able to activate cA-PK within its domain, but under appropriate conditions of phosphodiesterase (PDE) activity, it would be unable to diffuse from its domain.

A purely kinetic model can also explain selective activation of cA-PK without requiring that adenylate cyclase be compartmentalized. Selective diffusion of cyclic AMP could be produced without physical separation of hormone receptors and adenylate cyclase catalytic units if different hormones activate the individual molecules of adenylate cyclase differentially. Adenylate cyclase activity and cyclic AMP synthesis and loss may be in such balance that only at high cyclic AMP synthetic rates at each catalytic unit will cyclic AMP diffuse into distant intracellular compartments. Slow synthesis of cyclic AMP would allow complete degradation by PDE; only with rapid synthesis would PDE activities be saturated and sufficient cAMP survive to diffuse away from membrane-bound PDE and into areas containing the selectively activatable cA-PK. Given this hypothesis, only certain hormones could stimulate local cyclic AMP concentrations above the threshold necessary for diffusion to the compartmentalized cA-PK before being hydrolyzed by localized phosphodiesterase.

This kinetic theory can explain how $PGE_2$ activates rat calvarial osteoblast cA-PK type II selectively (Livesey *et al.*, 1982); type II kinase might exist in a local compartment (e.g., plasma membrane), while type I exists outside the diffusion range of PGE-stimulated cyclic AMP synthesis. PTH activates both isozymes; in this case, PTH may cause adenylate cyclase to be activated at a greater rate, thus synthesizing cyclic AMP more rapidly. This could allow for a greater diffusion range before cyclic AMP is hydrolyzed. Similarly, the kinetic hypothesis put forward here can account for the observations of Hayes and Brunton that only isoproterenol activates particulate cA-PK by assuming (without good data for or against the assumption) that the membranes containing adenylate cyclase and cA-PK are separate and that cyclic AMP diffusion to the particulate cA-PK must occur. The kinetic model predicts that only isoproterenol stimulates adenylate cyclase in a way allowing cyclic AMP to diffuse to the membrane-bound cA-PK. Note that the compartments in which cA-PK isozymes are held need not be compartments with physical walls. The isozymes merely need to be held on membranes, or on various elements of the cytoskeleton, in different locations within a single cytoplasm.

A biochemical model describing how such kinetic compartmentation could occur can be drawn from the facts known about the adenylate cyclase system, with specific hypotheses made where facts are lacking. The adenylate cyclase activation model based upon experiments with S49 lymphoma cells and turkey erythrocytes has recently been reviewed by Gilman (1984) and Schramm and Selinger (1984). Hormone–receptor interactions accelerate the rate at which cyclic AMP is synthesized by accelerating the rate at which GTP binds to the intermediary GTP-binding regulatory protein, $G_s$. GTP activates $G_s$ by dissociating the active $\alpha$ subunit from the inhibitory $\beta$ unit. Activated $G_{s\alpha}$ increases the rate at which cyclic AMP is synthesized by the catalytic unit ($C_{ac}$). The stoichiometries of these interactions are unknown; it is also unknown whether all $G_s$ are alike or whether there are different $G_s$, each coupled to one receptor type. The event terminating catalytic unit activation is also unclear, i.e., whether GTP hydrolysis itself terminates $G_s$ activation. Indeed, whether an activated $G_s$ becomes deactivated only after binding and activating $C_{ac}$ has yet to be established, although experiments by Brandt *et al.* (1983) show that reconstitution of hormone-stimulated GTPase activity into a lipid bilayer requires only $G_s$ and a hormone receptor without any need for $C_{ac}$. It is probable that the total amount of $G_s$ is not rate limiting in cells, but rather that the activation rate of $G_s$ controls adenylate cyclase activity. Hormones increase the rate at which GTP binds $G_s$, although whether all hormones do so at equal rates has not been investigated systematically.

Hormone–receptor interactions may also lead to adenylate cyclase inhibition through activation of a similar though distinct GTP binding protein, $G_i$ (Gilman, 1984). Hormone-activated receptors can increase the rate at which GTP binds to the $\alpha$ subunit of $G_i$, leading to the dissociation of $\alpha$ and $\beta$ subunits. The activated $G_i$ may inhibit in two ways, although whether each potential mechanism operates *in vivo* has yet to be established. $G_{i\alpha}$ may directly inhibit $C_{ac}$, and the $G_{i\beta}$ dissociated from activated $G_i$ may bind and thus deactivate free $G_{s\alpha}$. Pertussis toxin, by catalyzing ADP-ribosylation of $G_{i\alpha}$, prevents the hormonal activation of $G_i$. This toxin thus reduces inhibitory activity and can increase adenylate cyclase activity.

Many hormones, including $\alpha_2$-adrenergic agonists and somatostatin, undoubtedly activate $G_i$, since their activity to reduce adenylate cyclase activity is inhibited by pertussis toxin. In a few instances it is now known that a single agonist acting at a single pharmacological class of receptors can activate both $G_s$ and $G_i$ and therefore stimulate as well as inhibit adenylate cyclase. The best studied example of this phenomenon is provided by Asano *et al.* (1984), who showed that reconstitution of $\beta$-adrenergic receptors and $G_i$ together into phospholipid vesicles allows isoproterenol-stimulated activation of $G_i$, albeit with slightly less efficiency than isoproterenol activation of similarly reconstituted $\beta$-receptors with $G_s$.

Kinetic compartmentation can be modeled in several plausible ways. It is presumed that if any hormone-specific compartmentation of cyclic AMP effect occurs, it must be given its specificity by the initial hormone–receptor interaction. We hypothesize that different hormonally activated receptors interact with a single population of $G_s$ that in turn interacts with a single population of $C_{ac}$. $C_{ac}$ activity is further hypothesized to exist either at only two rates (basal or activated; model 1) or at three rates (basal, singularly activated, or doubly activated; model 2). A schematic representation of these models is presented in Fig. 4. Note that while we have drawn $R_2$ with two activation sites for $G_s$, it could also be hypothesized that one site more active at $R_2$ than at $R_1$ exists. We further hypothesize that for kinetic compartmentation, there must be differences in the way each hormone–receptor complex interacts with $G_s$, and that this in and of itself determines the hormone-specific interaction of a single class of $G_{s\alpha}$ with a single $C_{ac}$ population. There must be a particular (probability) lifetime to each $G_{s\alpha}$–$C_{ac}$ interaction. If the $G_{s\alpha}$ deactivation rate is faster than activation by one hormone-activated receptor, but slower than activation by another, and presuming $G_{s\alpha}$ can be deactivated before interacting with $C_{ac}$, then the percentage of activated $G_{s\alpha}$ that reaches and activates $C_{ac}$ would be different for the two hormones. Unbinding of $G_{s\alpha}$ from $C_{ac}$ would terminate the activation, and both models require that a period would then be necessary before another $G_{s\alpha}$–$C_{ac}$ interaction occurs with a freshly activated $G_{s\alpha}$ before another cyclic AMP synthetic pulse could begin.

Differential hormone activation of $G_s$ might also be provided by the ability of a single agonist to regulate both $G_s$ and $G_i$. The relative efficiency of any one activated receptor to activate each $G_s$ and $G_i$ may determine the activation state of $G_s$ and thus ultimately of $C_{ac}$. Two hormones may produce different net $G_s$ activation by producing different degrees of $G_i$ activation without necessarily producing different rates of $G_s$ activation. Direct effects of $G_{i\alpha}$ on $C_{ac}$ may also contribute.

The total cyclic AMP synthesized locally under stimulation by any hormone would depend on the fraction of $C_{ac}$ activated in each microenvironment by $G_{s\alpha}$ during any unit time. The two models differ only in the requirement for the size of this microenvironment. Model 1 requires that a microenvironment consist of at least a few $C_{ac}$ units; model 2, which requires that each $C_{ac}$ be activatable in two stages, does not require more than one $C_{ac}$ unit in each microenvironment. These models assume collision coupling of the components of adenylate cyclase without any compartmentation of the components; all cellular hormone receptors are free to interact with each $G_s$ and $C_{ac}$.

Steady-state adenylate cyclase activity would be the sum of many pulses of many $C_{ac}$ units, but in the microenvironment of each $C_{ac}$ unit (model 2) or small $C_{ac}$ unit cluster (model 1), the pulsatile cyclic AMP synthesis could lead to kinetic compartmentation. Only at stimulated

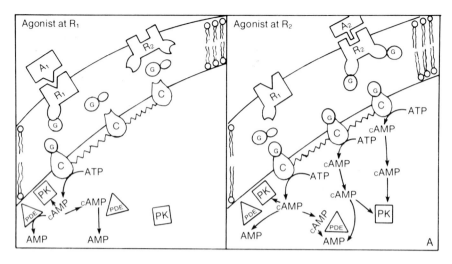

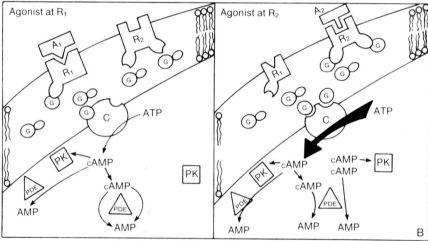

FIG. 4. Schematic representations of two models for selective activation of cyclic AMP-dependent protein kinase (PK). Model 1 (A) requires that several adenylate cyclase catalytic units ($C_{ac}$) are clustered and that one hormone-activated receptor is better able to activate $G_s$ than another. Schematically, receptor 1 ($R_1$) is drawn with one site for $G_s$ activation, while $R_2$ has two sites. It matters not whether $R_2$ has more sites or if each site is more efficient, but hormone-bound $R_2$ must activate more $G_s$ subunits per unit time than $R_1$. Under these conditions, membrane-bound cA-PK will be activated by either hormone. However, only when many $C_{ac}$ units within a cluster are activated simultaneously will sufficient cAMP be synthesized to occupy membrane-bound and soluble phosphodiesterase (PDE), permitting cAMP to diffuse to and thus activate cytoplasmic cA-PK. Model 2 (B) differs only in that $C_{ac}$ need not cluster to achieve different local cAMP synthesis rates. It is hypothesized in model 2 that the rate at which $C_{ac}$ synthesizes cAMP is directly dependent instead upon how many activated $G_s$ units simultaneously interact with it. Only with hormone 2 is the $G_s$ activation rate sufficient to drive cAMP synthesis maximally. Other features are as in model 1.

synthetic rates greater than some threshold would cyclic AMP diffuse from each $C_{ac}$ microenvironment before being eliminated by membrane-bound PDE hydrolysis or egress through the membrane. In model 1, rapid hormonal activation of $G_s$ would increase the probability that multiple $C_{ac}$ units within a microenvironment would be activated together before deactivation of each $G_{s\alpha}$; in model 2 the probability that two activated $G_{s\alpha}$ would together fully activate a $C_{ac}$ would be enhanced. The large cyclic AMP pulses generated in each microenvironment would allow more cyclic AMP to be delivered to intracellular cA-PK (albeit in short pulses) than would lower synthetic rates within the microenvironment stimulated by the hormone producing slower activation.

These models are fully consistent with experimental observations. Both homologous and heterologous desensitization can be accounted for without making any predictions concerning mechanism. Further, despite the necessarily quantal adenylate cyclase activation with these models, the overall cellular response would show the normal graded dose–response relationship to hormones. In either model, more hormone would activate additional receptors, which would lead to a greater number of $C_{ac}$ microenvironments becoming activated. This would produce normal log dose–response curves of hormone-activated adenylate cyclase.

In those tissues wherein two hormones combined activate adenylate cyclase no greater than either hormone alone, this model predicts that each hormone-activated receptor can activate $G_s$ fully, or that all $C_{ac}$ units are activatable by the $G_{s\alpha}$ affected by a single class of hormone-activated receptors. In either model, the faster activating hormone–receptor complex would dominate $G_s$ activation, and activation of all cA-PK forms would be expected. This prediction has been tested only in cardiomyocytes (Buxton and Brunton, 1983) in which isoproterenol and PGE combined activate particulate cA-PK like isoproterenol alone.

The two kinetic models presented are only the ones we believe most plausible; others are possible. If multiple classes of $G_s$ exist, one for each receptor, additional specificity can be built into the system. In this case, each receptor and thus hormone-specific $G_s$ would stimulate a single class of $C_{ac}$ at different rates. Individual $C_{ac}$ units could each constitute a microenvironment, and other features would be like model 2.

Whether such kinetic compartmentation occurs in cells is unknown. It is, however, possible, given the proper mix of adenylate cyclase and phosphodiesterase (or efflux) activities. Less complex schemes have previously been modeled more explicitly by several authors (Erneux *et al.*, 1980; Reynolds, 1982; Fell, 1980). Most important to understanding this hypothesis is an analysis by Fell (1980). He made some reasonable assumptions about the rates of a membrane-bound adenylate cyclase and low $K_m$ phosphodiesterase, of a soluble high $K_m$ phosphodiesterase, and of cyclic AMP diffusion into the interior of the cell. Under one simulation, Fell found that there could be 35 times as much cyclic AMP at the center of a hypothetical cell than at the membrane; other assumptions could lead to no more intracellular cyclic AMP than found at the intracellular membrane border. Given differential rates of adenylate cyclase activity (at least moment to moment) stimulated by each of two hormones and selective localization of adenylate cyclase and phosphodiesterase to membrane or cytosolic compartments, one can see that there may be quite different concentrations of cyclic AMP at intracellular sites without need for physical barriers to maintain compartmentation of the cyclic nucleotide. Selective activation of cA-PK isozymes compartmentalized by association with cytoplasmic proteins can be accomplished without physically compartmentalized cyclic AMP.

## 2. *Colocalization of Components and Interaction among Them*

Both physical and kinetic mechanisms can produce compartmentation of second messenger effect under appropriate conditions. Further, compartmentation of any one second messenger system can produce *de facto* compartmentation of others in many cases, due to the high degree of interaction among second messenger systems.

Examples of dually regulated processes are well known. Phosphorylase kinase is activated both by direct binding of $Ca^{2+}$ to integral calmodulin and by phosphorylation by cA-PK (Cohen *et al.*, 1978). Myosin light-chain kinase is activated by $Ca^{2+}$-calmodulin; the affinity with which myosin light-chain kinase binds calmodulin is decreased by prior phosphorylation of the enzyme by cA-PK (Adelstein *et al.*, 1978). Calcineurin, the $Ca^{2+}$-calmodulin-regulated protein phosphatase 2b, dephosphorylates the phospho-$R^{II}$ subunit of cA-PK (Klee *et al.*, 1983). Lamban, when phosphorylated by either cA-PK or a calmodulin-dependent protein kinase (LePeuch *et al.*, 1979), mediates $Ca^{2+}$ transport into cardiac sarcoplasmic reticulum (which then regulates how much $Ca^{2+}$ is available for cytoplasmic second messenger actions). Phosphatase 1 dephosphorylates proteins phosphorylated by both cA-PKs and $Ca^{2+}$-regulated protein kinases. The inhibitor of phosphatase

1, $I_1$, inhibits only when it is itself phosphorylated by cA-PK (Ingebritsen et al., 1983).

Cyclic nucleotides and calmodulin also interact in processes that regulate cyclic AMP concentration. Adenylate cyclase in some cell types, particularly neuronal, is regulated at least in part by calmodulin (Brostrom et al., 1975). The regulatory impact calmodulin makes in this situation is not known. However, adenylate cyclase from a Drosphila learning mutant, rutabaga, is biochemically characterized by the inability of calmodulin to stimulate its otherwise "normal" adenylate cyclase (Livingstone et al., 1984). Drosophila learning may thus be linked to effects of calmodulin on its adenylate cyclase. Calmodulin also impacts on cyclic AMP degradation. One phosphodiesterase isozyme is activated by calmodulin (Beavo et al., 1982). Thus, both synthesis and degradation of cyclic nucleotides can be regulated by calmodulin in certain cell types.

Some evidence also exists to link protein kinase C with adenylate cyclase. Protein kinase C is activated by phorbol esters, and phorbol esters reduce adenylate cyclase activity stimulated by glucagon or cholera toxin in rat hepatocytes [assayed with intact cells or membrane adenylate cyclase (Heyworth et al., 1984)]. In the latter study, phorbol esters reduced membrane adenylate cyclase activity by up to 20%, but only upon addition of $Ca^{2+}$, phosphatidyl serine, and ATP. Sibley et al. (1984) reported a 38% inhibition of duck erythrocyte adenylate cyclase activity by phorbol esters with concomitant phosphorylation, and thereby, they believe, regulation of $\beta$-adrenergic receptors.

The enzymes regulated by calmodulin and protein kinase C interact, since $Ca^{2+}$ is the second messenger used by each. Additionally, substrates have been found which are phosphorylated by both calmodulin kinases and protein kinase C, although the regulatory implications of these phosphorylations are not known (Nestler and Greengard, 1983).

The interactions between the second messenger systems are such that compartmentation of one system can effectively compartmentalize the actions of another second messenger system. If cA-PK action on myosin light-chain kinase were compartmentalized such that only a subset of the light-chain kinase could be phosphorylated, then the calmodulin effect would be compartmentalized as well. Calmodulin would stimulate the nonphosphorylated enzyme preferentially, effectively compartmentalizing calmodulin stimulation to the non-cA-PK-affected compartment, even though calmodulin is itself ubiquitous.

### 3. Synthesis and Action of Variant Forms of cA-PK Regulatory Subunits

Consistent with the role $R^I$ and $R^{II}$ play in inhibiting the kinase activity of the C subunit in the absence of cAMP, the cellular concentration of $R^I$ plus $R^{II}$ is generally equivalent to C. However, growth and hormones can induce changes in the molecular form of R and in the cellular content of R independent of C. Studies using the MCF-7 human breast cancer cell line (Kapoor and Cho-Chung, 1983) suggest that there is a complex relationship between the cell growth state, on the one hand, and the nuclear levels of $R^I$ subunits and the nuclear levels and form of the $R^{II}$ subunits, on the other. Cells grown in culture show both $R^I$ and $R^{II}$ in the nuclei during the initial stages of growth, with $R^{II}$ being localized specifically in the nucleolar region. After 3 days, when the cells form characteristic rosettes, the nuclear content of both $R^I$ and $R^{II}$ increased dramatically. Once a confluent monolayer was formed after 6 days of growth, nuclear $R^I$ and $R^{II}$ content fell to below baseline.

In studies by Kapoor *et al.* (1983), MCF-7 cells grown as tumors in nude mice required estrogen for growth. Nuclei isolated from growing tumors and precipitated with anti-$R^{II}$ sera contained the cAMP binding proteins with molecular weights of 34,000 and 44,000. After estrogen removal, the tumors regressed and new species of cAMP binding proteins precipitated by anti-$R^{II}$ appeared, with molecular weights of 50,000 and 52,000. These are the molecular weights that would be expected for undegraded and fully active $R^{II}$. Experimental $R^{II}$ isolation using protease inhibitors or purified undegraded $R^{II}$ added to cell extracts showed that the low apparent molecular weights of $R^{II}$ in the growing MCF-7 tumors were not due to proteolysis during nuclear preparation.

Richards and Rolfes (1980) and Richards *et al.* (1984) showed that follicle-stimulating hormone treatment of estrogen-primed ovarian graulosa cells caused selective 10- to 20-fold increases in the concentration of the $R^{II}$ subunit, with no corresponding change in $R^I$ or in the assayable amount of cAMP-dependent protein kinase activity. A cAMP binding protein identified in purified granulosa cell nuclei showed a molecular weight characteristic of $R^{II}$ or a modified form of $R^{II}$. Their data suggested that a cAMP binding protein (probably $R^{II}$) may control genomic events in differentiating granulosa cells.

There have been several reports that differential increases in $R^I$ develop in neuroblastoma–glioma hybrid cells, a model system for nerve tissue. Treatment of neuroblastoma–glioma hybrid cells with dibutyryl-cAMP causes an increase in intracellular content of $R^I$, while no significant changes occur in $R^{II}$ or in cAMP-dependent protein kinase activity (Walter *et al.*, 1979, 1981; Lohmann *et al.*, 1983). Treatment with $PGE_1$ or 3-isobutyl-1-methylxanthine, both of which increase cAMP content, mimicked the effect of dibutyryl-cAMP. The results obtained showed that the concentrations of $R^I$ and C were regulated independently in the neuroblastoma × glioma hybrid cells. Since dibutyryl-cAMP in the growth medium causes the cells to reduce their rate of division and produce long neurite-like extensions (Hemprecht, 1976), the high content of free $R^I$ concomitant with cell growth changes suggests that $R^I$ may be important in regulation of growth and differentiation in the tumor cells.

An $R^I$-like cAMP binding protein (R') has been found in neuroblastoma cells (Prashad, 1981). Dibutyryl-cAMP markedly stimulates the synthesis of R', but has no effect on $R^I$. R' did not bind to the C subunit of cAMP-dependent protein kinase, suggesting R' may have another function in the cell.

In a recent report by Robinson-Steiner *et al.* (1984), $R^{II}$'s of mammals were classified into six different forms based on SDS electrophoresis in Tris-glycine buffer and on steric exclusion (gel filtration) chromatography. Some of the differences in $R^{II}$ form appeared to correlate with species, but different forms of $R^{II}$ were found within one species and even within a single tissue. Two $R^{II}$'s were identified in bovine lung, bovine brain, rat adipose tissue, and *Erythrocebus patas* (monkey) heart. Several lines of evidence indicated that the diverse forms of $R^{II}$ were not derived from each other by proteolysis or through other post-translational modifications. Different forms of $R^{II}$ did not differ in interaction with cAMP and the C subunit. The rates of autophosphorylation were also similar. No important functional difference in these forms of $R^{II}$ were identified, but it is of course possible that the appropriate functional assay has yet to be developed.

The available data do not explain the existence of multiple forms of $R^{II}$, the function of R', or differentially increased concentration of $R^I$ or $R^{II}$ subunits without increased C. It is tempting to speculate that the novel forms of R which appear coincident with synthetic regulation of other proteins are themselves regulatory for a function other than protein kinase activity. Similarly, free R synthesized independent of C suggests independent function of R (although it is equally possible that the free R merely acts as a cyclic AMP buffer system to damp hormonal activation of cA-PK activity). Detailed knowledge of the compartmentation of these cyclic AMP binding proteins should provide insight into their potential function as second messengers in cellular regulation.

## III. Future Technology

### A. Site-Specific Antisera

Further understanding of the biological significance of compartmentalized second messenger systems will require more selective probes for the relevant molecules. FITC-coupled protein kinase inhibitor protein (Fletcher and Byus, 1982; Byus and Fletcher, 1982) has allowed cytofluorescent localization of free cA-PK catalytic unit without interference by concurrent holoenzyme detection. Presumptive sites of catalytic action can thus be determined. No similar probes are currently available for selective detection of either cA-PK holoenzyme to the exclusion of dissociated subunits or dissociated regulatory units alone. Such probes would improve our ability to detect hormone-dependent alterations of cA-PK activation state at any site. This capability might be especially valuable for understanding altered immunocytochemically localized cA-PK in nuclei of trophically stimulated cells, since each subunit could serve a distinct function in nuclear regulation.

Cyclic AMP-dependent protein kinase holoenzyme must be structually different from its separated subunits. The association site between the two subunit types must be outwardly directed only in the dissociated units, being hidden by each other in the holoenzyme. Additionally, fluorescence resonance studies indicate that there are conformational changes in the subunits upon binding cyclic AMP or each other (Smith *et al.*, 1981). It should be possible to produce antiserum probes to detect each of the conformationally different forms of the regulatory units. Unfortunately, previous attempts to do so have failed. No antisera have been produced which fully distinguish subunits from holoenzyme. Kapoor *et al.* (1979) found that one polyclonal antiserum raised to bovine $R^I$ recognized cyclic AMP-bound $R^I$ ~10-fold less well than depleted $R^I$, but insufficient supplies of the one bleed with this property precluded much investigation of this antiserum. Nevertheless, existence of such an antiserum, even with only 10-fold specificity, indicates that it should be possible to find others.

Several techniques may potentially allow one to direct antiserum production with the requisite specificity. The fact that no polyclonal or monoclonal antibody produced to date shows much specificity of this type indicates that the relevant sites are poor antigens. Techniques to enhance the immunogenicity of these sites must therefore be undertaken. One possible way to obtain specific antisera with selectivity for a single subclass of antigenic sites (epitopes) is by immunization with synthetic antigens. One may develop thereby an antiserum directed against a specific epitope and possibly an antiserum specific for a single site on the chosen protein. Alternatively, affinity purification of polyclonal antisera with a synthetic peptide of the desired site may accomplish the same purpose.

Synthetic peptide antigens have been used over the past 20 years to provide immunologists with clues to those properties of peptides that make good epitopes. Anderer (1963) first showed that immunization with a peptide could provide antisera capable of recognizing the intact parent protein. He showed that the C-terminal hexapeptide of tobacco mosaic virus coupled to bovine albumin could be used to elicit antisera recognizing the native viral protein.

Use of synthetic peptide antigens as tools to obtain antisera of defined specificity began about 5 years ago. Antisera raised in rabbits to large T antigen of simian virus 40 (SV40) recognize both large T antigen and small T antigen, presumably at their homologous region. Walter et al. (1980) showed that immunization of rabbits with synthetic peptides of the sequences found in each end of SV40 large T antigen produced antisera which recognized exclusively large T antigen.

Studies by Atassi and associates (Schmitz et al., 1983) have shown that the synthetic peptide used for immunization need not itself be an antigenic determinant (epitope) in the native molecule to induce production of antisera recognizing the intact protein. They have mapped all natural antigenic sites in sperm whale myoglobin. Two peptides (1–6 and 121–127) predicted to lie on the surface of the native molecule, but known not to be natural epitopes, were synthesized. Each, used in the free (unconjugated) form to immunize mice, elicited antisera and ultimately monoclonal antibodies which recognized specifically both the immunizing peptide and intact myoglobin by solid-phase radioimmunoassay.

Recent work by Niman et al. (1983) also indicates that antibodies raised against synthetic peptides frequently recognize the parent protein as well. On the other hand, not every peptide elicits antisera which recognize the native parent molecule. Even known antigenic sites may not be good antigens. Van Eldik et al. (1983) found that the major epitope of performic acid-oxidized calmodulin (peptide 137–143), presented to rabbits as the synthetic peptide coupled to keyhole limpet hemocyanin, elicits antisera recognizing only the immunizing or similar peptides and not native calmodulin in radioimmunoassay. These investigators did not determine whether the anti-peptide sera could recognize denatured calmodulin.

We have been attempting to raise antisera specific for dissociated cA-PK regulatory subunits in our own laboratories. In collaboration with Dr. Bruce Kemp, we have immunized rabbits with synthetic peptide 92–101 of bovine $R^{II}$ coupled to KLH. Antisera from each of three rabbits recognize the immunizing peptide and denatured rat $R^{II}$ using the Western transfer technique. The antisera, however, do not recognize $R^{II}$ without denaturing in detergent. Specificity of the antisera for the peptide-containing region of $R^{II}$ is indicated by the observation that the antisera recognize intact $R^{II}$ but not the 39,000-Da fragment of $R^{II}$ that lacks the region of the immunizing peptide.

Immunization of rabbits with the same peptide adsorbed to polyvinylpyrrolidone (Worobec *et al.*, 1972) proved less successful. Although all four rabbits immunized with PVP-$R^{II}$ peptide 94–101 developed antisera recognizing the peptide strongly, none of the antisera recognized native or denatured intact bovine $R^{II}$. Reduced conformational freedom of the peptide adsorbed to the polymer may have contributed to this lack of recognition.

## B. NONDESTRUCTIVE TISSUE PREPARATION

The detection of proteins and other molecules at the ultrastructural level by immunocytochemical techniques has been hindered by the severely reduced antigenicity of proteins in tissues treated with standard fixatives, especially glutaraldehyde. To circument this problem, the immunocytochemist has tried to utilize the lowest percentage of chemical fixative that maintains tissue preservation and allows the detection of the antigen. Usually the fraction of total antigenic sites detected is rather low (Sternberger, 1979).

We have developed recently (Linner and Steiner, unpublished observations) a procedure for the ultrastructural detection of proteins and water-soluble small molecules that we believe has great promise. Linner (unpublished observation) developed a tissue-drying procedure that utilizes low temperatures and high vacuum, so that water remains in a vitreous form without crystalizing. The water can then be sublimated out of the tissue by slow warming. Our preliminary results with a variety of tissues, including rat brain, skeletal muscle, liver, and kidney, indicate that ultra-thin sections of tissue can be obtained apparently free of ice crystal damage. Sections of unfixed tissues viewed at the ultrastructural level are virtually identical to sections of tissue prepared by fixation with glutaraldehyde.

These tissue sections should be superb for immunocytochemistry because the antigenic determinants of the proteins in the tissue have not been perturbed by fixation. We are starting experiments to test the adequacy of these tissue sections for immunocytochemistry. We are optimistic that this technological development will allow us to detect by electron microscopy cyclic nucleotides, protein kinase subunits, calmodulin, and other molecules involved in second messenger action. This development will help us to test our hypothesis of compartmentalized function of these messenger systems in hormone action.

## REFERENCES

Adelstein, R. S., Conti, M. A., Hathaway, D. R., and Klee, C. B. (1978). Phosphorylation of smooth muscle myosin light chain kinase by the catalytic subunit of adenosine 3':5'-monophosphate-dependent protein kinase. *J. Biol. Chem.* **253**, 8374–8350.

Alemany, S., Tung, H. Y. L., Shenolikar, S., Pilkis, S. J., and Cohen, P. (1984). Antibody to protein phosphatase 2A as a probe of phosphatase structure and function. *Eur. J. Biochem.* **145**, 51–56.

Anderer, F. A. (1963). Preparation and properties of an artificial antigen immunologically related to tobacco mosaic virus. *Biochim. Biophys. Acta* **71**, 246–248.

Arfmann, H.-A., Haase, E., and Schroter, H. (1981). High mobility group proteins from CHO cells and their modifications during cell cycle. *Biochem. Biophys. Res. Commun.* **101**, 137–143.

Ariano, M. A. (1983). Distribution of components of the guanosine 3',5'-phosphate system in rat caudate-putamen. *Neuroscience* **10**, 707–723.

Asano, T., Katada, T., Gilman, A. G., and Ross, E. M. (1984). Activation of the inhibitory GTP-binding protein of adenylate cyclase, $G_i$, by $\beta$-adrenergic receptors in reconstituted phospholipid vesicles. *J. Biol. Chem.* **259**, 9351–9354.

Barber, R., and Butcher, R. W. (1983). The egress of cyclic AMP from metazoan cells. *Adv. Cyclic Nucleotide Res.* **15**, 119–138.

Beale, E. G., Hartley, J. L., and Granner, D. K. (1982). $N^6,O^{2'}$-Dibutyryl-cyclic AMP and glucose regulate the amount of messenger RNA coding for hepatic phosphoenolpyruvate carboxykinase (GTP). *J. Biol. Chem.* **257**, 2022–2028.

Beavo, J. A., Hanson, R. S., Harrison, S. A., Hurwitz, R. L., Martins, T. J., and Mumby, M. C. (1982). Identification and properties of cyclic nucleotide phosphodiesterases. *Mol. Cell. Endocrinol.* **28**, 387–410.

Bloom, F. E., Hoffer, B. J., Battenberg, E. R., Siggins, G. R., Steiner, A. L., Parker, C. W., and Wedner, H. J. (1972). Adenosine 3',5'-monophosphate is localized in cerebellar neurons: Immunofluorescence evidence. *Science* **177**, 436–438.

Boney, C., Fink, D., Schlichter, D., Carr, K., and Wicks, W. D. (1983). Direct evidence that the protein kinase catalytic subunit mediates the effects of cAMP on tyrosine aminotransferase synthesis. *J. Biol. Chem.* **258**, 4911–4918.

Bonner, W. M. (1978). Protein migration and accumulation in nuclei. *In* "The Cell Nucleus" (H. Busch, ed.), Vol. 4, pp. 97–148. Academic Press, New York.

Brandt, D. R., Asano, T., Pedersen, S. E., and Ross, E. M. (1983). Reconstitution of catecholamine-stimulated guanosinetriphosphatase activity. *Biochemistry* **22**, 4357–4362.

Brostrom, C. O., Huang, Y.-C., Breckenridge, B. McL., and Wolff, D. J. (1975). Identification of a calcium-binding protein as a calcium-dependent regulator of brain adenylate cyclase. *Proc. Natl. Acad. Sci. U.S.A.* **72**, 64–68.

Browne, C. L., Lockwood, A. H., Su, J.-L., Beavo, J. A., and Steiner, A. L. (1980). Immunofluorescent localization of cyclic nucleotide-dependent protein kinases on the mitotic apparatus of cultured cells. *J. Cell Biol.* **87**, 336–345.

Browne, C. L., Lockwood, A. H., and Steiner, A. L. (1982). Localization of the regulatory subunit of type II cAMP-dependent protein kinase on the cytoplasmic microtubule network of cultured cells. *Cell Biol. Int. Rep.* **6**, 19–28.

Buxton, I. L. O., and Brunton, L. L. (1983). Compartments of cyclic AMP and protein kinase in mammalian cardiomyocytes. *J. Biol. Chem.* **258**, 10233–10239.

Byus, C. V., and Fletcher, W. H. (1982). Direct cytochemical localization of catalytic subunits dissociated from cAMP-dependent protein kinase in Reuber H-35 hepatoma cells. II. Temporal and spatial kinetics. *J. Cell Biol.* **93**, 727–734.

Byus, C. V., Klimpel, G. R., Lucas, D. O., and Russell, D. H. (1978). Ornithine decarboxylase induction in mitogen-stimulated lymphocytes is related to the specific activation of type I adenosine cyclic 3′,5′-monophosphate-dependent protein kinase. *Mol. Pharmacol.* **14**, 431–441.

Byus, C. V., Hayes, J. S., Brendel, K., and Russell, D. H. (1979). Regulation of glycogenolysis in isolated rat hepatocytes by the specific activation of type I cyclic AMP-dependent protein kinase. *Mol. Pharmacol.* **16**, 941–949.

Cimbala, M. A., Lamers, W. H., Nelson, K., Monahan, J. E., Yoo-Warren, H., and Hanson, R. W. (1982). Rapid changes in the concentration of phosphoenolpyruvate carboxykinase mRNA in rat liver and kidney. Effects of insulin and cyclic AMP. *J. Biol. Chem.* **257**, 7629–7636.

Clegg, J. S. (1984). Properties and metabolism of the aqueous cytoplasm and its boundaries. *Am. J. Physiol.* **246**, R133–R151.

Cohen, P. (1980). The role of calcium ions, calmodulin and troponin in the regulation of phosphorylase kinase from rabbit skeletal muscle. *Eur. J. Biochem.* **111**, 563–574.

Cohen, P., Burchell, A., Foulkes, J. G., Cohen, P. T. W., Vanaman, T. C., and Nairn, A. C. (1978). Identification of the $Ca^{2+}$ dependent modulator protein as the fourth subunit of rabbit skeletal muscle phosphorylase kinase. *FEBS Lett.* **92**, 287–291.

Cohen, P., Nimmo, G. A., Shenolikar, S., and Foulkes, J. G. (1979). The role of inhibitor-1 in the cyclic AMP-mediated control of glycogen metabolism in skeletal muscle. *In* "Cyclic Nucleotides and Protein Phosphorylation in Cell Regulation" (E. G. Krause, ed.), pp. 161–169. Pergamon, Oxford.

Corbin, J. D., Keely, S. L., and Park, C. R. (1975). The distribution and dissociation of cyclic adenosine 3′,5′-monophosphate-dependent protein kinases in adipose, cardiac, and other tissues. *J. Biol. Chem.* **250**, 218–225.

Dabauvalle, M. C., and Franke, W. W. (1984). Karyophobic proteins. *Exp. Cell Res.* **153**, 308–325.

Davies, J. I., and Williams, P. A. (1975). Quantitative aspects of the regulation of cellular cyclic AMP levels. I. Structure and kinetics of a model system. *J. Theor. Biol.* **53**, 1–30.

DeRobertis, E. (1983). Nucleocytoplasmic segregation of proteins and RNAs. *Cell* **32**, 1021–1025.

Dingwall, C., Sharnick, S. V., and Laskey, R. A. (1982). A polypeptide domain that specifies migration of nucleoplasmin into the nucleus. *Cell* **30**, 449–458.

Dopere, F., and Stalmans, W. (1982). Release and activation of phosphorylase phosphatase upon rupture of organelles from rat liver. *Biochem. Biophys. Res. Commun.* **104**, 443–450.

Doskeland, S. O., and Ogreid, D. (1981). Binding proteins for cyclic AMP in mammalian tissues. *Int. J. Biochem.* **13**, 1–19.

Engel, W. K. (1961). Cytological localization of glycogen in cultured skeletal muscles. *J. Histochem. Cytochem.* **9**, 38–42.

Erneux, C., Boeynaems, J.-M., and Dumont, J. E. (1980). Theoretical analysis of the consequences of cyclic nucleotide phosphodiesterase negative cooperativity. Amplification and positive cooperativity of cyclic AMP accumulation. *Biochem. J.* **192**, 241–246.

Falbriard, J.-G., Posternak, T., and Sutherland, E. W. (1967). Preparation of derivatives of adenosine 3′,5′-phosphate. *Biochim. Biophys. Acta* **148**, 99–105.

Fallon, E. F., Agrawal, R., Furth, E., Steiner, A. L., and Cowden, R. (1974). Cyclic guanosine and adenosine 3′,5′-monophosphates in canine thyroid; localization by immunofluorescence. *Science* **184**, 1089–1091.

Feldherr, C. M., and Pomerantz, J. (1978). Mechanism for the selection of nuclear polypeptides in *Xenopus* oocytes *J. Cell Biol.* **78**, 168–175.

Feldherr, C. M., Cohen, R. J., and Ogburn, J. A. (1983). Evidence for mediated protein uptake by amphibian oocyte nuclei. *J. Cell Biol.* **96**, 1486–1490.

Fell, D. A. (1980). Theoretical analyses of the functioning of high- and low-$K_m$ cyclic nucleotide phosphodiesterases in the regulation of the concentration of adenosine 3′,5′-cyclic monophosphate in animal cells. *J. Theor. Biol.* **84**, 361–385.

Flandroy, L., Cheung, W. Y., and Steiner, A. L. (1983). Immunofluorescent localization of cGMP, cGMP-dependent protein kinase, calmodulin and cAMP in the rat uterus. *Cell Tissue Res.* **233**, 639–646.

Fleischer, N., Rosen, O. M., and Reichlin, M. (1976). Radioimmunoassay of bovine heart protein kinase. *Proc. Natl. Acad. Sci. U.S.A.* **73**, 54–58.

Fletcher, W. H., and Byus, C. V. (1982). Direct cytochemical localization of catalytic subunits dissociated from cAMP-dependent protein kinase in Reuber H-35 hepatoma cells. I. Development and validation of fluorescinated inhibitor. *J. Cell Biol.* **93**, 719–726.

Foulkes, J. G., Cohen, P., Strada, S. J., Everson, W. V., and Jefferson, L. S. (1982). Antagonistic effects of insulin and β-adrenergic agonists on the activity of protein phosphatase inhibitor-1 in skeletal muscle of the perfused rat hemicorpus. *J. Biol. Chem.* **257**, 12493–12496.

Gilman, A. G. (1970). A protein binding assay for adenosine 3′,5′-cyclic monophosphate. *Proc. Natl. Acad. Sci. U.S.A.* **67**, 305–312.

Gilman, A. G. (1984). G proteins and dual control of adenylate cyclase. *Cell* **36**, 577–579.

Goldstein, L. (1958). Localization of nucleus specific protein as shown by transplantation experiments in amoeba proteus. *Exp. Cell Res.* **15**, 635–637.

Gurdon, J. B. (1968). Changes in somatic cell nuclei inserted into growing and maturing amphibian oocytes. *J. Embryol. Exp. Morphol.* **20**, 401–414.

Gurdon, J. B. (1970). Nuclear transplantation and the control of gene activity in animal development. *Proc. R. Soc. London Ser. B* **176**, 303–314.

Hamprecht, B. (1976). Neuron models. *Angew. Chem. Int. Ed. Engl.* **15**, 194–206.

Harper, J. F., and Steiner, A. L. (1983). Immunofluorescence localization of calmodulin in unfixed frozed tissue sections. *In* "Methods in Enzymology" (A. R. Means and B. W. O'Malley, eds.), Vol. 102, Part G, pp. 122–135. Academic Press, New York.

Harper, J. F., Cheung, W. Y., Wallace, R. W., Huang, H.-L., Levine, S. N., and Steiner, A. L. (1980). Localization of calmodulin in rat tissues. *Proc. Natl. Acad. Sci. U.S.A.* **77**, 366–370.

Harper, J. F., Wallace, R. W., Cheung, W. Y., and Steiner, A. L. (1981). ACTH stimulated changes in the immunocytochemical localization of cyclic nucleotides, protein kinases, and calmodulin. *Adv. Cyclic Nucleotide Res.* **14**, 581–591.

Harrison, J. J., Schwoch, G., Schweppe, J. S., and Jungmann, R. A. (1982). Phosphorylative modification of histone H1 subspecies following isoproterenol and $N^6,O^{2′}$-dibutyryl-cyclic AMP stimulation of rat C6 glioma cells. *J. Biol. Chem.* **257**, 13601–13609.

Hathaway, D. R., Adelstein, R. S., and Klee, C. B. (1981). Interaction of calmodulin with myosin light-chain kinase and cAMP-dependent protein kinase in bovine brain. *J. Biol. Chem.* **256**, 8183–8189.

Hayes, J. S., Brunton, L. L., Brown, J. H., Reese, J. B., and Mayer, S. E. (1979). Hormonally specific expression of cardiac protein kinase activity. *Proc. Natl. Acad. Sci. U.S.A.* **76**, 1570–1574.

Hayes, J. S., Brunton, L. L., and Mayer, S. E. (1980). Selective activation of particulate cAMP-dependent protein kinase by isoproterenol and prostaglandin $E_1$. *J. Biol. Chem.* **255**, 5113–5119.

Hayes, J. S., Bowling, N., King, K. L., and Boder, G. B. (1982). Evidence for selective regulation of the phosphorylation of myocyte proteins by isoproterenol and prostaglandin $E_1$. *Biochim. Biophys. Acta* **714**, 136–142.

Heyworth, C. M., Whetton, A. D., Kinsella, A. R., and Houslay, M. D. (1984). The phorbol ester, TPA inhibits glucagon-stimulated adenylate cyclase activity. *FEBS Lett.* **170**, 38–42.

Hofmann, F., Bechtel, P. J., and Krebs, E. G. (1977). Concentrations of cyclic AMP-dependent protein kinase subunits in various tissues. *J. Biol. Chem.* **252**, 1441–1447.

Ingebritsen, T. S., and Cohen, P. (1983). The protein phosphatases involved in cellular regulation. 1. Classification and substrate specificities. *Eur. J. Biochem.* **132**, 255–261.

Ingebritsen, T. S., Stewart, A. A., and Cohen, P. (1983). The protein phosphatases involved in cellular regulation. 6. Measurement of type 1 and type 2 protein phosphatases in extracts of mammalian tissues; an assessment of their physiological roles. *Eur. J. Biochem.* **132**, 297–307.

Iynedjian, P. B., and Hanson, R. W. (1977). Increase in level of functional messenger RNA coding for phosphoenolpyruvate carboxykinase (GTP) during induction by cyclic adenosine $3',5'$-monophosphate. *J. Biol. Chem.* **252**, 655–662.

Jamrich, M., Greenleaf, A. L., and Bautz, E. K. F. (1977). Localization of RNA polymerase in polytene chromosomes of *Drosophila melanogaster. Proc. Natl. Acad. Sci. U.S.A.* **74**, 2079–2083.

Johnson, E. M., and Allfrey, V. G. (1972). Differential effects of cyclic adenosine-$3',5'$-monophosphate on phosphorylation of rat liver nuclear acidic proteins. *Arch. Biochem. Biophys.* **152**, 786–794.

Jungmann, R. A., Christensen, M. L., Schweppe, J. S., Mednieks, M. I., and Spielvogel, A. M. (1976). Cyclic AMP-mediated nuclear translocation of cytoplasmic cAMP-dependent protein kinases: Identity of the nuclear and cytoplasmic enzymes. *In* "Cyclic Nucleotides and the Regulation of Cell Growth" (M. Abou-Sabe, ed.), pp. 225–251. Dowden, Hutchinson, & Ross, Stroudsburg, Pennsylvania.

Jungmann, R. A., Mednieks, M. I., and Schweppe, J. S. (1980). Nuclear compartmentation of protein kinase and the regulation of gene expression. *In* "Cell Compartmentation and Metabolic Channeling" (L. Nover, F. Lynen, and K. Mothes, eds.), pp. 415–426. Elseveir, Amsterdam.

Jungmann, R. A., Derda, D. F., Kelley, D. C., Miles, M. F., Milkowski, D., and Schweppe, J. S. (1983a). Regulation of lactate dehydrogenase gene expression. *Curr. Top. Biol. Med. Res.* **7**, 161–174.

Jungmann, R. A., Kelly, D. C., Miles, M. F., and Milkowski, D. M. (1983b). Cyclic AMP regulation of lactate dehydrogenase. Isoproterenol and $N^6,O^{2'}$-dibutyryl-cyclic AMP increase the rate of transcription and change the stability of lactate dehydrogenase A subunit messenger RNA in rat C6 glioma cells. *J. Biol. Chem.* **258**, 5312–5318.

Jurgensen, S. (1984). Inhibition of the Mg(II)-ATP-dependent phosphatase by cAMP-dependent protein kinase regulatory subunit. *Fed. Proc., Fed. Am. Soc. Exp. Biol.* **43**, 1899.

Kapoor, C. L., and Cho-Chung, Y. S. (1983). Compartmentalization of regulatory subunits of cyclic adenosine 3',5'-monophosphate-dependent protein kinases in MCF-7 human breast cancer cells. *Cancer Res.* **43**, 295–302.

Kapoor, C. L., and Steiner, A. L. (1982). Immunocytochemistry of cyclic nucleotides and their kinases. *Handb. Exp. Pharmacol.* **58/I** 333–354.

Kapoor, C. L., Beavo, J. A., and Steiner, A. L. (1979). Radioimmunoassay for the regulatory subunit of type I cAMP-dependent protein kinase. *J. Biol. Chem.* **254**, 12427–12432.

Kapoor, C. L., Grantham, F., and Cho-Chung, Y. S. (1983). Appearance of 50,000- and 52,000-dalton cAMP receptor proteins in the nucleoli of regressing MCF-7 human breast cancer upon estrogen withdrawal. *Cell Biol. Int. Rep.* **7**, 937–946.

Keely, S. L., Corbin, J. D., and Park, C. R. (1975). On the question of translocation of heart cAMP-dependent protein kinase. *Proc. Natl. Acad. Sci. U.S.A.* **72**, 1501–1504.

Kempner, E. S., and Miller, J. H. (1968a). The molecular biology of *Euglena gracilis*. IV. Cellular stratification by centrifuging. *Exp. Cell Res.* **51**, 141–149.

Kempner, E. S., and Miller, J. H. (1968b). The molecular biology of *Euglena gracilis*. V. Enzyme localization. *Exp. Cell Res.* **51**, 150–156.

Klee, C. B., Krinks, M. H., Manalan, A. S., Cohen, P., and Stewart, A. A. (1983). Isolation and characterization of bovine brain calcineurin: A calmodulin-stimulated protein phosphatase. *In* "Methods in Enzymology" (A. R. Means and B. W. O'Malley, eds.), Vol. 102, Part G, pp. 227–244. Academic Press, New York.

Klockmann, U., and Deppert, W. (1983). Acylation: A new posttranslational modification specific for plasma membrane associated simian virus 40 large T antigen. *FEBS Lett.* **151**, 257–259.

Klumpp, S., Steiner, A. L., and Schultz, J. E. (1983). Immunocytochemical localization of cyclic GMP, cGMP-dependent protein kinase, calmodulin, and calcineurin in *Paramecium tetraurelia. Eur. J. Cell Biol.* **32**, 164–170.

Koide, Y., Earp, H. S., Ong, S.-H., and Steiner, A. L. (1978). Alterations in the intracellular distribution of cGMP and guanylate cyclase activity during rat liver regeneration. *J. Biol. Chem.* **253**, 4439–4445.

Koide, Y., Beavo, J. A., Kapoor, C. L., Spruill, W. A., Huang, H.-L., Levine, S. N., Ong, S.-L., Bechtel, P. J., Yount, W. J., and Steiner, A. L. (1981). Hormonal effects on the immunocytochemical location of 3',5'-cyclic adenosine monophosphate-dependent protein kinase in rat tissues. *Endocrinology* **109**, 2226–2238.

Kuo, J. F., and Greengard, P. (1969). Cyclic nucleotide-dependent protein kinases. IV. Widespread occurrence of adenosine 3',5'-monophosphate-dependent protein kinase in various tissues and phyla of the animal kingdom. *Proc. Natl. Acad. Sci. U.S.A.* **64**, 1349–1355.

Laks, M. S., Harrison, J. J., Schwoch, G., and Jungmann, R. A. (1981). Modulation of nuclear protein kinase activity and phosphorylation of histone H1 subspecies during the prereplicative phase of rat liver regeneration. *J. Biol. Chem.* **256**, 8775–8785.

Lamers, W. H., Hanson, R. W., and Meisner, H. M. (1982). cAMP stimulates transcription of the gene for cytosolic phosphoenolpyruvate carboxykinase in rat liver nuclei. *Proc. Natl. Acad. Sci. U.S.A.* **79**, 5137–5141.

Lanford, R. E., and Butel, J. S. (1980). Biochemical characterization of nuclear and cytoplasmic forms of SV40 tumor antigens encoded by parental and transport-defective mutant SV40-adenovirus 7 hybrid viruses. *Virology* **105**, 314–327.

Lawrence, J. C., Jr., Hiken, J. F., DePaoli-Roach, A. A., and Roach, P. J. (1983). Hormonal control of glycogen synthase in rat hemidiaphragms: Effects of insulin and epinephrine on the distribution of phosphate between two cyanogen bromide fragments *J. Biol. Chem.* **258**, 10710–10719.

LePeuch, C. J., Haiech, J., and Demaille, J. G. (1979). Concerted regulation of cardiac sarcoplasmic reticulum calcium transport by cyclic adenosine monophosphate-dependent and calcium-calmodulin-dependent phosphorylations. *Biochemistry* **18,** 5150–5157.

Lillie, R. D. (1947). Malt diastase and ptyalin in place of saliva in the identification of glycogen. *Stain Technol.* **22,** 76–70.

Livesey, S. A., Kemp, B. E., Re, C. A., Partridge, N. C., and Martin, T. J. (1982). Selective hormonal activation of cyclic AMP-dependent protein kinase isoenzymes in normal and malignant osteoblasts. *J. Biol. Chem.* **257,** 14983–14987.

Livesey, S. A., Collier, G., Zajac, J. D., Kemp, B. E., and Martin, T. J. (1984). Characteristics of selective activation of cyclic AMP-dependent protein kinase isoenzymes by calcitonin and prostaglandin $E_2$ in human breast cancer cells. *Biochem. J.* **244,** 361–370.

Livingstone, M. S., Sziber, P. P., and Quinn, W. G. (1984). Loss of calcium/calmodulin responsiveness in adenylate cyclase of rutabaga, a *Drosophila* learning mutant. *Cell* **37,** 205–215.

Lohmann, S. M., Schwoch, G., Reiser, G., Port, R., and Walter, U. (1983). Dibutyryl-cAMP treatment of neuroblastoma–glioma hybrid cells results in selective increase in cAMP-receptor protein (R-I) as measured by monospecific antibodies. *EMBO J.* **2,** 153–159.

Marcum, J. M., Dedman, J. R., Brinkley, B. R., and Means, A. R. (1978). Control of microtubule assembly–disassembly by calcium-dependent regulator protein. *Proc. Natl. Acad. Sci. U.S.A.* **75,** 3771–3775.

Masters, C. (1984). Interactions between glycolytic enzymes and components of the cytomatrix. *J. Cell Biol.* **99,** 222s–225s.

Mastro, A. M., and Keith, A. D. (1984). Diffusion in the aqueous compartment. *J. Cell Biol.* **99,** 180s–187s.

Means, A. R., and Dedman, J. R. (1980). Calmodulin—An intracellular calcium receptor. *Nature (London)* **285,** 73–77.

Meyer, F., Heilmeyer, L. M. G., Haschke, R. H., and Fischer, E. H. (1970). Control of phosphorylase activity in a muscle glycogen particle. *J. Biol. Chem.* **245,** 6642–6648.

Mitchell, S. J., and Kleinsmith, L. J. (1983). Nuclear protein kinases. *In* "Chromosomal Nonhistone Proteins" (L. S. Hnilica, ed.), Vol. 3, pp. 131–171. CRC Press, Boca Raton, Florida.

Moore, P. B., and Dedman, J. R. (1982). Calcium binding proteins and cellular regulation. *Life Sci.* **31,** 2937–2946.

Murdoch, G. H., Franco, R., Evans, R. M., and Rosenfeld, M. G. (1983). Polypeptide hormone regulation of gene expression. Thyrotropin-releasing hormone rapidly stimulates both transcription of the prolactin gene and the phosphorylation of a specific nuclear protein. *J. Biol. Chem.* **258,** 15329–15335.

Murtaugh, M. P., Steiner, A. L., and Davies, P. J. A. (1982). Localization of the catalytic subunit of cAMP-dependent protein kinase in cultured cells using a specific antibody. *J. Cell Biol.* **95,** 64–72.

Nahas, N., Juhl, H., and Esmann, V. (1984). Chromatographic characteristics and subcellular localization of synthase phosphatase, phosphorylase phosphatase and histone phosphatase in human polymorphonuclear leukocytes. *Mol. Cell. Biochem.* **58,** 147–156.

Nemenoff, R. A., Blackshear, P. J., and Avruch, J. (1983). Hormonal regulation of protein dephosphorylation. Identification and hormonal regulation of protein phosphatase inhibitor-1 in rat adipose tissue. *J. Biol. Chem.* **258,** 9437–9443.

Nestler, E. J., and Greengard, P. (1983). Protein phosphorylation in the brain. *Nature (London)* **305**, 583–588.

Ng, K. W., Livesey, S. A., Larkins, R. G., and Martin, T. J. (1983). Calcitonin effects on growth and on selective activation of type II isoenzyme of cyclic adenosine 3',5'-monophosphate-dependent protein kinase in T 47D human breast cancer cells. *Cancer Res.* **43**, 794–800.

Niman, H. L., Houghten, R. A., Walker, L. E., Reisfeld, R. A., Wison, I. A., Hogle, J. M., and Lerner, R. A. (1983). Generation of protein-reactive antibodies by short peptides is an event of high frequency: Implications for the structural basis of immune recognition. *Proc. Natl. Acad. Sci. U.S.A.* **80**, 4949–4953.

Nishizuka, Y. (1984). Turnover of inositol phospholipids and signal transduction. *Science* **225**, 1365–1370.

Noguchi, T., Diesterhaft, M., and Granner, D. (1982). Evidence for a dual effect of dibutyryl-cyclic AMP on the synthesis of tyrosine aminotransferase in rat liver. *J. Biol. Chem.* **257**, 2386–2390.

Ong, S.-H., Whitley, T. H., Stowe, N. W., and Steiner, A. L. (1975). Immunohistochemical localization of 3',5'-cyclic AMP and 3',5'-cyclic GMP in rat liver, intestine and testis. *Proc. Natl. Acad. Sci. U.S.A.* **72**, 2022–2026.

Ortez, R. A., Sikes, R. W., an Sperling, H. G. (1980). Immunohistochemical localization of cyclic GMP in goldfish retina. *J. Histochem. Cytochem.* **28**, 263–270.

Paine, P. L. (1984). Diffusive and nondiffusive proteins *in vivo*. *J. Cell Biol.* **99**, 185s–195s.

Parker, P. J., Caudwell, F. B., and Cohen, P. (1983). Glycogen synthase from rabbit skeletal muscle; effect of insulin on the state of phosphorylation of the seven phosphoserine residues *in vivo*. *Eur. J. Biochem.* **130**, 227–234.

Porter, K. R., Berkerle, M., and McNiven, M. (1983). The cytoplasmic matrix. *Mod. Cell Biol.* **2**, 259–302.

Potter, J. D., and Johnson, J. D. (1982). Troponin. *In* "Calcium and Cell Function" (W. Y. Cheung, ed.), Vol. 2, pp. 145–169. Academic Press, New York.

Prashad, N. (1981). Induction of free cyclic-AMP-binding protein by dibutyryl-cyclic AMP in neuroblastoma cells. *Cold Spring Harbor Conf. Cell Prolif.* **8**, 159–178.

Pryzwansky, K. B., Steiner, A. L., Spitznagel, J. K., and Kapoor, C. L. (1981). Compartmentalization of cyclic AMP during phagocytosis by human neutrophilic granulocytes. *Science* **211**, 407–410.

Reynolds, C. H. (1982). Simulations of the roles of multiple cyclic nucleotide phosphodiesterases. *Biochem. J.* **202**, 125–132.

Richards, J. S., and Rolfes, A. I. (1980). Hormonal regulation of cyclic AMP binding to specific receptor proteins in rat ovarian follicles. Characterization by photoaffinity labeling. *J. Biol. Chem.* **255**, 5481–5489.

Richards, J. S., Haddox, M., Tash, J. S., Walter, U., and Lohmann, S. (1984). Adenosine 3',5'-monophosphate-dependent protein kinase and granulosa cell responsiveness to gonadotropins. *Endocrinology* **114**, 2190–2198.

Robinson-Steiner, A. M., Beebe, S. J., Rannels, S. R., and Corbin, J. D. (1984). Microheterogeneity of type II cAMP-dependent protein kinase in various mammalian species and tissues. *J. Biol. Chem.* **259**, 10596–10605.

Robison, G. A., Butcher, R. W., and Sutherland, E. W. (1971). "Cyclic AMP." Academic Press, New York.

Rosenfeld, M. G., Amara, S. G., Birnberg, N. C., Mermod, J.-J., Murdoch, G. H., and Evans, R. M. (1983). Calcitonin, prolactin, and growth hormone gene expression as model systems for the characterization of neuroendocrine regulation. *Recent Prog. Horm. Res.* **39**, 305–351.

Saffer, J. D., and Glazer, R. I. (1982). The phosphorylation of high-mobility group proteins 14 and 17 and their distribution in chromatin. *J. Biol. Chem.* **257**, 4655–4660.

Sarkar, D., Erlichman, J., and Rubin, C. S. (1984). Identification of a calmodulin-binding protein that copurifies with the regulatory subunit of brain protein kinase II. *J. Biol. Chem.* **259**, 9840–9846.

Scheidtmann, K. H., Schickendanz, J., Walter, G., Lanford, R. E., and Butel, J. S. (1984). Differential phosphorylation of cytoplasmic and nuclear variants of simian virus 40 large T antigen encoded by simian virus 40 adenovirus hybrid viruses. *J. Virol.* **50**, 636–640.

Schmitz, H. E., Atassi, H., and Atassi, M. Z. (1983). Production of monoclonal antibodies to surface regions that are non-immunogenic in a protein using free synthetic peptide as immunogens: Demonstration with sperm-whale myoglobin. *Immunol. Commun.* **12**, 161–175.

Schramm, M., and Selinger, Z. (1984). Message transmission: Receptor controlled adenylate cyclase system. *Science* **225**, 1350–1356.

Schwoch, G. (1978). Differential activation of type I and type II adenosine 3',5'-cyclic monophosphate-dependent protein kinases in liver of glucagon-treated rats. *Biochem. J.* **170**, 469–477.

Schwoch, G., Hamann, A., and Hilz, H. (1980). Antiserum against the catalytic subunit of adenosine 3',5'-cyclic monphosphate-dependent protein kinase. Reactivity toward various protein kinases. *Biochem. J.* **192**, 223–230.

Shenolikar, S., and Steiner, A. L. (1984). Immunological approach to the study of hormone action: Regulation of the phosphorylation state of protein phosphatase inhibitor-1 by hormones. *Adv. Cyclic Nucleotide Res.* **17**, 405–415.

Sibley, D. R., Nambi, P., Peters, J. R., and Lefkowitz, R. J. (1984). Phorbol diesters promote β-adrenergic receptor phosphorylation and adenylate cyclase desensitization in duck erythrocytes. *Biochem. Biophys. Res. Commun.* **121**, 973–979.

Sigel, P., and Pette, D. (1969). Intracellular localization of glycogenolytic and glycolytic enzymes in white and red rabbit skeletal muscle. *J. Histochem. Cytochem.* **17**, 225–229.

Siggins, G. R., Battenberg, E. F., Hoffer, B. J., Bloom, F. E., and Steiner, A. L. (1973). Non-adrenergic stimulation of cyclic adenosine monophosphate in rat Purkinje neurons: An immunocytochemical study. *Science* **179**, 585–588.

Smith, J. W., Steiner, A. L., Newberry, W. M., and Parker, C. W. (1971). Cyclic adenosine 3',5'-monophosphate in human lymphocytes. Alterations after phytohemagglutinin stimulation. *J. Clin. Invest.* **50**, 432–441.

Smith, S. B., White, H. D., Siegel, J. B., and Krebs, E. G. (1981). Cyclic AMP-dependent protein kinase I: Cyclic nucleotide binding, structural changes, and release of the catalytic subunits. *Proc. Natl. Acad. Sci. U.S.A.* **78**, 1591–1595.

Spielvogel, A. M., Mednieks, M. I., Eppenberger, U., and Jungmann, R. A. (1977). Evidence for the identity of nuclear and cytoplasmic adenosine-3',5'-monophosphate-dependent protein kinase from porcine ovaries and nuclear translocation of the cytoplasmic enzyme. *Eur. J. Biochem.* **73**, 199–212.

Spruill, A., and Steiner, A. (1976). Immunohistochemical localization of cyclic nucleotides during testicular development. *J. Cyclic Nucleotide Res.* **2**, 225–239.

Spruill, W. A., Hurwitz, D. R., Lucchesi, J. C., and Steiner, A. L. (1978). Association of cyclic GMP with gene expression of polytene chromosomes of *Drosophila melanogaster*. *Proc. Natl. Acad. Sci. U.S.A.* **75**, 1480–1484.

Steiner, A. L., Kipnis, D. M., Utiger, R., and Parker, C. (1969). Radioimmunoassay for the measurement of adenosine 3',5'-cyclic phosphate. *Proc. Natl. Acad. Sci. U.S.A.* **64**, 367–373.

Steiner, A. L., Parker, C. W., and Kipnis, D. M. (1972). Radioimmunoassay for cyclic nucleotides. I. Preparation of antibodies and iodinized cyclic nucleotides. *J. Biol. Chem.* **247**, 1106–1113.

Steiner, A. L., Ong, S.-H., and Wedner, H. J. (1976). Cyclic nucleotide immunocyto-chemistry. *Adv. Cyclic Nucleotide Res.* **7**, 115–155.

Steiner, A. L., Koide, Y., Earp, H. S., Bechtel, P. J., and Beavo, J. A. (1978). Compart-mentalization of cyclic nucleotides and cyclic AMP-dependent protein kinases in rat liver: Immunocytochemical demonstration. *Adv. Cyclic Nucleotide Res.* **9**, 691–705.

Sternberger, L. A. (1979). "Immunocytochemistry," 2nd Ed. Wiley, New York.

Tallant, E. A., Wallace, R. W., and Cheung, W. Y. (1983). Purification and radioimmu-noassay of calmodulin-dependent protein phosphatase from bovine brain. *In* "Meth-ods in Enzymology" (A. R. Means and B. W. O'Malley, eds.), Vol. 102, Part G, pp. 244–256. Academic Press, New York.

Theurkauf, W. E., and Vallee, R. B. (1982). Molecular characterization of the cAMP-dependent protein kinase bound to microtubule-associated protein 2. *J. Biol. Chem.* **257**, 3284–3290.

Tolkovski, A. M. and Levitzki, A. (1978). Coupling of a single adenylate cyclase to two receptors: Adenosine and catecholamine. *Biochemistry* **17**, 3811–3817.

Ullmann, A., and Danchin, A. (1983). Role of cyclic AMP in bacteria. *Adv. Cyclic Nucleo-tide Res.* **15**, 1–53.

Uno, I., Ueda, T., and Greengard, P. (1977). Adenosine 3',5'-monophosphate-regulated phosphoprotein system of neuronal membranes. II. Solubilization, purification, and some properties of an endogenous adenosine 3'-5'-monophosphate-dependent pro-tein kinase. *J. Biol. Chem.* **252**, 5164–5174.

Van Eldik, L. J., Watterson, D. M., Fok, K.-F., and Erickson, B. W. (1983). Elucidation of a minimal immunoreactive site of vertebrate calmodulin. *Arch. Biochem. Biophys.* **277**, 522–533.

Walsh, D. A., Perkins, J. P., and Krebs, E. G. (1968). An adenosine 3',5'-monophosphate-dependent protein kinase from rabbit skeletal muscle. *J. Biol. Chem.* **243**, 3763–3774.

Walsh, D. A., Ashby, C. D., Gonzalez, C., Calkins, D., Fischer, E. H., and Krebs, E. G. (1971). Purification and characterization of a protein inhibitor of adenosine 3',5'-monophosphate-dependent protein kinases. *J. Biol. Chem.* **246**, 1977–1985.

Walter, G., Scheidtmann, K.-H., Carbone, A., Laudano, A. P., and Doolittle, R. F. (1980). Antibodies specific for the carboxy- and amino-terminal regions of simian virus 40 large tumor antigen. *Proc. Natl. Acad. Sci. U.S.A.* **77**, 5197–5200.

Walter, U., Costa, M. R. C., Breakefield, X. O., and Greengard, P. (1979). Presence of free cyclic AMP receptor protein and regulation of its level by cyclic AMP in neuroblas-toma–glioma hybrid cells. *Proc. Natl. Acad. Sci. U.S.A.* **76**, 3251–3255.

Walter, U., De Camilli, P., Lohmann, S. M., Miller, P., and Greengard, P. (1981). Regula-tion and cellular localization of cAMP-dependent and cGMP-dependent protein ki-nases. *Cold Spring Harbor Conf. Cell Prolif.* **8**, 141–157.

Walton, G. M., Spiess, J., and Gill, G. N. (1982). Phosphorylation of high mobility group 14 protein by cyclic nucleotide-dependent protein kinases. *J. Biol. Chem.* **257**, 4661–4668.

Wang, K. C., Wong, H. Y., Wang, J. H., and Lam, H.-Y. P. (1983). A monoclonal antibody showing cross-reactivity toward three calmodulin-dependent enzymes. *J. Biol. Chem.* **258**, 12110–12113.

Weber, I. T., Takio, K., Titani, K., and Steitz, T. A. (1982). The cAMP-binding domains of the regulatory subunit of cAMP-dependent protein kinase and the catabolite gene activator protein are homologous. *Proc. Natl. Acad. Sci. U.S.A.* **79**, 7679–7683.

Wedner, H. J., Hoffer, B. J., Battenberg, E., Steiner, A. L., Parker, C. W., and Bloom, F. E. (1972). A method for detecting intracellular cyclic adenosine monophosphate by immunofluorescence. *J. Histochem. Cytochem.* **20**, 293–295.

Wedner, H. J., Bloom, F. E., and Parker, C. W. (1975). The role of cyclic nucleotides in lymphocyte activation. *In* "Immune Recognition" (A. S. Rosenthal, ed.), pp. 337–357. Academic Press, New York.

Whitley, T. H., Stowe, N. W., Ong, S.-H., Ney, R. L., and Steiner, A. L. (1975). Control and localization of rat adrenal cyclic guanosine 3′,5′-monophosphate: Comparison with adrenal cyclic adenosine 3′,5′-monophosphate. *J. Clin. Invest.* **56**, 146–154.

Wood, J. G., Wallace, R. W., Whitaker, J. N., and Cheung, W. Y. (1980). Immunocytochemical localization of calmodulin and heat-labile calmodulin-binding protein (CaM-BP$_{80}$) in basal ganglia of mouse brain. *J. Cell Biol.* **84**, 66–76.

Worobec, R. B., Wallace, J. H., and Huggins, C. G. (1972). Angiotensin–antibody interaction. I. Induction of the antibody response. *Immunochemistry* **9**, 229–238.

Wynshaw-Boris, A., Lugo, T. G., Short, J. M., Fournier, R. E. K., and Hanson, R. W. (1984). Identification of a cAMP regulatory region in the gene for rat cytosolic phosphoenolpyruvate carboxykinase (GTP). Use of chimeric genes transfected into hepatoma cells. *J. Biol. Chem.* **259**, 12161–12169.

Zeilig, C. E., Langan, T. A., and Glass, D. B. (1981). Sites in histone H1 selectivity phosphorylated by guanosine 3′,5′-monophosphate-dependent protein kinase. *J. Biol. Chem.* **256**, 994–1001.

Zeller, R., Nyffenegger, T., and DeRobertis, E. M. (1983). Nucleocytoplasmic distribution of snRNPs and stockpiled snRNA-binding proteins during oogenesis and early development in *Xenopus laevis. Cell* **32**, 425–434.

Zor, U. (1983). Role of cytoskeletal organization in the regulation of adenylate cyclase-cyclic adenosine monophosphate by hormones. *Endocr. Rev.* **4**, 1–21.

# Autoimmune Endocrine Disease

# JOHN B. BUSE

*Duke University Medical Center*
*Durham, North Carolina*

# GEORGE S. EISENBARTH

*Joslin Diabetes Center*
*Brigham and Women's Hospital*
*New England Deaconess Hospital*
*Harvard Medical School*
*Boston, Massachusetts*

## I. Introduction

Many different definitions of autoimmune disease exist (Table I). From a pathophysiological point of view, autoimmune disease represents physiology altered as a direct result of antibodies or lymphocytes reacting with "self" antigens. From an immunological point of view, autoimmune disease should be transferable with antibodies or lymphocytes, and the disease process should be reenacted in normal trans-

253

TABLE I

CRITERIA FOR AN AUTOIMMUNE DISEASE

1. Autoantibodies and lymphocytes reactive with normal tissue or tissue components resulting in altered physiology
2. Transfer of disease with lymphocytes or antibody
3. Reenactment of immunologically mediated tissue destruction in normal transplanted tissue in the absence of rejection
4. Cure or prevention with immunotherapy

planted tissue without evidence of tissue rejection. From a clinical point of view, autoimmune disease should be preventable or curable with immunotherapy. Over the past decade, it has become clear that many prevalent endocrinologic diseases are caused by disordered immune function (Type I diabetes, Graves' disease, thyroiditis). In addition, less common autoimmune endocrine illnesses are of importance both because of the morbidity of the illness (e.g., Addison's disease, primary gonadal failure, idiopathic hypoparathyroidism) and because of the reagents and understanding of normal physiology they provide (e.g., diabetes secondary to anti-insulin receptor antibodies). As the study of endocrine autoimmunity as well as other autoimmune diseases has progressed, many common themes link these various illnesses.

One important theme is that multiple genes usually contribute to the development of autoimmunity and one or more of these genes are in the region of the major histocompatibility complex (MHC). The MHC (HLA of man, H-2 of mouse, RT1 of rats) consists of about 4–6 million base pairs of genome and is known to contain genes that code for three classes of glycoprotein molecules important in immune function as well as other molecules such as the enzyme 21-hydroxylase (Steinmetz and Hood, 1983). Class I HMC antigens are classic transplantation antigens (HLA-A, -B, and -C of humans and H-2K, D, and L of mice) and restrict the recognition of foreign antigens such as viruses or neoantigens by cytotoxic T lymphocytes (Zinkernagel and Doherty, 1980). Class II MHC antigens (HLA-DR, -DC, and -SB of humans; H2 IA and IE of mice) are required for antigen presentation and lymphocyte interactions and are associated with immune responsiveness to foreign antigens (Benacerraf, 1981). Class III molecules are components of the complement cascade. Because of the central role of the MHC in the normal immune system, it is not surprising that the MHC plays a role in the susceptibility of individuals to autoimmune endocrine disease.

A second common theme in autoimmune endocrine disease is that immunodeficiency, at times dramatic but often subtle, predisposes to autoimmunity. In several animals models of autoimmunity, dramatic immunodeficiencies are present. Recognizing the immunodeficiencies has allowed investigators to understand more readily the pathophysiology and genetics of these disorders and has facilitated development of effective immunotherapy. In human autoimmune endocrine disease, the role of immunodeficiency is poorly documented for the majority of diseases, but subtle "immune deficiencies" are beginning to be recognized. It is hoped that characterization of these deficiencies will lead to better understanding of the nature of autoimmune endocrine disease as well as allow for safer immunotherapy.

A third common theme is that because of the nature of the regulation of the immune system, many cells (B, T, Fc receptor bearing non-B, non-T lymphocytes, and macrophages) and their products (antibodies and lymphokines) are involved in autoimmunity.

A final theme is that active autoimmunity is a chronic process which often exists long before the relatively acute presentation of illness and that often several immunoendocrinopathies can present in the same patient at different times. Usually there are subclinical endocrine abnormalities which precede the presentation of disease (i.e., loss of insulin secretion in response to intravenous glucose, elevations of TSH, ACTH, FSH, or LH).

There are three major pathogenic mechanisms in autoimmune endocrine disease. The most common cause of disease is the destruction of a specific gland or cell type (Type I diabetes mellitus, thyroiditis, idiopathic primary adrenal insufficiency, idiopathic hypoparathyroidism, primary gonadal insufficiency, and hypophysitis). The next most common cause of autoimmune endocrine disease results from antibody interactions with cell surface receptors either mimicking hormone action (Graves' disease, hypoglycemia with anti-insulin receptor antibodies) or blocking receptor function (atrophic hypothyroidism and insulin resistance secondary to anti-insulin receptor antibodies). Finally, antibodies can bind directly to hormones or ions, decreasing "free" hormone or ion concentrations and causing thereby disease or distorted laboratory tests. No matter what immune mechanism is involved in a given immunoendocrinopathy, cells of the immune system and their products must be involved, and these are available for study in making diagnoses or monitoring therapy.

A general sequence of "pathologic" stages associated with autoimmunity begins with genetic susceptibility, followed by a triggering environmental influence (often hypothetical), followed by active autoimmunity (both cellular and humoral) leading to clinical disease. In this review, we will discuss these stages as they are currently understood in individual autoimmune endocrine diseases while emphasizing the general themes mentioned above. A better understanding of autoimmune endocrine disease should allow (1) prediction of the development of autoimmune endocrine disease before end-stage cellular destruction or metabolic decompensation, and (2) tailoring and monitoring immunotherapies to prevent or cure these immunoendocrinopathies.

## II. Autoimmune $\beta$-Cell Insufficiency (Type I Diabetes Mellitus)

### A. The BB Rat

We will begin our review of autoimmune endocrine disease with a detailed discussion of the BB rat because it is an extensively studied animal model which demonstrates the role of genetics, immunodeficiency, and autoimmunity in endocrine disease. The BB rat strain was developed by selective breeding after diabetes spontaneously appeared in a commercial outbred colony of Wistar-derived rats (Chappel and Chappel, 1983). In the BB rat strain, ~60% of animals develop diabetes mellitus which rapidly progresses to ketoacidosis and death if not treated with exogenous insulin. Their disease is of autoimmune etiology as it is characterized by (1) lymphocytic and macrophage inflammation of pancreatic islets, (2) circulating antibodies which precede the development of diabetes and bind to isolated rat islets, (3) progressive and selective destruction of the vast majority of insulin-producing $\beta$ cells, (4) the ability to transfer diabetes to immunodeficient animals with concanavalin A-activated splenic lymphocytes, (5) selective immune destruction of $\beta$ cells in transplanted islets, and (6) the ability to prevent the development of diabetes with multiple forms of immunotherapy. In addition, from neonatal life onward BB rats also exhibit a profound lymphopenia with an almost total lack of circulating T lymphocytes despite a grossly normal thymus.

### 1. Genetics

At least two genes contribute to the development of diabetes of the BB rat. One is autosomal recessive with 100% penetrance and determines the T cell immunodeficiency of the BB rat. The second is linked to the rat MHC (Jackson *et al.*, 1984a). Colle and co-workers (1983)

have implicated a third diabetogenic gene which is autosomal dominant and determines a lymphocytic inflammation of pancreatic acinar
tissue. These three genes are not linked.

Studies of the inheritance of the *RT1* complex of the BB rat indicate
that the diabetogenic MHC-linked gene (termed *RT1-DM*) most likely
acts in a codominant fashion with the probability of an animal becoming overtly diabetic being highest in *RT1-DM* homozygotes, low in
*RT1-DM* heterozygotes, and nil in animals lacking in *RT1-DM*. The
actual diabetogenic RT1 gene product is unknown and only inheritance of the whole histocompatibility complex is followed in current
breeding studies. It is therefore possible that the few diabetic animals
which are *RT1* heterozygotes may actually represent crossover events
between the serologic markers of the *RT1* complex and *RT1-DM* gene,
and *RT1-DM* is strictly recessive.

To further study *RT1-DM*, we have examined restriction fragment-
length polymorphisms in BB rats and in a control strain (BBN). These
two strains were coderived from the same original outbred colony by
selecting for (BB) or against the development of diabetes (BBN). Restriction polymorphism analysis involves using specific DNA probes
and restriction enzymes to distinguish different chromosome types in a
population. The DNA probes we utilized are copies of either messenger
RNA or nuclear DNA which code for major histocompatibility proteins.
These probes were developed by scientists studying the major histocompatibility region of man and mouse and cross-react with rat DNA.
The DNA probes replicate in bacterial plasmids and prior to use for
restriction polymorphism analysis are purified and radioactively labeled. Using a class II MHC probe (Fig. 1), we are able to detect four
different chromosome types in the control BBN population, and only
one of these chromosomes, which we have named type IIa, is found
among BB rats and in BB-derived rat strains (Buse *et al.*, 1984a,b).
With use of a class I probe, many different polymorphic chromosome
types are evident in the control BBN population, all having an 8.5-
kilobase (kb) *Eco*Ri band. In contrast, neither BB rats nor members of
BB-derived rat strains have this 8.5-kb *Eco*RI band [including the W-
line rat which was derived from a BB substrain and lacks the lymphopenia gene, but by breeding studies appears to carry *RT1-DM* (Like
and Rossini, 1984)]. Type IIa homozygous BBN rats can share all other
class I bands with BB rats only differing at the 8.5-kb band. Initial
breeding studies involving mating of rats known to bear genes yielding
certain restriction fragment types indicate that all IIa chromosomes
independent of their class I polymorphisms are diabetogenic and that
RT1-DM is likely a class II or class II-associated gene.

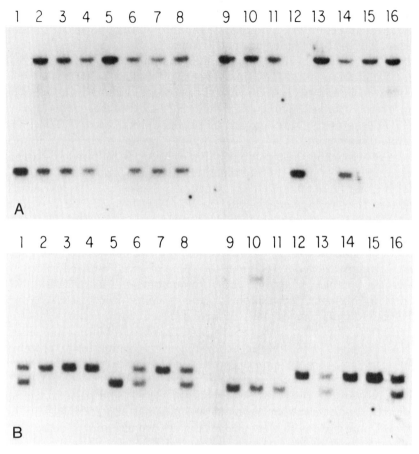

Fɪɢ. 1. Autoradiogram of a Southern blot of BBN (lanes 1–8 and 12–16) and BB (lanes 9–11) rat tail DNA after digestion with restriction enzymes *Eco*RI (A) and *Bam*HI (B) and hybridization with [32]P-labeled class II MHC (A-α) probe. We have called the upper *Eco*RI band "a" and the lower "b" and the upper *Bam*HI band "I" and the lower "II." Thus, the three BBs and the BBN in lane 5 are IIa homozygotes. The BBN in lane 15 is an Ia and the BBn in lane 12 is an Ib. The BBN in lane 1 is an Ib/IIb heterozygote. The chromosome types are inherited by simple Mendelian genetics.

## 2. *Immunodeficiency*

The importance of the BB rat's profound T cell lymphopenia in the pathogenesis of diabetes is reflected in the fact that immunotherapies such as blood transfusions, lymphocyte infusions, and bone marrow transplants, which partially reverse the immunodeficiency, prevent the development of diabetes (Naji *et al.*, 1981,1983; Benjamin *et al.*,

1984; Rossini *et al.*, 1984a), and that diabetes can be transferred from acutely diabetic BB rats with concanavalin A-activated splenic lymphocytes only to immunocompromised rats (splenectomy and antilymphocyte serum treated, high-dose cyclophosphamide treated, neonatally thymectomized normal rats, as well as young BB rats) (Koevary *et al.*, 1983a,b; Like *et al.*, 1983a).

The immunodeficiency of the BB rat is profound. The BB rat exhibits an almost total lack of circulating defined T cells (Jackson *et al.*, 1981,1983; Poussier *et al.*, 1982; Elder and Maclaren, 1983; Maclaren *et al.*, 1983). This decrease in the absolute number of T lymphocytes is apparent in both the helper/inducer (as defined by monoclonal antibody W3/25) and the cytotoxic/suppressor (as defined by monoclonal antibody OX8) populations of T cells. A decrease in the ratio of W3/25- to OX8-positive cells in BB rats 75- to 115-days old also has been noted by Elder and Maclaren (1983), but these changes in ratios were not related to the development of diabetes and seem relatively inconsequential compared to the >90% reduction in total T cells identified with the T cell-specific monoclonal antibody OX19 (Jackson and Eisenbarth, 1984). Absolute B lymphocyte numbers are normal in the BB rat when compared to controls (Jackson *et al.*, 1981; Poussier *et al.*, 1982; Elder and Maclaren, 1983). Other formed elements in blood are normal except for one report of increased numbers of polymorphonuclear cells (Elder and Maclaren, 1983) and one report of a high incidence of eosinophilia (Wright *et al.*, 1983). Similar T cell deficiency, though not as dramatic as for peripheral blood, has been reported for thoracic duct lymphocytes, lymph node, and spleen (Poussier *et al.*, 1982; Bellgrau *et al.*, 1982; Naji *et al.*, 1983).

Histologically there is T cell depletion in the white pulp of the spleen and the cortical areas of lymph nodes (Elder and Maclaren, 1983; Naji *et al.*, 1983). In addition, there seems to be a greater depletion of OX8-positive cells as compared to W3/25-positive cells in lymph nodes of BB rats (Like *et al.*, 1983b).

The thymus of the BB rat is grossly normal histologically (Elder and Maclaren, 1983; Buse *et al.*, 1983). BB thymocytes are apparently normal expressing the immature T cell phenotyping (OX19, W3/25, and OX8 positive). Poussier *et al.* (1982) reported decreased numbers of thymocytes in BB rats as compared to controls, a finding we cannot confirm (Jackson *et al.*, 1981). This discrepancy may be due to the well-known effect of stress or infection causing thymic involution coupled with the BB rat's susceptibility to infection. With use of monoclonal antibodies which react with neuroendocrine epithelial cells (BB-TECS and A2B5) and stromal reticular cells (DM-TECS) of the thymus, the nonlymphoid portion of the BB thymus is also grossly normal (Buse *et al.*, 1983; Jackson *et al.*, 1984b). Also, BB rats have increased levels of thymic hormones thymosin $\alpha_1$ and $\beta_4$, possibly reflecting a form of end-organ failure wherein the lack of circulating mature T cells results in decreased feedback inhibition of thymic hormone production (Buse *et al.*, 1983; Jackson *et al.*, 1984b).

The T cell deficits of the BB rat are functionally apparent. BB rats poorly reject skin grafts across both major and minor histocompatibility differences (Elder and Maclaren, 1983; Naji *et al.*, 1983), one way mixed lymphocyte responses are decreased (Bellgrau *et al.*, 1982; Elder and Maclaren, 1983; Naji *et al.*, 1983) and BB splenic and peripheral blood responses to mitogens are profoundly depressed (Elder and Ma-claren, 1983; Jackson *et al.*, 1983; Rossini *et al.*, 1983a). However, BB rats show no evidence of anti-pancreatic $\beta$-cell immunity (Rossini *et al.*, 1983a). Bellgrau *et al.* (1982) found decreased mitogen responsive-ness of BB thoracic duct lymphocytes, but normal responsiveness among lymph node cells. Thymic lymphocytes have been reported to proliferate normally to concanavalin A by one group (Elder and Ma-claren, 1983) and deficiently by another (Jackson *et al.*, 1983). Prud'homme *et al.* (1984a) have shown that high numbers of activated suppressor macrophages may cause the decreased mitogen responsive-ness of BB splenocyte isolates and, furthermore, that BB macrophages are capable of suppressing normal rat mitogenic responses. This effect is partially reversible with indomethacin and is not due to deficient IL-1 production or IL-2 consumption. B lymphocyte function has not been studied *in vitro*, but circulating $\gamma$-globulin levels are normal in the BB rat (Elder and Maclaren, 1983).

The T cell lymphopenia of BB rats is inherited in an autosomal recessive fashion. The nature of the genetic defect which causes the T cell immunodeficiency is not known. Neonatal bone marrow transplan-tation, blood transfusions, or T cell infusion seem to reverse some of the T cell deficiencies observed in BB rats (Naji *et al.*, 1983; Rossini *et al.*, 1983a,1984a), and T cells derived from transplanted bone marrow are responsible for the improved immune function (Naji *et al.*, 1983). Studies by Benjamin *et al.* (1984) have shown that bone marrow cells from normal rats depleted of T cells (anti-T cell antibody plus comple-ment) do not decrease the incidence of diabetes when transplanted into neonatal BB rats. Furthermore, young (<45-days old) BB rats which are irradiated and then reconstituted with normal T cell-depleted bone marrow do not develop diabetes and have normal T cell subsets. These results would indicate that transplanted mature T cells can normalize T cell function in the BB rat.

As a consequence of their immunodeficiency, BB rats are highly susceptible to infection (especially mycoplasma pneumonia), granulomas, lymphoid hyperplasia, and lymphoma (Seemayer *et al.*, 1982a; Wright *et al.*, 1983, Yale and Marliss, 1984).

### 3. *Triggering Events*

The diabetes of the BB rat seems to develop independent of the influence of horizontally transmitted infectious agents, as the expected number of rats develop diabetes when raised in a germ-free environment after sterile cesarean delivery (Rossini *et al.*, 1979). Such gnotobiotic rats were free of bacteria or parasites on smears and showed no detectable antibodies against any recognized rat viruses. Virus particles have not been detected on electron microscopy in the pancreas of diabetic rats (Marliss *et al.*, 1981). Furthermore, Rossini *et al.* (1983b) have shown that hypophysectomy, castration, vagotomy, agents protective against $\beta$-cytotoxins, and stress had no effect on the incidence of diabetes. Rossini *et al.* (1983b) also found no effect of diet on the incidence of diabetes using high carbohydrate (68% by weight), high fat (45% by weight), or high protein (64% by weight) diets. Scott and Trick (1983) found a decreased incidence of diabetes in rats fed a semipurified diet relatively high in fat, as did Elliott and Martin (1984) using a semisynthetic diet in which natural proteins were replaced with amino acids. It is possible that these "purified" or "synthetic" diets lack some nutrient leading to further immunosuppression of the BB rat, thereby preventing diabetes. There was evidence of malnutrition in animals receiving the artificial diet. It is known that protein deprivation, calorie deprivation, or single-nutrient deficiency can cause immunodeficiency (Beisel *et al.*, 1981).

### 4. *Active Autoimmunity*

*a. Prediabetic Physiology.* Sixty percent of BB rats develop ketosis-prone diabetes mellitus between 60 and 120 days of age (Like *et al.*, 1982a). Diabetes is preceded by mononuclear cell infiltration of pancreatic islets with progressive selective destruction of the insulin producing $\beta$ cells (Nakhooda *et al.*, 1976, 1978; Like *et al.*, 1982a; Marliss *et al.*, 1981; Tannenbaum *et al.*, 1981a,b; Seemayer *et al.*, 1982b; Logothetopoulos *et al.*, 1984) and by the development of islet cell surface antibodies (Dyrberg *et al.*, 1982,1983, 1984; Pollard *et al.*, 1983; Baekkeskov *et al.*, 1983; Martin and Logothetopoulos, 1984; Poussier *et al.*, 1983). The prediabetic period is characterized physiologically by normal oral glucose tolerance testing within 4 days of the onset of hyperglycemia and abnormal oral glucose tolerance tests no greater than 11 days before the onset of hyperglycemia (Nakhooda *et al.*, 1978). Some BB rats display persistently impaired glucose tolerance characterized by (1) decreased glucose response to oral and intraperitoneal glucose and intraperitoneal arginine and tolbutamide, (2) fasting hypoinsulinemia, (3) decreased insulin response to glucose and tolbutamide, (4) suppression of both early and late insulin response to intravenous glucose, (5) normal glucagon secretion, and (6) an association with significant mononuclear cell inflammation of pancreatic islets (Nakhooda *et al.*, 1983). In some cases of persistent impaired glucose tolerance, there was a progression to overt diabetes, and in ~3% of animals, impaired glucose tolerance was transient.

*b. Cellular Autoimmunity.* From transfer studies and immunohistopathology of the pancreases of diabetic BB rats, it seems likely that cellular immune effector mechanisms are largely responsible for the destruction of $\beta$ cells. Histologically, mononuclear cell infiltration of pancreatic islets begins 2 to 3 weeks before the onset of diabetes (Logothetopoulos *et al.*, 1984.)

In Fig. 2, a normal islet from a nondiabetic BB rat is shown in the upper left panel. In the upper right panel massive acute mononuclear cell inflammation of a pancreatic islet is shown. In the lower left panel, an end-stage islet is seen with disruption of normal islet architecture and continued presence of inflammation. In the lower right panel, the islet has been stained with anti-glucagon antibody, demonstrating the virtual absence of insulin-producing cells (which comprise the bulk of normal islet cell mass) and the selectivity of the autoimmune process with sparing of glucagon-producing cells in the destruction of islet cells. All islets of long-term diabetic rats are such "end-stage" islets.

The mononuclear cells infiltrating the islets consist of Ia-positive cells (macrophages and activated T lymphocytes reacting with anti-Ia monoclonal OX4), antigen W3/25-positive cells (T cells associated with helper and inducer function), and OX8-positive cells (T cells associated with suppressor and cytotoxic functions) in order of decreasing frequency. B lymphocytes are seen infrequently in the inflamed islets (Like *et al.*, 1983a). Macrophages from BB rats have been reported to have strong cytostatic effects on tumor cells and can inhibit insulin secretion by a rat insulinoma line (Prud'homme *et al.*, 1984a). Whether macrophages in the islets of BB rats are acting as antigen-presenting cells, or are present as a result of lymphokine production, or are directly involved in the $\beta$-cell destruction is still open to question. T cell cultures which express the helper T cell-associated W3/25 antigen and which proliferate in the presence of islet cell antigens and MHC-matched accessory cells have been produced (Prud'homme *et al.*, 1984b).

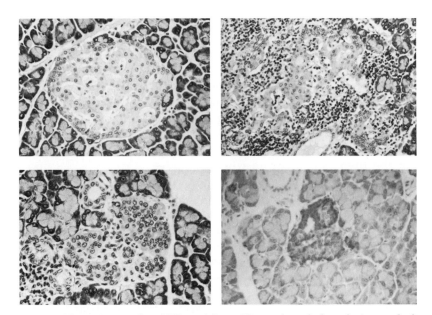

Fɪɢ. 2. Photomicrographs of BB rat islets of Langerhans before, during, and after active autoimmune destruction of insulin-producing $\beta$ cells. Upper right panel demonstrates the intense mononuclear cell infiltration (lymphocytes and monocytes) of an islet. Lower left panel shows an end-stage pseudoatrophic islet with disrupted architecture and few remaining mononuclear cells. The lower right panel shows immunoperoxidase staining of such a pseudoatrophic islet with anti-glucagon demonstrating the preponderance of glucagon-secreting $\alpha$ cells as opposed to the normal preponderance of insulin-producing $\beta$ cells. These pictures were kindly provided by Dr. A. A. Like (University of Massachusetts Medical Center, Worcester, Massachusetts).

The best evidence for T cell-mediated effector mechanism being involved in the pathogenesis of diabetes in the BB rat comes from transfer experiments carried out by Koevary *et al.* (1983a). In this model, 5–10 × 10⁷ concanavalin A-activated spleen cells from acutely diabetic BB rats transfer diabetes to 30-to 40-day-old rats in 90% of cases ~12 days after transfer (normally diabetes does not develop in BB rats less than 60 days of age). Additionally, transfer of diabetes could be effected in immunosuppressed normal rat strains (Koevary *et al.*, 1983b; Like *et al.*, 1983b). Further studies by Koevary and co-workers have shown that T cell depletion of the concanavalin A-activated spleen cells decreases the efficiency of transfer of disease.

An interesting question arises in trying to understand cell-mediated autoimmunity in the BB rat. How does one explain the apparent role of circulating T cells in the pathogenesis of diabetes when there is an almost total lack of T cells and T cell function? The answer may lie in the observation that the lymphocytes accumulating in the islets are the same subsets deficient in the circulation, and alteration of circulatory T cell dynamics is not equivalent to a total T cell deficiency.

Occasional BB rats have high numbers of W3/13[+], OX19[-], W3/25[-], OX8[-] "large" cells in their peripheral blood (Jackson et al., 1984a). By fluorescent cell sorting these circulating cells are polymorphonuclear lymphocytes (unpublished observations). Benjamin et al. (1984) report that all BB rats have mononuclear cells of this phenotype in the spleen, while control rats do not.

In the thymus of BB rats when compared to controls, we find increased numbers of "large" thymocytes which are selectively enriched for W3/13, 6B2 (thymic differentiation antigen), and OX8 and depleted for OX19 and W3/25 (Jackson et al., 1984b). Cantrell et al. (1982) find that rat natural killer cells express W3/13 and/or OX8 (cells that kill target cells usually virally infected or neoplastic without evidence of previous sensitization) and morphologically appear as large granular lymphocytes. Horowitz and Bakke (1984) have ascribed a large number of functions to a subset of cells (large granular lymphocytes) they term L cells, including natural killer function, antibody-dependent cellular cytotoxicity, and non-T non-B suppression. It is possible that a whole range of cytotoxic and regulatory functions is represented in the BB's W3/13[+], OX8[+], OX19[-], W3/25[-] mononuclear cell subset and that these cells are increased due to the absence of normal T cell function. One additional finding relevant to this discussion is that BB rats transplanted with isolated and purified islet cells under the kidney capsule destroy transplanted $\beta$ cells in parallel with destruction of their own pancreas in a non-MHC-restricted fashion in the absence of tissue rejection (Weringer and Like, 1984). Classical T cell mechanisms are MHC restricted, and this finding may reflect activity of the BB's W3/13[+], OX8[+], OX19[-], W3/25[-] subset, though other explanations are possible.

c. Humoral Autoimmunity. Serum antibodies reacting with islet cell surface antigens have been detected in BB rats using indirect immunofluorescence and a [125]I-labeled protein A radioligand assay (Pollard et al., 1983; Dyrberg et al., 1982,1983,1984). Neither of these assays can distinguish prediabetic or diabetic BB rats from nondiabetic BB rats. A control showing lack of binding to an irrelevant cell type, such as fibroblasts, has not been reported. With use of the [125]I-labeled protein A radioligand assay, islet cell surface antibodies may be detected and/or show peak values either before or after the onset of diabetes, impaired glucose tolerance, or mononuclear cell inflammation of pancreatic islets (Dyrberg et al., 1984). BB rat sera contain antibodies which in the presence of complement can be cytotoxic to islet cells (Martin and Logothetopoulos, 1984) as well as suppressive of insulin release (Poussier *et al.*, 1983). Sera from BB rats immunoprecipitate a 64,000-Da protein from rat islets or insulinoma cells which is similar in molecular size to protein precipitated by some human diabetic sera (Baekkeskov *et al.*, 1983). Approximately 30% of sera from a control strain also precipitates this 64,000-Da molecule. Antibodies binding to frozen sections of islets have not been detected in the BB rat.

Antibodies binding to lymphocytes have also been found in BB rats by Dyrberg *et al.* (1982,1983,1984) using the [125]I-labeled protein A assay, and they are negatively correlated with peripheral blood lymphocytes counts in animals with islet inflammation. Antibodies cytotoxic to lymphocytes in the presence of guinea pig complement are reported to exist in approximately one-third of BB rats (Elder and Maclaren, 1983), though these findings were not confirmed (Guttmann *et al.*, 1983).

Using indirect immunofluorescence on thin sections of rat tissues, Elder *et al.* (1982) detected antibodies reacting with gastric parietal cells in about 50% of BB rats without relation to diabetes. This finding was associated with lymphocytic gastritis, squamous metaplasia, and some loss of gastric mucosal cells without evidence of overt pernicious anemia (Like *et al.*, 1982a,b; Sternthal *et al.*, 1981). Antibodies against smooth muscle have also been demonstrated without relation to any histopathology (Elder *et al.*, 1982; Like *et al.*, 1982a,b). None of the antibodies has been shown to react with islet cell cytoplasm, anterior pituitary, adrenal, testes, or red blood cells (Elder *et al.*, 1982; Like *et al.*, 1982a,b; Maclaren *et al.*, 1983). Thus, the BB rat shows evidence of limited polyglandular autoimmunity without true polyglandular failure.

## 5. *Immunotherapy*

The diabetes of the BB rat can be prevented with a range of immunotherapies, including immunosuppression via anti-lymphocyte serum plus glucocorticoids (Like *et al.*, 1979), thymectomy (Like *et al.*, 1982c), whole body irradiation (Like *et al.*, 1979), total lymphoid irradiation (Rossini *et al.*, 1984b), or cyclosporine therapy (Like *et al.*, 1983c; Laupaucis *et al.*, 1983; Stiller *et al.*, 1983a). Immunoenhancing therapies that appear to reverse the T cell immunodeficiency of the BB rat also prevent the development of diabetes, and they include bone marrow transplantation (Naji *et al.*, 1981,1983; Benjamin *et al.*, 1984), blood transfusions (Rossini *et al.*, 1983a), and lymphocyte infusions (Rossini *et al.*, 1984a). Only anti-lymphocyte serum plus glucocorticoids can reverse the diabetes of the BB rat (Like *et al.*, 1983c). Naji and co-workers (1981) have shown that after anti-lymphocyte therapy with reversal of diabetes, in 30% of cases diabetes recurs after cessation of immunotherapy, and that islets transplanted into diabetic rats are destroyed by recurrence of the autoimmune disease process in the absence of immunosuppressive therapy.

## B. OTHER ANIMAL MODELS OF TYPE I DIABETES MELLITUS

The other animal models of Type I diabetes mellitus are less well studied than the BB rat or do not fulfill all the criteria for autoimmune disease listed in Table I. However, they do provide some insight into the genetics of autoimmunity, the role of immunodeficiency, and possible triggering mechanisms in Type I diabetes mellitus.

The NOD mouse is a new model of autoimmune $\beta$-cell insufficiency developed by Makino and co-workers (1980). Lymphocytic inflammation of pancreatic islet cells precedes the onset of diabetes which develops in 80% of females and 20% of males. In crosses of NOD mice with inbred strains, two nonlinked genes seem to be necessary for the development of diabetes, though the nature of these is not known (M. Hattori, personal communication). Immunologically, the NOD mouse is not normal, but its abnormalities in cellular immune function are much milder than in the BB rat (Kataoka *et al.*, 1984). Prior to the development of complete $\beta$-cell destruction, the pancreas of the NOD mouse loses the insulin secretory response to glucose, but responds to other secretagogues. Islet cell antibodies are found at high frequency in mice with insulitis (Kataoka *et al.*, 1984). The NOD mouse holds great promise for future understanding of autoimmune endocrine disease, as the reagents for study of the mouse immune system far exceed those available for the rat.

Several other mouse strains exhibit spontaneous mononuclear cell infiltrates of pancreatic islets with or without glucose intolerance (though none develop ketosis-prone diabetes). Kolb *et al.* (1980) describe infiltrates of lymphocytes in pancreatic islets, but not acinar tissue in 80% of NZB mice, 50% of MR1 mice, 50% of NZB×NZW mice, and <20% of BXSB mice. Furthermore, they found that all NZB mice and 20–50% of animals in the three other strains exhibited glucose intolerance without fasting hyperglycemia. All four strains have immunologic disorders leading to a lupus-like autoimmune disease. However, Seemayer and Colle (1984) could not demonstrate either inflammation of islets or glucose intolerance in NZB mice. It is intriguing that these four mouse strains exhibit an age-dependent loss in the ability to produce functional interleukin-2 or T cell growth factor (Dauphinee *et al.*, 1981), and at least *in vitro* low levels of interleukin-2 are necessary to generate cytotoxic T lymphocytes while high levels of interleukin-2 are necessary to generate suppressor T cells (Ting *et al.*, 1984). (Both decreased levels of interleukin-2 production and suppressor cell activity are reported for human autoimmune disease, as will be discussed later.)

The *db/db* mouse, which was initially characterized because of its development of diabetes associated with insulin resistance, acquires a T cell and a thymic immunodeficiency and eventual β-cell destruction (Debray-Sachs *et al.*, 1983; Dardenne *et al.*, 1984). This animal model may represent a transition from type II diabetes to autoimmune β-cell destruction, causing type I diabetes.

## C. TYPE I DIABETES OF MAN

Type I diabetes mellitus (insulin-dependent diabetes mellitus, formerly termed juvenile onset diabetes) meets all the criteria for an autoimmune disease listed in Table I except for transfer of disease with cells or antibody. The disease process is characterized by inflammation of pancreatic islets with lymphocytes and monocytes, with progressive selective destruction of the insulin-producing β cells. This process is associated with antibodies reacting with the surface and cytoplasm of islet cells. The autoimmune disease process is repeated in an accelerated form in pancreatic transplants from normal monozygotic twins in their diabetic twin mates; this process can be prevented by immunotherapy.

### 1. *Genetics*

The importance of heredity on the development of Type I diabetes mellitus is apparent from twin data. In the largest series of diabetes in identical twins, ~50% were concordant for the development of diabetes before the age of 40 (Barnett *et al.*, 1981) as opposed to a 12% concordance rate in nonidentical twins (Harvald and Hauge, 1963). These studies almost certainly are biased toward concordance, and the true rate of concordance in monozygotic twins is probably in the range of 20–30%. Nevertheless, there clearly is a genetic influence on the development of diabetes.

The genetics of Type I diabetes in man is less well understood than that of the BB rat. Type I diabetes is associated with MHC antigens HLA DR3 and DR4 (Rimoin and Rotter, 1984; Nerup *et al.*, 1984; Raum *et al.*, 1984; Wolf *et al.*, 1983). DR antigens are polymorphic serologically defined class II MHC antigens analogous to Ia antigens of mouse. Ninety-eight percent of Caucasians with Type I diabetes express DR3 or DR4 versus 60% of the general population. The relative risk (ratio of the frequency of a marker in diabetes to the frequency of the marker in control population) is 5 for DR3-positive individuals, 7 for DR4-positive individuals, and 14 for individuals who are both positive for DR3 and DR4. Approximately 50% of Type I diabetic patients are DR3/4 heterozygotes. Identical twins expressing both DR3 and DR4 are more often concordant for diabetes than twins expressing either DR3 or DR4 (Johnston *et al.*, 1983), suggesting that DR3 and DR4 or their associated linked diabetogenic genes are synergistic in producing diabetes and therefore represent at least two diabetogenic genes.

In family studies, specific HLA alleles are of less importance than sharing HLA alleles with the diabetic proband in defining the risk of developing diabetes (Gorsuch *et al.*, 1982). Approximately 20% of siblings who are HLA identical to a diabetic sibling develop diabetes by age 40, while siblings who share only one HLA haplotype with the diabetic proband have a 5% chance of diabetes, and those who share neither HLA haplotype have the same risk of developing diabetes as the general population (Fig. 3).

Some investigators (Bottazzo and Doniach, 1976; Irvine, 1978; Rotter and Rimoin, 1978) have proposed to subdivide Type I diabetes into HLA-DR3 and HLA-DR4 variants. Diabetic patients who are DR3 positive have a tendency toward more associated autoimmune disease, persistent islet cell antibodies, higher residual $\beta$-cell function at the time of diagnosis, and less frequent anti-insulin antibodies after the initiation of therapy than diabetic patients who are DR4 positive. However, there are little data to suggest that the mechanism of $\beta$-cell

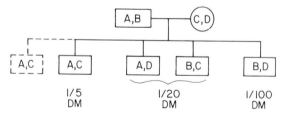

FIG. 3. Schematic of the inheritance of HLA haplotypes (father A, B; mother C, D) in relation to the development of Type I diabetes where one sibling has diabetes mellitus (DM) and carries the A haplotype of the father and the C haplotype of the mother. Adapted from data of Gorsuch *et al.* (1982).

destruction or the course of disease is different in DR3-positive versus DR4-positive diabetes.

Efforts have been made to subtype HLA-DR3- and HLA-DR4-positive diabetic patients and controls to more clearly define a diabetogenic genotype. Approximately 60% of the population at large expresses either DR3 or DR4 antigens, though less than 5 in 1000 develop Type I diabetes. Owerbach *et al.* (1983) have studied restriction fragment-length polymorphism using a human class II MHC gene probe and find restriction fragments positively and negatively associated with DR4-positive diabetics when compared to controls. Another approach has been to examine "extended haplotypes." The HLA region encodes many defined polymorphic markers which can be detected in an individual serum or on cells, including the class I classic transplantation antigens expressed on all nucleated cells (HLA-A, -B, and -C), class II "immune-associated" antigens present on endothelial cells, B lymphocytes, activated T lymphocytes and macrophages (HLA-DR -DC, and -SB), and class III molecules important in complement activation (C2, C4A, C4B, and properidin factor B). Also, the HLA complex is linked to a polymorphic serum enzyme glyoxalase. Alleles of these markers are often found associated in individuals or racial groups more frequently than would be expected from their relative frequencies in the population at large, and such groupings of distinct markers are termed extended haplotypes. Extended haplotypes can exist because of very tight linkage or physical proximity on human chromosome 6 of the genes which encode these markers, resulting in nonrandom distribution of these markers relative to each other (linkage dysequilibrium). There seem to be diabetogenic as well as nondiabetogenic forms of DR3 and DR4 extended haplotypes (Raum *et al.*, 1984; Marcelli-Barge *et al.*, 1984; Mustonen *et al.*, 1984; McCluskey *et al.*, 1983; Contu *et al.*, 1982). Furthermore, it seems likely that if DR3 and DR4 (at least as currently defined) are diabetogenic, there are other important linked genes at other loci in linkage dysequilibrium.

In both population and family studies, the excess of DR3 and DR4 in Type I diabetes is seen with a concomitant decrease in DR1, 2, 5, W6, 7, and W10. Of these, DR2, 5, and 7 are the DR haplotypes found in lowest frequency in the diabetic population when compared to controls. This observation could be due to a diabetes resistance gene in linkage dysequilibrium, a negative-linkage dysequilibrium with the DR3 and DR4 susceptibility gene, or could merely be secondary to the increased frequency of DR3 and DR4. Deschamps *et al.* (1984) have studied 66 HLA-genotyped families with Type I diabetes and at least one HLA-DR2-positive parent. Transmission of DR2 as well as DR5 and DR7 was decreased in diabetic siblings and random in unaffected siblings, but this was due to overtransmission of DR3 and DR4. Forty-five percent of the diabetic patients were neither DR3 nor DR4. Extended haplotype analysis revealed a DR2 containing "diabetic" haplotypes present in 19% of "nondiabetic haplotypes," but only 4% of "diabetic DR2s." Similarly, Cohen *et al.* (1984) have described a restriction fragment polymorphism detected with a DC β-chain DNA probe, which is strongly correlated with DR2 in the general population, but absent among DR2-positive diabetic patients. Bach *et al.* (1982) showed that the common cellularly defined DW haplotypes associated with HLA-DR2 were absent in all of five DR2-positive diabetic patients. These results reveal a heterogeneity in DR2 in the diabetic population, but do not elucidate the nature of the apparent DR2 "nonsusceptibility" or "resistance" evident on a population level.

Despite the high frequency of DR3 and DR4 and the relative paucity of DR2 in Type I diabetes, the course and nature of the destruction of β cells seem to be identical in both populations. Even DR2/DR1 individuals can develop slowly progressive β-cell destruction in association with islet cell antibodies. In one family we have studied, two of three HLA-identical siblings (DR2/DR1) display Type I diabetes, and the third HLA-identical sibling (islet cell antibody positive) has lost first-phase insulin secretion (evidence of β-cell destruction, to be discussed later).

HLA-linked genes seem to account for the bulk of the inheritable predisposition toward Type I diabetes as the incidence of diabetes in HLA-identical siblings (~20%) approaches that of identical twins. Studies to define diabetogenic loci outside of the MHC have met with only limited success except perhaps for reported associations between diabetes and a polymorphic locus near the insulin gene on chromosome 11 (Bell *et al.*, 1984) and enzyme polymorphisms mapping to chromosomes 1, 4, and 9 (Hodge *et al.*, 1983).

In 1981, Dr. Rotter proposed that the genetics of human Type I diabetes was "no longer a nightmare, but still a headache." There have been many proposed modes of inheritance of Type I diabetes, ranging from autosomal recessive to dominant with one or multiple genes and with single or up to three alleles (reviewed in Rotter, 1981). The major stumbling blocks in understanding the genetics of Type I diabetes are a lack of precise knowledge of the penetrance of Type I diabetes and a lack of phenotypic markers for the genes which predispose toward diabetes other than the presence of disease itself. The existence of linkage dysequilibrium and many different alleles at each genetic locus of the MHC make it difficult to determine which genes are truly diabetogenic. It is hoped that with population-based ascertainment of twin pairs with diabetes, disease penetrance will be more clearly defined. Studies are under way to develop tests to identify phenotypic markers, such as the lymphopenia of BB rats, which will allow simplification of possible modes of inheritance. With more extensive study of the MHC and its linked genes (which, like 21-hydroxylase, need not have classic MHC function), the nature and mechanism of the MHC association of Type I diabetes may be better understood. Despite the importance of MHC typing to diabetes research, currently it has little clinical utility. A majority of the general population expresses HLA-DR3 or -DR4, while only 0.3% develops diabetes. And even in a family, being HLA identical to a diabetic sibling only confers a 20% risk of developing diabetes, and as much as 36 years can elapse between the development of Type I diabetes in one twin and his or her identical twin (Srikanta *et al.*, 1983a,b).

At this time the hypothesis we favor is that DR4 and perhaps DR3 as immune response genes contribute to the development of diabetes, but that there is another gene (? recessive) in the MHC region contributing to susceptibility.

### 2. *Immunodeficiency*

Patients with Type I diabetes do not have a defect in the immune system as dramatic as the BB rat. However, there are intriguing studies suggesting that there may be more subtle abnormalities in immune system parameters between diabetics, prediabetics, and/or identical twins of patients with Type I diabetes and normal controls.

Vergani *et al.* (1983) have measured the levels of the fourth component of complement (C4) in non-insulin-dependent diabetics, Type I diabetics, and controls. They report low serum C4 in patients with both recent onset and long-standing diabetes when compared to both controls and non-insulin-dependent diabetics. This occurred in the absence of low C3 levels or evidence of C4 consumption. Additionally, there was a linear correlation in serum C4 values between twins both concordant and discordant for diabetes. As was pointed out by Dawkins *et al.* (1983), these results may be due to the known association of Type I diabetes with DR3-extended MHC haplotypes, including C4 null alleles and a proposed inverse relationship between serum C4 levels and the number of C4 null alleles. Ruuska *et al.* (1984) report low erythrocyte C3b receptor levels associated with low C3 and C4 levels in Type I diabetes. This finding has also been described in other HLA-DR3-related illnesses, including systemic lupus erythematosus and Sjogren's syndrome.

Hoddinott *et al.* (1982) examined immunoglobulin levels in Type I diabetes. Among 129 patients, he found 2 were completely IgA deficient and 1 had complete IgG deficiency. Additionally, excluding those three cases, there were low IgG levels in diabetics when compared to controls with nondiabetic first-degree relatives having intermediate IgG levels. In both the diabetic populations and healthy first-degree relatives, 10% of cases had serum IgG concentrations greater than two standard deviations below the mean for the control distribution. This abnormality was unrelated to HLA type.

Recently, Zier and co-workers (1984) described decreased production of T cell growth factor interleukin-2 *in vitro* by lymphocytes from Type I diabetics. Lymphocytes were isolated, stimulated with a lectin, and the culture supernatants harvested. The content of "interleukin-2" was then determined in a bioassay using a cell line whose growth is stimulated by interleukin-2. Type I diabetics with recent onset and long-standing disease had depressed interleukin-2 production in contrast to normals and Type II diabetics. We do not know whether interleukin-2 deficiency develops prior to overt diabetes or in genetically susceptible individuals. Studies of five pairs of identical twins discordant for diabetes suggest the deficiency associated with diabetes is not genetically determined (unpublished observations).

### 3. *"Triggering" Events*

Since less than 50% of monozygotic twins are concordant for Type I diabetes (Barnett *et al.*, 1981), it has been hypothesized that some environmental event must contribute to the development of disease. It is now apparent that immunoglobulin and T cell receptor diversity is generated by several mechanisms (somatic cell mutations) involving "random" gene rearrangements. Therefore, even at birth identical twins are not identical, at least as far as the immune system is concerned.

The search for environmental triggers for the development of Type I diabetes has been disappointing. This may relate to the emphasis of studies on evaluating the immediate prediabetic period. Ingestion of Vacor, a rat poison, causes Type I diabetes and a severe peripheral neuropathy (Karam *et al.*, 1980). There have been a few case reports of diabetes developing in association with overwhelming viral infection (Yoon *et al.*, 1979), but recent pathologic study reveals chronic $\beta$-cell destruction had preceded the acute infection (Gepts, 1984) in that case report. If acute $\beta$-cell destruction leading to Type I diabetes occurs, it is probably an extremely rare event.

A search has begun for environmental agents which may lead to chronic $\beta$-cell destruction. The most interesting findings to date relate to congenital rubella in which ~20% of children develop overt diabetes years after the congenital infection (Rubenstein et al., 1982). These children with diabetes express HLA alleles DR3 and DR4 (Rubenstein et al., 1982), but apparently do not develop anti-cytoplasmic islet cell antibodies (Clarke et al., 1984). In addition, these children have a high prevalence of autoimmune thyroid disease (Clarke et al., 1984). It is not known whether the virus produces autoimmunity by target gland damage or through effects on the developing immune system. Another reported congenital influence on the development of diabetes has been the ingestion of "smoked/cured mutton" containing N-nitroso compounds (Helgason et al., 1981, 1982). An increased incidence of diabetes was seen in offspring (by epidemiologic study of man and toxicologic studies in mice) rather than the individuals ingesting the mutton.

### 4. Active Autoimmunity

Antibodies reacting with the cell surface or cytoplasm of all islet cells have been described (Table II). The only assay that to date has provided clinically important prognostic information in nondiabetic relatives is the measurement of antibodies reacting with nonfixed frozen sections of normal human pancreas (Irvine et al., 1980; Irvine, 1980; Gorsuch et al., 1981; Srikanta et al., 1983a,b; Kanatsuna et al., 1982). In this assay, sera from patients with Type I diabetes or their relatives are incubated with pancreatic sections and the binding of antibody detected with fluorescein-conjugated anti-human antibodies. Sera containing high titers of anti-islet antibodies produce fluorescence limited to islet cells. Measurement of anti-islet antibodies by indirect immunofluorescence is not a routine assay. It is a qualitative test extremely dependent on the pancreatic substrate. Pancreases obtained at autopsy are useless and even pancreases obtained from cadaveric donors vary in their suitability. Attempts at improving the assay using fixed tissue lead to a loss of specificity (Yagihashi et al., 1982). Adding an extra step of complement fixation with subsequent tests with fluorescent anti-complement antibodies may increase specificity by decreasing sensitivity (Bottazzo et al., 1980). These technical difficulties have limited widespread availability of assays for cytoplasmic anti-islet antibodies, but a number of clinical research laboratories have screened thousands of relatives for anti-islet antibodies.

Strongly positive anti-islet antibodies reacting with the cytoplasm of unfixed islet cells are found in ~2% of relatives of Type I diabetics (Riley and Maclaren, 1984). These antibodies characteristically pre-

TABLE II

ANTI-ISLET ANTIBODY ASSAYS

| Assay | Reference |
|---|---|
| 1. Anti-"cytoplasmic" islet antibodies indirect immunofluorescence with | |
|   A. Frozen sections of normal pancreas, fluorescein anti-human antibody | Irvine (1980); Gorsuch et al. (1981); Srikanta et al. (1983a); Riley and Maclaren (1984). |
|   B. Frozen sections of normal pancreas, complement fixation, fluorescein anti-complement antibody | Bottazzo et al. (1980) |
|   C. Sections of Bouin's fixed pancreas | Yagihashi et al. (1982) |
| 2. Anti-surface islet cell antibodies | |
|   A. Cytotoxicity normal rat islet cells ($^{51}$Cr release) | Dobersen et al. (1980) |
|   B. Cytotoxicity rat insulinoma (RINm5F) cells ($^{51}$Cr release) | Eisenbarth et al., (1981) |
|   C. Cytotoxicity normal rat islets cells in monolayer (ethidium bromide uptake) | Dobersen and Scharff (1982) |
|   D. Indirect immunofluorescence living islet cells | Lernmark et al. (1978) |
|   E. $^{125}$I-labeled protein A radioassay using normal rat islets cells | Huen et al. (1983) |
|   F. $\beta$-cell specific surface assays | Dobersen et al. (1980); Adams and Kennedy (1967) |
| 3. Immunoprecipatation assays | |
|   A. Antibodies to insulin | Palmer et al. (1983) |
|   B. Antibodies to glycoproteins | Baekkeskov et al. (1982) |

cede by years the onset of overt diabetes, though as many as 30% of patients developing Type I diabetes do not show detectable anti-islet antibodies with the current crude assays (Srikanta et al., 1984a). Some individuals may express anti-islet antibodies for more than a decade without developing diabetes, and in some individuals antibodies may disappear. The finding that antibodies disappear may be more apparent than real. Variation in assay sensitivity and interassay variation using different pancreases is a particular problem with low-titer antisera (Marner et al., 1983). Development of quantitative assays will probably precede commercially reliable assays. This will depend on isolation and characterization of the target islet antigens. Both glycoproteins and glycolipids are potential candidate antigens, and we and others are currently engaged in making and using monoclonal antibodies and polyclonal antisera to isolate potential target antigens (Baekkeskov et al., 1982; Eisenbarth et al., 1982, 1983b).

It is likely that cell-mediated immunity rather than autoantibodies is the major determinant of $\beta$-cell destruction. Activated T cells transfer the diabetes of the BB rat (Koevary et al., 1983a), and despite numerous attempts, no one has transferred overt diabetes to animals with anti-islet antibodies, though anti-islet antibodies inhibit in vitro insulin release (Kanatsuna et al., 1982).

In vitro studies of T cells of Type I diabetics reveal several abnormalities including production of migration inhibition factor in response to islet antigens (Nerup et al., 1971), cytotoxicity against an islet cell tumor (Huang and Maclaren 1976), in vitro inhibition of insulin release (Boitard et al., 1981), and decreased suppressor activity (Horita et al., 1982; Verghese et al., 1981).

Recently, monoclonal antibodies have been used to quantitate T cell subsets. In contrast to the BB rat where an autosomal recessive gene produces a profound T cell lymphopenia and contributes to the development of diabetes (Guttman et al., 1983; Jackson et al., 1981,1984a), dramatic abnormalities of resting T cells in Type I diabetes of man have not been defined (Jackson et al., 1982; Mascart-Lemone et al., 1982; Selam et al., 1979; Gupta et al., 1982; Buschard et al., 1983). Four groups have reported an increase in the percentage of cells expressing activation antigens (Jackson et al., 1982; Haywood and Herberger, 1984; Pozzilli et al., 1982; Leslie et al., 1984). In particular, an elevation of cells bearing the Ia or DR antigen can be detected with monoclonal antibodies reacting with the nonpolymorphic backbone of these molecules (e.g., monoclonal L243). These "activated" T cells also express the interleukin-2 receptor and incorporate [³H]thymidine (Haywood and Herberger, 1984). In one report they express transferrin receptors (monoclonal 5E9) and the 4F2 activation antigen (Pozzilli et al., 1982). Ia-positive T cells, similar to islet cell antibodies, precede the development of diabetes in the majority, but not in all patients. Both anti-islet antibodies and Ia-positive T cells usually disappear after the development of overt hyperglycemia (Jackson et al., 1982). Activated T cells are found in a series of DR3-associated autoimmune endocrine diseases (Jackson et al., 1984c; Rabinowe et al., 1984a) and states of immune activation, such as mononucleosis.

## 5. Progressive $\beta$-Cell Insufficiency

Islet cell antibodies reacting with the cytoplasm of unfixed pancreas have prognostic significance. This assay in combination with endocrine testing can be used to predict which relatives are at high risk for the development of overt diabetes or which adult patients will progress to insulin dependence. The prognostic significance of other current assays is unknown and in most instances is limited by a lack of specificity [e.g., thyroiditis patients have antibodies reacting with the surface of islet cells (Lernmerk *et al.*, 1978), Bouin's fixed pancreas reacts with sera from patients with polyclonal activation (Eisenbarth and Crump, 1981), Ia-positive T cells are present in many organ-specific autoimmune diseases (Jackson *et al.*, 1982, 1984c; Rabinowe *et al.*, 1984a)].

In the screening of relatives for cytoplasmic islet cell antibodies, it has been rare to detect an islet cell antibody-negative individual who subsequently develops these antibodies (Srikanta *et al.*, 1983a,b). Coincident with the development of islet cell antibodies, insulin secretion progressively declines in the majority of patients. We have observed a slow and progressive decrement in insulin release on intravenous glucose stimulation in all relatives we have studied who have developed overt Type I diabetes (Srikanta *et al.*, 1983a,b,1984a,b). Loss of the first-phase insulin response to intravenous glucose is progressive once insulin release falls below the tenth percentile for normal subjects, and this abnormality precedes hyperglycemia by years. Insulin secretion in response to intravenous glucose can be profoundly abnormal (lower than the response of more than 400 tests in normal individuals) at a time when oral glucose tolerance testing is normal. At a time when there is essentially no secretory response to intravenous glucose, rapid responses are evident to intravenous glucagon, arginine, or tolbutamide (Ganda *et al.*, 1984). Such a selective loss in response to intravenous glucose can be produced by partial pancreatectomy of rats (Weir *et al.*, 1981), and we suspect that in pre-Type I diabetes it reflects progressive β-cell destruction. Insulin release can also be normal and stable for years despite presence of anti-islet antibodies (Srikanta *et al.*, 1983a,b).

Usually at the time of diagnosis of overt diabetes the great majority of β cells have been destroyed (Gepts, 1982). Pseudoatrophic islets consisting of A and D cells with no β cells are frequent. In the identical twin transplants performed by Sutherland and co-workers, islet lymphocytic infiltration correlated with presence of β cells within an islet. There was no infiltration in islets containing only A and D cells (pseudoatrophic islets) (Sutherland *et al.*, 1984).

## 6. *Immunotherapy*

The increasing evidence that Type I diabetes is an autoimmune disease, and in particular a slow autoimmune disease, has led to initial trials of immune intervention with drugs such as cyclosporin A (Stiller *et al.*, 1983b,1984), anti-thymocyte globulin (Eisenbarth *et al.*, 1983a), prednisone (Jackson *et al.*, 1982; Elliott *et al.*, 1981), and azathioprine (Leslie and Pyke, 1980). None of the trials to date has been randomized and double blinded (Rabinowe and Eisenbarth, 1984). In our own studies with anti-thymocyte globulin, we concluded that extension of the honeymoon phase which occurred with this drug was not of sufficient clinical benefit in light of its side effects, including fever, rash, and severe transient thrombocytopenia. Prednisone given after the onset of diabetes (perhaps related to its inherent property of creating insulin resistance) is ineffective clinically, though C-peptide secretion may be higher with its administration. The most promising studies are with cyclosporin A. At the end of 1 year of therapy approximately one-half of initially diabetic subjects no longer required insulin and HbA1 was near normal (Stiller *et al.*, 1983b,1984). However, these subjects were not normal and were similar to pre-Type I diabetics in showing the insulin secretory defect to intravenous glucose challenge. Larger randomized trials of cyclosporin A to determine efficacy in relation to safety are just beginning.

Cyclosporin A is being tested in a series of autoimmune diseases and is being used for the first time without other immunosuppressive drugs. A major side effect of immunosuppression in transplant patients where multiple immunosuppressive drugs are used has been the development of lymphomas. It has recently been reported that these lymphomas disappear with reduction or discontinuation of immunosuppression (Starzl *et al.*, 1984). This suggests that such lymphomas are responsive to T cell suppression. Other side effects of cyclosporin A are a dose-dependent nephro- and hepatotoxicity, and the dilantin-like side effects of gingival hyperplasia, hirsutism, and paresthesias. The manner in which cyclosporin will be used to treat autoimmunity may obviate the most serious side effects. Nevertheless, until randomized trials of this drug are completed in Type I diabetes, it should *not* be used clinically because uncontrolled use may do more harm than good and because this drug may have to be given for life if permanent reversal of diabetes is the goal.

## III. THYROIDITIS

### A. CLASSIFICATION

The term thyroiditis refers to inflammation of the thyroid gland (DeGroot *et al.*, 1984). In this review we will not discuss infectious thyroiditis (bacteria, mycobacteria, fungi, protozoa, or flatworms), involvement of the thyroid by systemic inflammatory diseases (e.g., sarardosis and amyloidosis), and Reidel's thyroiditis where there is

TABLE III
THYROIDITIS

| Type | Pathology | Time course | Symptoms |
|------|-----------|-------------|----------|
| Infectious | Infection | Acute, subacute | Painful |
| Hashimoto's | Lymphocytes | Chronic | — |
| de Quervain's | Giant cells | Subacute | Painful |
| Subacute | | | |
| lymphocytic | Lymphocytes | Subacute | — |
| Reidel's | Sclerosis | Chronic | — |

sclerosing connective tissue growth (at times extending outside of the thyroid). The diseases we will discuss include de Quervain's thyroiditis (termed subacute thyroiditis), Hasimoto's thyroiditis with a goitrous and atrophic variant, and subacute lymphocytic thyroiditis (termed painless thyroiditis). Subacute lymphocytic thyroiditis is histologically similar to Hashimoto's thyroiditis, but its clinical course resembles the "painful" de Quervain's thyroiditis (Table III). A syndrome of postpartum transient thyrotoxicosis is similar to subacute lymphocytic thyroiditis. Both postpartum transient thyrotoxicosis and subacute thyroiditis often have a transient thyrotoxic phase followed by hypothyroidism and finally, for most patients, normal thyroid function. In contrast to Graves' disease, the uptake of radioactive iodine is suppressed in all forms of subacute thyroiditis with hyperthyroidism. In these diseases, it is preformed thyroid hormone which is released, as compared to enhanced synthesis of thyroxine in Graves' disease with attendant iodine uptake and organification.

## B. ANIMAL MODELS

The obese strain of chicken is an extensively studied animal model of Hashimoto's thyroiditis which spontaneously develops hypothyroidism (Cole, 1966; Rose *et al.*, 1976). Similar to Type I diabetes of the BB rat, multiple genes and lymphocyte subsets contribute to the destruction of thyroid follicular cells of these animals. The obese strain of chickens was developed from the Cornell strain on the basis of the recognition of hereditary hypothyroidism. In current strains more than 90% of chickens develop spontaneous autoimmune thyroiditis. In birds a single organ, the bursa of Fabricius, contains the progenitors of B cells, and thus, the importance to the autoimmune process of both B cells (bursa derived) and T cells (thymus derived) in the obese chicken can be readily studied. Early bursectomy (at day 19 *in ovo* and at hatching) delays and markedly decreases the severity of thyroiditis (Cole, 1968; Wick *et al.*, 1970). Injection of autologous bursa cells to bursectomized animals restores the susceptibility to thyroiditis. The importance of bursa-derived cells to the development of thyroiditis is probably related to their production of anti-thyroglobulin antibodies. [Such antibodies increase thyroiditis in genetically susceptible animals (Jaroszewski *et al.*, 1978).] Though the bursa-derived cells are necessary for the development of thyroiditis, they do not genetically determine thyroiditis susceptibility (Polley *et al.*, 1981). Polley and co-workers crossed the obese strain of chickens (OS) with control Cornell strain (CS) chickens. The resulting $F_1$ animals (OS × CS) were bursectomized and then bursa cells from OS, CS, and $F_1$ animals injected into the $F_1$ bursectomized chicks. Thyroiditis developed independent of whether bursa cells from thyroiditis-susceptible or -resistant strains (CS) were utilized.

Thymus-derived or T cells are also necessary for the development of thyroiditis (Pontes de Carvalho *et al.*, 1981), but in contrast to bursa cells, thymic cells do genetically determine the development of spontaneous autoimmune thyroiditis. Though thymectomy alone enhances thyroiditis (Welch *et al.*, 1973), thymectomy plus administration of anti-thymocyte serum abrogates the development of thyroiditis (Pontes de Carvalho *et al.*, 1981). Livezey and co-workers (1981) depleted CS chicks of T cells by neonatal thymectomy and irradiation. After reconstitution with OS or CS thymocytes, all animals showed normal T cell function, but only animals which received T cells from susceptible (OS) chickens developed thyroiditis.

The specific genes producing thyroiditis in obese strain chickens are unknown, but there is evidence that multiple independent genes contribute to disease susceptibility. One gene is linked to the histocompatibility region, and animals homozygous for the obese strain histocompatibility haplotype have the most severe spontaneous thyroiditis. Multiple thymic abnormalities have also been reported in obese strain chickens, including abnormal response to minor histocompatibility antigens with accelerated rejection of skin allografts (Jakobisiak *et al.*, 1976), increased radiolabeled thymidine uptake by thymocytes (Livezey *et al.*, 1981), and a deficiency in thymic nurse cells (Boyd *et al.*, 1984).

What determines the targeting to the thyroid in the autoimmune process of the obese chicken? It has been proposed that an independent gene(s) results in an abnormality of thyroid function which in the presence of an abnormal immune system leads to autoimmune thyroid disease. Sundick and Wick (1976) transplanted embryonic obese strain and normal thyroid glands onto the chorioallentoic membrane of normal chicken embryos and observed increased $^{131}$T uptake of the OS thyroid gland. In addition, in very young OS chickens prior to evidence of active autoimmunity, radioactive iodine uptake cannot be suppressed with exogenous thyroid hormone (Sundick et al., 1979). Obese strain thyroid cells also grow more slowly in vitro than Cornell strain thyroid cells (Truden et al., 1983). Current evidence suggests that at least two genes, one in the MHC influencing immune function and another influencing thyroid function, combine to produce disease. There is additional evidence of non-MHC genes contributing to disease susceptibility by effects on immune function (Boyd et al., 1983).

Wick and co-workers (1982) studied effect of cyclosporin A on the development of thyroiditis in the obese chicken. In marked contrast to the BB rat where cyclosporin A prevents diabetes, in the obese chicken if the drug is given after hatching, it does not alter antibody titers or thyroid inflammation. Cyclosporin administration prior to hatching exacerbates the disease.

In addition to the obese chicken, spontaneous autoimmune thyroiditis has been observed in dogs (Mizejewski et al., 1971), the Buffalo rat strain (Noble et al., 1976), and the BB rat (Sternthal et al., 1981). In rats a number of seemingly unrelated drugs exacerbate the thyroiditis of genetically susceptible animals, such as methylcholanthrene and carbon tetrachloride in Buffalo rats (Silverman and Rose, 1975a,b; Glover and Reuber, 1967), progesterone in thymectomized and irradiated PVG/C rats (Ahmed et al., 1983), and iodine in the BB rat (Sternthal et al., 1981). This influence of iodine in genetically susceptible BB rats is of particular interest in light of similar effects in man. In addition, neonatal thymectomy (Silverman and Rose, 1974) and injection of a thyroid extract with incomplete Freund's adjuvant in BUF rats, but not normal rats, greatly increases thyroiditis (Silverman and Rose, 1975b). Many additional rat strains develop thyroiditis when thyroid extracts are administered with complete Freund's adjuvant (Lillehoj and Rose, 1981).

The experimental induction of autoimmune thyroiditis has been extensively studied in mice. A gene(s) in the MHC is an important determinant of disease (Rose and Kong, 1983; Beisel et al., 1982; Vladutiu, 1983). Though all mice can produce significant titers of anti-thyroglobulin antibodies after injection of murine thyroglobulin with complete Freund's adjuvant, only mice of the $H$-$2$ haplotypes $H$-$2^k$ and $H$-$2^s$ develop severe thyroiditis, while $H$-$2^b$ and $H$-$2^d$ mice are resistant. Both $I$-$A$ subregion genes (class II) and class I genes interact to determine thyroiditis (Rose and Kong, 1983). In addition, non-MHC genes influence induced thyroiditis (Beisel *et al.*, 1982). Similar to the thyroiditis of obese strain chickens, T cells in reconstitution experiments determine the immune response to thyroglobulin, while severe thyroiditis develops in reconstitution experiments of lethally irradiated mice whether the B cells are derived from responder or nonresponder mice (Vladutiu and Rose, 1975).

An important development in the study of experimental autoimmune thyroiditis has been the production of a T lymphocyte line specific for thyroglobulin which both produces and vaccinates against autoimmune thyroiditis in mice (Maron *et al.*, 1983). With the discovery of interleukin-2 (T cell growth factor), it has become possible to generate continuous T cell lines. Maron and co-workers (1983) immunized susceptible mice with thyroglobulin in complete Freund's adjuvant, isolated lymph node cells, stimulated these cells *in vitro* with thyroglobulin, and then propagated the cells with media containing interleukin-2. As few as $10^5$ of the resulting T cells injected into recipient mice produce severe thyroiditis. If mice were first immunized with the T cell line, thyroiditis could no longer be induced by the injection of thyroglobulin and complete Freund's adjuvant. Anti-thyroglobulin antibodies appeared unrelated to the development of thyroiditis or its prevention by T cell line immunization.

The obese chicken, Buffalo rat, BB rat, and the experimental autoimmune thyroiditis models resemble Hashimoto's thyroiditis. Imahori and Vladutiu (1983) have described an experimentally induced thyroiditis in two inbred strains of mice which resembles subacute (de Quervain's) thyroiditis. Mice of the RF and SJL strains injected with thyroglobulin develop granulomatous thyroiditis with giant cells, transient hyperthyroidism (with suppressed iodine uptake), a later hypothyroid phase, and eventually normal thyroid hormone concentrations. This animal model suggests that the histologic lesions of subacute thyroiditis can develop independent of viral infection.

## C. THYROIDITIS OF MAN

Familial aggregation of clinically overt Hashimoto's thyroiditis and anti-thyroid antibodies has been described (Hall *et al.*, 1962,1972). In a normal middle-aged rural population anti-thyroglobulin antibodies were found in 26% of siblings of probands with such antibodies versus 11% of probands lacking antibodies. Anti-microsomal antibodies were found in 32% of siblings with anti-microsomal antibodies versus 11% of those without. This high prevalence of anti-thyroid antibodies in an aged population without clinically overt thyroid disease is a common finding. Detection of antibodies correlates with histologic evidence of thyroid inflammation, but alone is a relatively poor predictor of the development of overt hypothyroidism (Gray *et al.*, 1983; Bjoro *et al.*, 1984; Lazarus *et al.*, 1984; Dissaint and Wemeau, 1982; Bonnyns *et al.*, 1982; Gordin and Lamberg, 1975; Gray *et al.*, 1983; Tunbridge *et al.*, 1981). Subjects with normal circulating thyroxine concentrations but with small elevations of thyroid-stimulating hormone (reflecting decreased thyroid reserve) and anti-microsomal anti-thyroid antibodies develop overt hypothyroidism at a rate of ~5% per year in the general as well as the diabetic populations (Tunbridge *et al.*, 1981; Gray *et al.*, 1983; Gordin and Lamberg, 1975). A combination of immunologic and endocrinologic abnormalities is the best predictor of subsequent overt disease.

The specific genetic abnormalities predisposing to Hashimoto's thyroiditis have not been defined. Similar to other autoimmune endocrine diseases, genes in the MHC and perhaps immunoglobulin allotypes (Uno *et al.*, 1981) are associated with disease susceptibility. The HLA-DR5 allele is found with increased frequency in patients with goiters and Hashimoto's thyroiditis (no HLA-A, -B, and -C association), while in patients without goiter (atrophic thyroiditis), there is an increased association with HLA-DR3 and HLA-B8 (Chopra *et al.*, 1977; Ludwig *et al.*, 1977; Irvine, 1978; Weissel *et al.*, 1980; Moens and Farid, 1978; Farid *et al.*, 1981).

This apparent genetic heterogeneity of Hashimoto's thyroiditis may relate to multiple different autoantibodies in thyroiditis patients, including antibodies which inhibit TSH binding, inhibit TSH activation of thyroid adenylate cyclase, stimulate adenylate cyclase (Konishi *et al.*, 1983; Bliddal *et al.*, 1982; Marriotti *et al.*, 1983), or react with thyroglobulin, second colloidal antigen, or microsomal thyroid antigens. Anti-microsomal antibodies react with the apical surface of the follicular epithelium (Khoury *et al.*, 1984). Access of antibody to the apical membrane of thyroid cells probably evolves upon disruption of thyroid follicular architecture (Khoury *et al.*, 1984).

In addition to these multiple autoantibodies, the pathologic hallmark of Hashimoto's thyroiditis is lymphocytic infiltration of the gland and damaged thyroid cells packed with mitochondria showing acidophilic staining character (Hurthle or Askanazy cells). The inflammatory infiltrate is composed of lymphocytes, plasma cells, and macrophages (Wall *et al.*, 1983; Jansson *et al.*, 1983,1984). Thin needle biopsy samples of the infiltrating cells reveal the majority of lymphocytes to be T cells with relatively less T8-positive cells (suppressor or cytotoxic) than in the peripheral circulation. In addition, there is an increased percentage of B lymphocytes. Presence of autoantibodies correlates with the lymphocytic inflammation (Baker et al., 1983).

de Quervain's (subacute) thyroiditis differs from Hashimoto's thyroiditis genetically, pathologically, in clinical findings, and in clinical course. The illness classically is associated with a tender slightly enlarged thyroid gland, an elevated erythrocyte sedimentation rate reflecting inflammation, a gland with granulomatous inflammatory changes (including giant cells clustered about degenerating thyroid follicles), transient thyrotoxicosis with low radioactive iodine uptake, then hypothyroidism, and finally in 90% of patients return to normal thyroid function. Anti-thyroglobulin and anti-microsomal antibodies are usually absent in contrast to Hashimoto's thyroiditis. The absence of anti-thyroglobulin antibodies and subacute clinical course of de Quervain's thyroiditis has led to the speculation that this illness is caused by viral infection (Volpe et al., 1967). Nevertheless, despite much study, no specific virus has been associated with the syndrome. In addition, studies of an experimental autoimmune animal model of the disease (Imahori and Vladutiu, 1983) and a characteristic HLA association (Bech et al., 1977; Nyulassay et al., 1977) suggest that this form of thyroiditis is due to specific genetic susceptibility. de Quervain's thyroiditis is associated with the HLA-B antigen Bw35 with a relative risk of 11.5 (Farid, 1981). This is a higher association with a single HLA allele than is found with any other autoimmune endocrine disease.

The immunogenetics of painless subacute thyroiditis (occurring spontaneously and postpartum) is not as well defined as de Quervain's thyroiditis. Whereas the Bw35 allele is found in 70% of patients with de Quervain's thyroiditis, only 24% of patients with transient postpartum thyrotoxicosis expressed this allele (versus 17% of controls). Though the series are small, DR3 appears to be associated with both postpartum and spontaneous painless thyroiditis and DR5 with postpartum thyroiditis (60% of patients versus 27% of controls), and there is one report of a DR4 association with postpartum thyroiditis (Farid et al., 1983; Lervang et al., 1984; Howe et al., 1982).

Given genetic susceptibility, what triggers the development of active thyroiditis? In both animal models and man the ingestion of large quantities of iodine is associated with autoimmune thyroid disease (Sternthal et al., 1981; Martino et al., 1984). The most dramatic association is with the drug amiodarone, an iodine-containing antiarrhythmic. Normal dietary iodine consumption in the United States ranges between 200 and 500 $\mu$g/day, while patients receiving amiodarone consume the equivalent of over 20 mg of free iodine per day. Martino and co-workers (1984) have evaluated autoimmune thyroid disease in a population receiving amiodarone with high (Massachusetts) and low (Italy) iodine consumption. They documented a remarkably high overall prevalence of autoimmune thyroid disease, with more hypothyroidism in Massachusetts and more hyperthyroidism in Italy. Anti-thyroglobulin and anti-microsomal antibodies were prevalent in patients on amiodarone, and there were low titers of antibodies blocking TSH binding. We have evaluated T cell subsets using the monoclonals T4 ("helper"), T8 ("suppressor/cytotoxic"), and a new monoclonal 3G5 which reacts with a complex ganglioside expressed on both T4 and T8 mature T cells (Rabinowe et al., 1984b) in patients taking amiodarone. The percentage of T4- and T8-positive cells were normal, while the percentage of 3G5 cells was increased with 60% of the patients on amiodarone being above the normal range. Of the 10 patients on amiodarone, one was overtly hypothyroid, one hyperthyroid, and a third had Graves' ophthalmopathy. It is likely that the iodine content of amiodarone triggers autoimmunity which causes overt disease in genetically susceptible subjects.

## IV. Idiopathic Adrenal Insufficiency/Primary Hypogonadism/Idiopathic Hypoparathyroidism/Autoimmune Polyglandular Syndrome Type I and Type II

In Addison's disease, autoantibodies (anti-adrenal antibodies and antibodies that cross-react with other steroid cells) are found (Betterle et al., 1983), and there is evidence of cell-mediated immunity directed against the adrenal (Nerup and Bendixen, 1969), and an elevated percentage of T cells expressing the Ia antigen (Rabinowe et al., 1984a). Anti-adrenal antibodies may predict the development of Addison's disease, but there can be a very long subclinical phase of adrenal destruction.

In patients with Addison's disease, premature ovarian failure in the absence of chromosomal abnormalities occurs in as many as 25% of women (Turkington and Lebovitz, 1967; Edmonds et al., 1973; Sotsiou et al., 1980; Doniach and Bottazzo 1981; Irvine et al., 1968; McNatty et al., 1975; Leer et al., 1980; Gloor and Hurlimann 1984). Autoimmune ovarian failure can also occur in the absence of Addison's disease. Three different immunofluorescent patterns of reaction of antibodies with corpus luteal cells of the ovary have been observed and suggest that there are three separate target antigens including anti-cell surface antibodies (McNatty *et al.,* 1975). Essentially all patients with gonadal autoantibodies also have adrenocortical antibodies (Elder *et al.,* 1981). Since the gonadal autoantibodies can be absorbed with powdered adrenal cortex, these antibodies are cross-reactive "steroidal cell" antibodies. In addition, antibodies to sperm and ova have been found in ~25% of patients with infertility (Doniach and Bottazzo 1981). Case reports of amenorrheic patients with presumed autoimmune oophoritis responding to prednisone immunosuppression exist, but "benefit" has for the most part been transient and not well documented (Coulam *et al.,* 1981). Testicular failure is much less common than ovarian failure in patients with polyendocrine autoimmunity (Eisenbarth and Jackson, 1981).

As found with thyroiditis, genetic analysis of Addison's disease has led to the recognition of disease heterogeneity. The combination of chronic mucocutaneous candidiasis, hypoparathyroidism, and Addison's disease has been termed type I autoimmune polyglandular syndrome, in contrast to a type II syndrome displaying neither candidiasis nor hypoparathyroidism (Neufeld *et al.,* 1981; Maclaren and Neufeld 1981; Eisenbarth and Jackson; 1981). The disease associations of these two syndromes and the major differences between the syndromes are listed in Table IV. The type I syndrome (mucocutaneous candidiasis,

TABLE IV
Autoimmune Polyglandular Syndromes

| Type I | Type II |
| --- | --- |
| Siblings affected | Multiple generations affected |
| No HLA Association | HLA-B8,DR3 associated |
| Onset in youth or infancy | Peak incidence ages 20–60 |
| One-third patients mucocutaneous candidiasis | No mucocutaneous candidiasis |
| Hypoparathyroidism | Rare, if every hypoparathyroidism |
| Addison's disease | Addison's disease |
| Primary hypothyroidism | Primary hypothyroidism |
| 5% Type I diabetes | 50% Type I diabetes |
|  | Graves' disease common |
|  | Myasthenia gravis |
| Malabsorption syndromes | Celiac disease |
| Primary hypogonadism | Primary hypogonadism |
| Vitiligo | Vitiligo |
| Pernicious anemia | Pernicious anemia |
| Alopecia | Alopecia |

hypoparathyroidism and Addison's disease) appears to be an auto-somal recessive disease with the common occurrence of multiply af-fected siblings. To our knowledge there are no reports of a parent and child with this syndrome. Mucocutaneous candidiasis and hypopara-thyroidism rarely if ever occur in the type II syndrome where Addi-son's disease associated with Type I diabetes and Graves' disease is common. In the type II syndrome multiple generations are usually affected. HLA typing also distinguishes the two syndromes. The type II polyglandular syndrome is HLA-B8,DR3 associated, while there is no HLA association with the type I syndrome (Eisenbarth and Jackson, 1981; Eisenbarth *et al.*, 1978, 1979; Anderson *et al.*, 1980; Farid *et al.*, 1980). Within type II families, disease often correlates with inheri-tance of specific HLA haplotypes, whereas this is not the case in a limited number of families studied with the type I syndrome (Eisen-barth and Jackson, 1981; Anderson *et al.*, 1980; Farid *et al.*, 1980).

In the type II polyglandular autoimmune syndrome, HLA associa-tions do not explain the variety of associated diseases in family mem-bers, the age range of disease onset in patients with multiple illnesses, or the lack of 100% concordance of twins for individual diseases. What appears to be inherited is a susceptibility to develop an organ-specific autoimmune disease rather than a specific illness. This point can be illustrated by a representative family (Eisenbarth *et al.*, 1978). The proband displayed five diseases (Addison's disease, myasthenia gravis, hypothyroidism, vitaligo, and premature menopause). Her mother and aunt were severely hypothyroid (diagnosed by family testing) and had alopecia totalis, which developed in childhood. Both siblings and a niece were hypothyroid and one sib had hypogonadism. All the affected family members shared an HLA-A1,B8 haplotype.

## V. Hypophysitis

Autoantibodies reacting with selective pituitary cells as well as lym-phocytic infiltration (rare case reports) of the pituitary with associated hypopituitarism have been described (Hume and Roberts, 1967; Goudie and Pinkerton 1957; Lock, 1975; Bottazzo and Doniach, 1978; Pouplard *et al.*, 1976). In addition, Bottazzo and co-workers (1980) have detected antibodies reacting with vasopressin-containing cells of the hypothalamus. The pathogenic significance of these abnormalities is not defined, but in polyendocrine patients pituitary insufficiency can coexist with autoimmune destruction of a primary gland (e.g., thyroid, adrenal, gonad).

## VI. Graves' Disease

Graves' disease is a systemic disorder involving multiple organs with variation in the extent of lesions and in the course of the disease. The hyperthyroidism (with or without diffuse goiter), exophthalmos, and pretibial myxedema of Graves' disease do not always occur simultaneously and may result from associated but separate autoimmune processes.

Graves' disease may be caused by interaction of multiple genes predisposing to autoimmunity. The exact concordance of monozygotic twins for Graves' disease has not been established, but there are many case reports describing concordant monozygotic twins (Hassan *et al.*, 1966). This lack of a population-based study of twins for concordance of Graves' disease makes it difficult to define the genetic "penetrance" of this disorder which is both familial and common (Farid *et al.*, 1977; Baldwin, 1978). At least three separate genetic loci may contribute to the development of Graves' disease: genes in the MHC (chromosome six), sex-linked genes (female-to-male ratio among patients is 6 or 8 to 1), and genes determining immunoglobulin heavy-chain allotypes (chromosome 14).

Similar to many organ-specific autoimmune diseases, Graves' disease is associated with HLA-DR3 (Farid *et al.*, 1979, 1983b; Grumet *et al.*, 1974). Because HLA alleles A1 and B8 are in linkage dysequilibrium (nonrandomly associated) with HLA-DR3, these alleles are also associated with Graves' disease. There is increasing evidence of immunogenetic heterogeneity of Graves' disease with an association of toxic diffuse goiter with both HLA-DR3 and HLA-DR5 (Schleusener *et al.*, 1983). The HLA-DR3-associated disease variant may include patients with ophthalmopathy and antibodies inhibiting TSH binding; neither ophthalmopathy nor TSH binding inhibiting antibodies are associated with HLA-DR5-linked disease (Schleusener *et al.*, 1983).

Since HLA-DR3 and -DR5 are found in less than 50% of affected patients and these alleles exist in 20–30% of the normal population, HLA typing cannot be used to categorize individuals. There is considerable controversy as to whether the HLA-DR3 correlates with remission rates. HLA-DR3-positive patients reportedly are more likely to display unremitting hyperthyroidism (McGregor *et al.*, 1980a; Irvine *et al.,* 1977; Dahlberg *et al.,* 1980). This controversy is not resolved, but may relate to the immunogenetic heterogeneity of Graves' disease. Patients positive for antibodies inhibiting TSH binding or for ophthalmopathy are less likely to remit if HLA-DR3 positive (Schleusener *et al.,* 1983), and patients without ophthalmopathy and inhibiting antibodies are less likely to remit if HLA-DR5 positive.

In a review of HLA typing of 43 sib pairs with Graves' disease (Farid *et al.,* 1983; Bech *et al.,* 1978), 63, 32, and 4.7% of sib pairs shared 2, 1, and no HLA haplotypes. This contrasts with an expected sharing of 25, 50, and 25%, if the HLA region were independent of Graves' disease. The proportions are remarkably similar to HLA haplotype sharing in sib pairs with Type I diabetes.

In addition to histocompatibility genes, genes determining immunoglobulin allotypes may be associated with Graves' disease (Pepper *et al.,* 1981; Nakao *et al.,* 1982; Uno *et al.,* 1981). Genetic differences among antibodies of the same class ($IgG_1$, $IgG_2$, $IgG_3$, IgM, IgA, IgD, IgE, light-chain $\kappa$ or $\lambda$) are referred to as allotypes. Allotypes are determined by amino acid sequence differences in constant regions of the immunoglobulin heavy or light chains and are given numeric or alphanumeric designations. For example, $IG_1$ can be subdivided into allotypes Glm 3, Glm 17, Glm 1, and Glm 2. Races differ in their expression of allotypes; some are very common for a given race (haplotype). Some have reported that Graves' disease is associated with specific Gm allotypes (Pepper *et al.,* 1981; Nakao *et al.,* 1982); others have not found such an association (Uno *et al.,* 1981). Even in the latter report on Japanese subjects who showed no increase in a specific Gm allotype, 14 of 15 sibs of patients with Graves' disease shared at lease one Gm allotype.

A hallmark of Graves' disease is autoantibodies which stimulate the thyroid. In 1956 Adams and Purves described an unusual thyroid stimulator in the serum of Graves' disease patients, and in 1958 McKenzie described a bioassay for thyrotropin which became the standard for measuring immunoglobulin stimulators of the thyroid (Long Acting Thyroid Stimulator—LATS) (McKenzie, 1958). This and other assays of abnormal immunoglobulins from patients with Graves' disease have been studied extensively (Table V). Increasing evidence suggests that antibodies binding to different classes of molecules (glycolipids, the glycoprotein TSH receptor) can produce dramatically different effects on the thyroid, including stimulation or inhibition of thyroid growth (Drexhage *et al.,* 1980,1981; Doniach *et al.,* 1982) and stimulation or inhibition of thyroid hormonogenesis (Endo *et al.,* 1978; Matsuura *et al.,* 1980; Orgiazzi *et al.,* 1976; Carayon *et al.,* 1983). Some of this

TABLE V

ASSAYS FOR AUTOANTIBODIES OF GRAVES' DISEASE[a]

| Basis of Each Measurement | Ref. | "Activity" measured | Acronym |
|---|---|---|---|
| 1. Release of radioiodine from prelabeled mouse thyroid glands | McKenzie (1958) | Long-acting thyroid stimulator | LATS |
| 2. Inhibition of binding of reference LATS activity to human thyroid protein | Adams and Kennedy (1967) | Long-acting thyroid stimulator protector | LATS-P |
| 3. Stimulation of intracellular colloid droplet formation in human thyroid slices | Onaya et al. (1973) | Human thyroid stimulator | HTS |
| 4. Inhibition of binding of radiolabeled bovine TSH to crude human thyroid membranes | Smith and Hall (1974) | Thyroid-stimulating immunoglobulin index | TSI |
| 5. Stimulation of adenylate cyclase in purified human thyroid membranes | Orgiazzi et al. (1976) | Human thyroid adenylate cyclase stimulator | HATCS |
| 6. Cyclic AMP accumulation in human thyroid slices | McKenzie and Zakarija (1978) | Thyroid-stimulating antibodies | TSAB |
| 7. Cyclic AMP accumulation in cultured human thyroid cells | Hinds et al. (1981; Ettienne-Deceef and Winard (1981) | — | — |
| 8. Cytochemical bioassay detecting an increase in lysosomal permeability in guinea pig thyroid segments | Bitensky et al. (1974) | — | — |
| 9. Radioimmunological measurement of release of T3 and T4 from porcine thyroid slices, mouse thyroid lobes or human thyroid fragment | Laurberg and Weeke (1975); Chapman et al. (1976) | — | — |

[a] From Farid et al. (1983b).

marked heterogeneity of Graves' immunoglobulins is being dissected by Kohn and co-workers using monoclonal antibodies reacting with thyroid membranes (Kohn et al., 1983; Valente et al., 1982; Ealey et al., 1984). These monoclonals (some produced by fusing lymphocytes from patients with Graves' disease) appear to recreate the heterogeneous effects of Graves' disease antibodies. The monoclonal antibodies can be divided into major groups based on inhibition of [125]I-labeled TSH binding. Antibodies which potently inhibit TSH binding react with the glycoprotein TSH receptor and inhibit TSH action. Antibodies that only minimally inhibit TSH binding react with complex gangliosides and are potent stimulators of thyroid adenylate cyclase and of naphthylamidase activity (Valente *et al.*, 1982). Monoclonal antibodies with a mixture of these properties have also been produced (Ealey *et al.*, 1984). A finding of particular significance is the inability of inhibitory antibodies (which can completely block TSH stimulation) to block the activity of monoclonal antibody stimulators. The existence of multiple circulating autoantibodies, all inhibiting TSH binding to some extent, but reacting with different molecules of the thyroid membrane, may explain the heterogeneity of the clinical course of Graves' disease and of neonatal hyperthyroidism and hypothyroidism (Zakarija and McKenzie, 1983).

In addition to studies of monoclonal autoantibodies in Graves' disease, monoclonal antibodies have been used to study the T cells of patients with Graves' disease. As with Type I diabetes no abnormality characteristic of resting T cell subsets has been defined (Jackson *et al.*, 1984c; Sridama *et al.*, 1982; Thielemans *et al.*, 1981; Wall *et al.*, 1983; Iwatani *et al.*, 1983). Wall and co-workers reported a marked increase in the percentage of mononuclear cells reacting with a monoclonal antibody to the Ia antigen in untreated Graves' hyperthyroidism, but thought the Ia-positive cells were mainly B lymphocytes (Wall *et al.*, 1983). In our own studies of purified T cells reacting with monoclonal L243 (anti-Ia), we found a 10-fold increase in the average number of circulating Ia-positive T cells and no difference in the number of B cells between patients with new onset Graves' disease when compared to controls, non-Graves' hyperthyroid patients, or long-term ablated Graves' disease (Fig. 4) (Jackson *et al.*, 1984c). Such an increase in Ia-positive T cells has been found in three HLA-DR3-associated diseases, Graves' disease, Type I diabetes, and idiopathic Addison's disease (Jackson *et al.*, 1982, 1984c; Rabinowe *et al.*, 1984a).

What environmental factors trigger the development of Graves' disease? Relatively little is known concerning such factors, but the expression by *Yersinia* of molecules resembling the "TSH receptor" (Weiss *et al.*, 1983) and the influence of pregnancy, iodine, and iodine-containing drugs are being studied (Martino *et al.*, 1984; Klein and Levey, 1983). Destruction of the thyroid (thyroidectomy, radioactive iodine) or treatment with methimizole decreases not only homonogenesis, but also the titer of autoantibodies and circulating Ia-positive T cells (Jackson *et al.*, 1984c; Muktar *et al.*, 1975; McGregor *et al.*, 1980). Whether iodine-containing drugs and thyroid ablation influence the development and maintenance of hyperthyroidism in part by their influence on the immune system is currently not known. It has recently been reported that thyroid follicular cells in Graves' disease patients or normal thyroid cells activated with lectins react with anti-

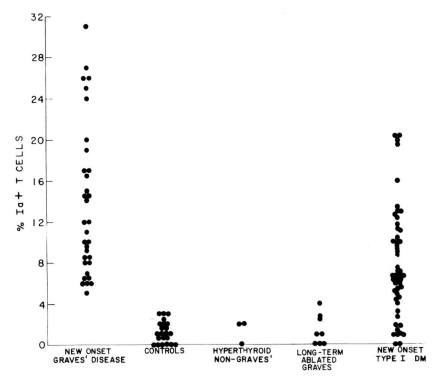

Fig. 4. Percentage of circulating T lymphocytes bearing the Ia surface antigen in patients with active untreated Graves' disease compared with normal individuals, patients with non-Graves' hyperthyroidism, and patients with Graves' disease of greater than 1-year duration who had been treated with surgery or [131]I. Patients with Type I diabetes of less than 4-months duration are also shown. From Jackson et al. (1984c).

Ia monoclonal antibodies (Pujol-Borrel et al., 1983). Thus, endogenous "activation" of thyroid follicular cells may enhance the autoimmune response to the thyroid.

Other manifestations of Graves' disease such as ophthalmopathy and pretibial myxedema may be independent but related autoimmune components of this illness. Ophthalmopathy is associated with extensive lymphocytic infiltrates of extraocular muscles (Wall et al., 1981). Investigators are evaluating antigens shared between thyroid and extraocular muscles, anatomical relationships between the thyroid and eye (Kriss and Medhi, 1979), and correlation of stimulation of cellular growth by Graves' immunoglobulins [e.g., fibroblast growth studied in pretibial myxedema (Cheung et al., 1978)]. To date there is no assay that can allow prediction of which patient will develop ophthalmopathy or in which patient it will progress. A series of immunotherapies to influence ophthalmopathy are being studied, including cyclosporin A. The efficacy of these therapies is currently poorly defined (Gorman, 1978).


## VII. ANTI-INSULIN RECEPTOR ANTIBODIES

Diseases characterized by antibodies to the insulin receptor are rare, with approximately 25 reported patients (Flier *et al.*, 1975; Kahn and Harrison, 1980). Antibodies to the insulin receptor have been found in patients who are euglycemic but have marked compensatory hyperinsulinism, patients with diabetes mellitus and extreme insulin resistance, and in patients with fasting hypoglycemia (Flier *et al.*, 1978; Taylor *et al.*, 1982). It is not known whether these differences in glycemia reflect heterogeneity of the autoantibodies or differences in physiologic response to similar autoantibodies. Since all anti-insulin receptor sera are insulinomimetic *in vitro* but desensitize tissue to the effects of insulin after prolonged exposure, it is likely that physiologic alterations underlie changes in glycemia (Dons *et al.*, 1983).

Approximately one-third of patients with anti-insulin receptor antibodies have an associated autoimmune illness, including systemic lupus erythematosis, Sjogren's syndrome, and ataxia telangiectasia (Kahn and Harrison, 1980). Anti-nuclear antibodies, elevated erythrocyte sedimentation rate, and hypocomplementemia are common.


## VIII. ANTIBODIES TO HORMONES AND IONS

### A. ANTI-INSULIN ANTIBODIES

Anti-insulin antibodies occur spontaneously without insulin therapy in at least two situations. The first is a subset of patients with Type I diabetes prior to insulin therapy, and these express such antibodies in low titer (Palmer *et al.*, 1983). In these patients anti-insulin antibodies may provide a quantitative assay of the disordered immunity prior to diabetes. In small number of patients initially described from Japan (Ichihara *et al.*, 1977) but recently reported from the United States (Goldman *et al.*, 1979), spontaneously occurring antibodies to insulin have been associated with hypoglycemia, at times reactive hypoglycemia. These patients show high concentrations of circulating insulin bound to antibodies, and the major differential is the exclusion of factitious insulin use. Specialized laboratory techniques can be used to distinguish the species specificity of antibodies if factitious use of porcine or bovine insulin is suspected. The cause of hypoglycemia in these patients is not completely defined, but may relate to sporadic release of insulin from a large pool of antibody-bound insulin.

## B. Anti-thyroid Hormone Antibodies

Both polyclonal and monoclonal antibodies reacting with thyroxine and triiodothyronine have been described (Robbins et al., 1956; Premachandra and Blumenthal, 1967; Ochi et al., 1972; Staeheli et al., 1975; Wu and Green, 1976; Karlsson et al., 1977; Hermann et al., 1977; Beck-Peccoz et al., 1984; Ginsberg et al., 1978; Inada et al., 1980; Rodriquez-Espinosa et al., 1980; Trimarchi et al., 1982; DeBaets et al., 1982; Moroz et al., 1983). Monoclonal anti-thyroid hormone antibodies have been found in a significant number of patients, including patients with Waldenstrom's macroglobulinemia and Graves' disease (Rodriquez-Espinosa et al., 1980; Trimarchi et al., 1982; DeBaets et al., 1982; Moroz et al., 1983). In most of the patients, the thyroid hormone binding antibodies do not cause disease, but produce elevations of circulating hormones. Treatment to lower hormone concentrations or reduction of thyroxine replacement in a patient with such antibodies can produce disease. In such patients determination of TSH in hypothyroid patients taking thyroxine or response of TSH to TRH can confirm clinical euthyroidism despite aberrant laboratory tests.

## C. Antibodies to Calcium

Similar to spontaneous antibodies to thyroid hormone, spontaneous autoantibodies to calcium (Soria et al., 1976; Jaffe and Mosher, 1979; Spira et al., 1980; Lingarde and Zetterval, 1973; Annesley et al., 1982) are not usually associated with disease except when this "artifactual" hypercalcemia is inappropriately treated. Ionized calcium is normal in these patients while calcium measured on an autoanalyzer can be markedly elevated (Annesley et al., 1982). Aggressive therapy to lower calcium can result in severe hypocalcemia, tetany, and seizures. The patients most often reported with such antibodies have multiple myeloma with a monoclonal antibody reacting with calcium. The finding of marked hypercalcemia in a patient with no symptoms related to hypercalcemia should prompt measurement of ionized calcium.

## IX. Summary

Despite obvious differences related to target organs and the target antigens within organs, there are remarkable similarities in time course and immunogenetics of the autoimmune endocrine disorders. These similarities extend even to the non-organ-specific autoimmune diseases such as Sjogren's syndrome and lupus erythematosus (Laskin *et al.*, 1982; Chused *et al.*, 1977). Each of the diseases can be divided into a series of stages beginning with genetic susceptibility. Usually the interactions of more than one gene [e.g., BB rat, NZB mouse (Laskin *et al.*, 1982), obese chicken, Type I diabetes, Graves' disease] produce disease susceptibility. One of the genes resides in the region of the major histocompatibility complex and other genes can profoundly influence immune function. Each single gene is usually "necessary" but not sufficient by itself to produce disease, and the same phenotype (e.g., adrenal cortical destruction) can result from different genetic abnormalities (Addison's disease of the type II and type I autoimmune polyglandular syndromes). Concordance rates of identical twins is usually less than 50% and siblings concordant for disease are often HLA identical, sometimes share one HLA haplotype, and rarely have neither HLA haplotype in common.

The lack of 100% concordance in identical twins has led to a search for "environmental" influences. Multiple drugs such as procainamide (Lahita *et al.*, 1979), hydralazine (Bjorck *et al.*, 1983), and aldomet (Petz, 1980) are known to induce autoantibodies and autoimmunity. Infectious agents can also precipitate the production of autoantibodies (Haspel *et al.*, 1983). In autoimmune endocrine disorders "triggering" agents have not been well defined, but include congenital rubella for diabetes and amiodarone or other iodine-containing medications for thyroid autoimmunity. It is likely that there are multiple triggering factors in some patients, and in some animal strains no trigger is necessary.

In each of the organ-specific autoimmune diseases, it appears that multiple molecules are antigenic targets. In Type I diabetes a subset of patients even produces antibodies to insulin prior to insulin therapy. Patients developing Type I diabetes produce other autoantibodies reacting with both the surface and cytoplasm of islet cells. In Graves' disease, autoantibodies to surface glycolipids, the glycoprotein TSH receptor itself, and perhaps other antigens may determine the clinical course (hyperthyroidism versus hypothyroidism with or without a goiter). In the organ-specific autoimmune diseases, in addition to autoantibodies, there are frequently T cell abnormalities such as the increase in Ia-positive T cells in Graves' disease, Type I diabetes, and Addison's disease. It is likely that cell-mediated immunity is responsible for tissue destruction.

The actual autoimmune destruction of an organ appears for most endocrine diseases to be remarkably slow. There is a long prodromal phase (measured in years) during which autoantibodies are present and sensitive endocrine tests reveal progressive endocrine dysfunction (e.g., TSH elevations prior to overt hypothyroidism, loss of first-phase insulin response to intravenous glucose prior to Type I diabetes). An exception to this chronic process is the rapid destruction of transplanted $\beta$ cells in identical twin pancreatic transplants. In these patients, diabetes recurs in weeks, not years, and appears to be secondary to an anamnestic immune response (Sutherland et al., 1984).

Despite a remarkable recent increase in understanding of basic immunology (Stastny et al., 1983; Rose, 1982; Yanagi et al., 1984), very few gene products contributing to the development of autoimmunity have been defined. Those genes that have been defined are all associated with immunodeficiency states such as nucleoside phosphorylase deficiency (Webster, 1982), which gives rise to a severe T cell abnormality and occasionally hemolytic anemia, complement deficiencies associated with forms of lupus erythematosus (Rynes, 1982), and C1-esterase deficiency of hereditary angioneurotic edema (Gelfand, 1982). In the BB rat an autosomal recessive gene produces a profound circulating T cell lymphopenia which in some manner contributes to the development of diabetes. The most effective and certainly the safest immunotherapies to prevent the Type I diabetes of the BB rat replace this T cell deficit (e.g., blood transfusions). When the actual gene products determining endocrine autoimmunity in man are elucidated, it is possible that some form of "replacement" therapy may prevent disease. Without such fundamental knowledge, therapies aimed at partial immunosuppression are being studied in Graves' ophthalmopathy and Type I diabetes. With so many immunologic, genetic, and pathogenic similarities, it is likely that lessons learned from study of immunotherapy in one of the organ-specific autoimmune diseases will be applicable to many of these related disorders.

ACKNOWLEDGMENTS

The authors greatly appreciate the patience and diligence of Ms. Patty Cronin in the preparation of this manuscript. We thank Dr. Arthur Like (University of Massachusetts Medical Center, Worcester, Massachusetts) for providing us with the photographs which comprise Fig. 1. This work was supported by grants from the NIH (GM-07171, AM-25778). Dr. Eisenbarth is the recipient of a Career Development Award from the Juvenile Diabetes Foundation.

# REFERENCES

Adams, D. D., and Kennedy, T. H. (1967). Occurrence in thyrotoxicosis of a gamma globulin which protects LATS from neutralization by an extract of thyroid gland. *J. Clin. Endocrinol. Metab.* **27,** 173–177.

Adams, D. D., and Purves, H. D. (1956). Abnormal responses in the assay of thyrotropin. *Proc. Univ. Otago Med. Sch.* **34,** 11–12.

Ahmed, S. A., Young, P. R., and Penhale, W. J. (1983). The effects of female sex steroids on the development of autoimmune thyroiditis in thymectomized and irradiated rats. *Clin. Exp. Immunol.* **54,** 351–358.

Anderson, P. B., Fein, S. H., and Frey, W. G., III (1980). Familial Schmidt's syndrome. *J. Am. Med. Assoc.* **244,** 2068–2070.

Annesley, T. M., Burritt, M. F., and Kyle, R. A. (1982). Artifactual hypercalcemia in multiple myeloma. *Mayo Clin. Proc.* **57,** 572–575.

Bach, F. M., Segall, M., Rich, S., and Barbosa, J. (1982). HLA and susceptibility to type I diabetes: Hypothesis. *Tissue Antigens* **20,** 28–32.

Baekkeskov, S., Nielsen, J. H., Marner, B., Bilde, T., Ludvigsson, J., and Lernmark, A. (1982). Autoantibodies in newly diagnosed diabetic children immunoprecipitate specific human islet cell proteins. *Nature (London)* **298,** 167–169.

Baekkeskov, S., Dyrberg, T., and Lernmark, A. (1983). A 64K protein immunoprecipitated from normal rat islets by antibodies from spontaneously diabetic BB rats. *Diabetologia* **25,** 138.

Baker, B. A., Gharib, H., and Markowitz, H. (1983). Correlation of thyroid antibodies and cytologic features in suspected autoimmune thyroid disease. *Am. J. Med.* **74,** 941–944.

Baldwin, D. B. (1978). Incidence of thyroid disorders in Connecticut. *J. Am. Med. Assoc.* **239,** 741–744.

Bankhurst, A. D., Torrigiani, G., and Allison, A. C. (1973). Lymphocytes binding human thyroglobulin in healthy people and its relevance to tolerance for autoantigens. *Lancet* **1,** 226–230.

Barnett, A. H., Eff, C., Leslie, R. D. G., and Pyke, D. A. (1981). Diabetes in identical twins. *Diabetologia* **20,** 87–93.

Bech, K., Nerup, J., Thomsen, M., Platz, P., Ryder, L. P., Svejgaard, A., Siersbaek-Nielsen, K., and Mølholm-Hansen, J. E. (1977). Subacute thyroiditis de Quervain: A disease associated with an HLA-B antigen. *Acta Endocrinol.* **86,** 504–509.

Bech, K., Lumholtz, B., Nerup, J., Thomsen, M., Platz, P., Ryder, L. P., Svejgaard, A., Siersbaek-Nielsen, K., Molholm-Hansen, J. E., and Larsen, J. H. (1978). HLA antigens in Graves' disease. *Acta Endocrinol.* **86,** 510–516.

Beck-Peccoz, P., Romelli, P. B., Cattaneo, M. G., Faglia, G., White, E. L., Barlow, J. W., and Stockigt, J. R. (1984). Evaluation of free thyroxine methods in the presence of iodothyronine-binding autoantibodies. *J. Clin. Endocrinol. Metab.* **58,** 736–739.

Beisel, W. R., Edelman, R., Nauss, K., and Suskind, R. M. (1981). Single-nutrient effects on immunologic functions. *J. Am. Med. Assoc.* **245,** 53–58.

Beisel, K. W., Kong, Y. M., Babu, S. J., David, C. S., and Rose, N. R. (1982). Regulation of experimental autoimmune thyoriditis: Influence of non-*H-2* genes. *J. Immunogenet.* **9,** 257–265.

Bell, G. I., Horita, A., and Karam, J. H. (1984). A polymorphic locus near the human insulin gene is associated with insulin-dependent diabetes mellitus. *Diabetes* **33,** 176–183.

Bellgrau, D., Naji, A., Silvers, W. K., Markmann, J. F., and Barker, C. F. (1982). Spontaneous diabetes in BB rats: Evidence for a T-cell dependent immune response defect. *Diabetologia* **23,** 359–364.

Benacerraf, B. (1981). Role of MHC gene products in immune regulation. *Science* **212,** 1229–1238.

Benjamin, D. C., Scott, J., Curnow, R. T., and Engelhard, V. H. (1984). Stem cells vs. differentiative environment defects in the BB rat. *Diabetes* **33** (Suppl. 1), 11A.

Betterle, C., Aanette, F., Zanchetta, R., Pedini, B., Trevison, A., Montero, F., and Rigon, F. (1983). Complement-fixing adrenal autoantibodies as a marker for predicting onset of idiopathic Addison's disease. *Lancet* **1** 1238–1240.

Bitensky, L., Aalaghband-Zadeh, J., and Chayen, J. (1974). Studies on thyroid stimulating hormone and the long-acting thyroid stimulating hormone. *Clin. Endocrinol.* **3,** 363–374.

Bjorck, S., Westberg, G., Svalander, C., and Mulec, H. (1983). Rapidly progressive glomerulonephritis after hydralizine. *Lancet* **2,** 42.

Bjoro, T., Gaarder, P. I., Smeland, E. B., and Kornstad, L. (1984). Thyroid antibodies in blood donors: Prevalence and clinical significance. *Acta Endocrinol.* **105,** 324–329.

Bliddal, H., Beck, K., Feldt-Rasmussen, U., Thomsen, M., Ryder, L. P., Hansen, J. M. Siersbaek-Nielsen, K., and Friis, T. (1982). Thyroid-stimulating immunoglobulins in Hashimoto's thyroiditis measured by radioreceptor assay and adenylate cyclase stimulation and their relationship to HLA-D alleles. *J. Clin. Endocrinol. Metab.* **55,** 995–998.

Boitard, C., Debray-Sachs, M., Pouplard, A., Assan, R., and Hamburger, J. (1981). Lymphocytes from diabetics suppress insulin release *in vitro. Diabetologia* **21,** 41–46.

Bonnyns, M., Vanhaelst, L., and Bastenie, P. A. (1982). Asymptomatic atrophic thyroiditis. *Horm. Res.* **16,** 338–344.

Bottazzo, G. F., and Doniach, D. (1976). Pancreatic autoimmunity and HLA antigens. *Lancet* **2,** 800.

Bottazzo, G. F., and Doniach, D. (1978). Pituitary autoimmunity: A review. *J. R. Soc. Med.* **71,** 433–436.

Bottazzo, G. F., Gorsuch, A. N., Dean, B. M., Cudworth, A. G., and Doniach, D. (1980). Complement-fixing islet cell antibodies in type I diabetes: Possible monitors of active beta cell damage. *Lancet* **1,** 668–672.

Bottazzo, G. F., Vandelli, G., and Mirakian, R. (1980). The detection of autoantibodies to discrete endocrine cells in complex endocrine organs. *In* "Autoimmune Aspects of Endocrine Disorders" (A. Pinchera, D. Doniach, G. F. Fenzi, and L. Baschieri, eds.), pp. 367–377. Academic Press, New York.

Boyd, R. L., Cole, R. K., and Wick, G. (1983). Genetically controlled severity of autoimmune thyroiditis in obese strain (OS) chickens is expressed at both the humoral and cellular effector mechanism level. *Immunol. Commun.* **12,** 263–272.

Boyd, R. L., Oberhuber, G., Hala, K., and Wick, G. (1984). Obese strain (OS) chickens with spontaneous autoimmune thyroiditis have a deficiency in thymic nurse cells. *J. Immunol.* **132,** 718–724.

Buschard, K., Ropke, C., Madsbad, S., Mehlsen, J., Sorensen, T. B., and Rygaard, J.

(1983). Alterations of peripheral T lymphocyte subpopulations in patients with insulin-dependent (type I) diabetes mellitus. *Clin. Lab. Immunol.* **10**, 127–131.

Buse, J. B., Srikanta, S., Haynes, B., and Eisenbarth, G. S. (1983). Type I diabetes mellitus: Monoclonal human and rat autoantibodies reacting with thymic endocrine epithelium. *Clin. Res.* **31**, 339A.

Buse, J. B., Ben-Nun, A., Klein, K. A., Eisenbarth, G. S., Seidman, J. G., and Jackson, R. A. (1984a). Specific class II gene polymorphism in BB rats. *Diabetes* **33**, 700–704.

Buse, J. B., Chaplin, D. D., Ben-Nun, A., Klein, K. A., Eisenbarth, G. S., Seidman, J. G., and Jackson, R. A. (1984b). Class I, II, and III major histocompatibility gene polymorphisms in BB rats. *Diabetologia* **22**, 77–79.

Cantrell, D. A., Robins, R. A., Brooks, C. G., and Baldwin, R. W. (1982). Phenotype of rat natural killer cells defined by monoclonal antibodies marking rat lymphocyte subsets. *Immunology* **45**, 97–103.

Carayon, P., Adler, G., Roulier, R., and Lissitzky, S. (1983). Heterogeneity of the Graves' immunoglobulins directed toward the thyrotropin receptor—Adenylate cyclase system. *J. Clin. Endocrinol. Metab.* **56**, 1202–1208.

Chapman, R. S., Malan, P. G., and Ekins, R. P. (1976). The effects of microunit doses of thyrotropin on iodothylinine release from mouse thyroid lobes *in vitro. In* "Thyroid Research" (J. Robbins and L. E. Braverman, eds.), pp. 217–220. American Elsevier, New York.

Chappel, C. I., and Chappel, W. R. (1983). The discovery and development of the BB rat colony: An animal model of spontaneous diabetes mellitus. *Metabolism* **32**, 8–10.

Cheung, H. S., Nicoloff, J. T., Kamiel, M. B., Spolter, L., and Nimni, M. E. (1978). Stimulation of fibroblast biosynthetic activity by serum of patients with pretibial myxedema. *J. Invest. Dermatol.* **71**, 12–17.

Chopra, I. J., Soloman, D. H., Chopra, U., Yoshihara, E., Teraski, P. I., and Smith, F. (1977). Abnormalities in thyroid function in relatives of patients with Graves' disease and Hashimoto's thyroiditis: Lack of correlation with inheritance of HLA-B8. *J. Clin. Endocrinol. Metab.* **45**, 45–54.

Chused, T. M., Kassan, S. S., Opelz, G., Moutsopoulos, H. M., and Terasaki, P. I. (1977). Sjogren's syndrome associated with HLA-DW3. *N. Engl. J. Med.* **296**, 895–897.

Clarke, W. L., Shaver, K. A., Bright, G. A., Rogal, A. D., and Nance, W. E. (1984). Autoimmunity in congenital rubella syndrome. *J. Pediatr.* **104**, 370–373.

Cohen, P., Cohen, O., Marcadet, A., Massart, C., Lathrop, M., Deschamps, I., Hors, J., Schuller, E., and Dausset, J. (1984). Class II HLA-DC beta-chain DNA restriction fragments differentiate among HLA-DR2 individuals in insulin-dependent diabetes and multiple sclerosis. *Proc. Natl. Acad. Sci. U.S.A.* **81**, 1774–1778.

Cole, R. K. (1966). Hereditary hypothyroidism in the domestic fowl. *Genetics* **53**, 1021–1033.

Cole, R. K., Kite, J. H., and Witebsky, E. (1968). Hereditary autoimmune thyroiditis in the fowl. *Science* **169**, 1357–1358.

Cole, R. K., Kite, J. H., Wick, G., and Witebsky, E. (1970). *Poultry Sci.* **49**, 839–848.

Colle, E., Guttmann, R. D., and Seemayer, T. (1981). Spontaneous diabetes mellitus syndrome in the rat. I. Association with the major histocompatibility complex. *J. Exp. Med.* **154**, 1237–1242.

Colle, E., Guttman, R. D., Seemayer, T. A., and Michel, F. (1983). Spontaneous diabetes mellitus syndrome in the rat. IV. Immunogenetic interactions of MHC and non-MHC interaction components of the syndrome. *Metabolism* **31** (Suppl. 1), 54–61.

Contu, L., Deschamps, I., Lestradet, H., Hors, J., Schmid, M., Busson, M., Benajam, A., Marcelli-Barge, A., and Dausset, J. (1982). HLA haplotype study of 53 juvenile insulin-dependent (I.D.D.) families. *Tissue Antigens* **20**, 123–140.

Coulam, C. B., Kempers, R. D., and Randall, R. V. (1981). Premature ovarian failure: Evidence for the autoimmune mechanism. *Fertil. Steril.* **36**, 238–240.

Dahlberg, P. A., Holmlund, G., Karlsson, F. A., and Safenberg, J. (1980). Predication of relapse in Graves' disease. *Lancet* **2**, 1144.

Dardenne, M., Savino, W., and Bach, J. (1984). Autoimmune mice develop antibodies to thymic hormone: Production of anti-thymulin monoclonal autoantibodies from diabetic (db/db) and B/W mice. *J. Immunol.* **133**, 740–743.

Dauphinee, J. M., Kipper, S. B., Wofsy, D., and Talal, N. (1981). Interleukin-2 deficiency is a common feature of autoimmune mice. *J. Immunol.* **127**, 2483–2487.

Dawkins, R. L., Uko, G., Christiansen, F. T., and Kay, P. H. (1983). Letter. *Br. Med. J.* **287**, 839.

DeBaets, M., Sels, J., van Breda Vriesman, P., Elewaut, A., Vermeulen, A., Williams, P., and Coenegracht, J. (1982). Monoclonal triiodothyroxine (T3) binding immunoglobulins in a euthyroid woman. *Clin. Chim. Acta* **118**, 293–301.

Debray-Sachs, M., Dardenne, M., Sai, P., Savino, W., Quiniou, M., Boillot, D., Gepts, W., and Assan, R. (1983). Anti-islet immunity and thymic dysfunction in the mutant diabetic C57BL/KsJ db/db mouse. *Diabetes* **32**, 1048–1054.

DeGroot, L. J., Larsen, P. R., Refetoff, S., and Stanbury, J. B. (1984). "The Thyroid and Its Diseases." Wiley, New York.

Deschamps, I., Goderel, I., Lestradet, H., Schmid, M., Busson, M., Cohen, D., and Hors, J. (1984). Segregation of HLA-DR2 among affected and non-affected offspring of 66 families with type I (insulin-dependent) diabetes. *Diabetologia* **27**, 80–82.

Dessaint, J. P., and Wemeau, J. L. (1982). Autoimmunity and hypothyroidism. *Horm. Res.* **16**, 329–337.

Dobersen, M. J., and Scharff, J. E. (1982). Preferential lysis of pancreatic beta cells by islet cell surface antibodies. *Diabetes* **31**, 459–462.

Dobersen, M. J., Scharff, B. S., Ginsberg-Fellner, F., and Notkins, A. L. (1980). Cytotoxic autoantibodies to beta cells in the serum of patients with insulin-dependent diabetes mellitus. *N. Engl. J. Med.* **303**, 1493–1498.

Doniach, D., and Bottazzo, G. F. (1981). Polyendocrine autoimmunity. *In* "Clinical Immunology Update" (E. C. Franklin, ed.), pp. 96–121. Am. Elsevier, New York.

Doniach, D., Chiovato, T., Hanafusa, T., and Bottazzo, G. F. (1982). The implications of "thyroid growth-immunoglobulins" (TGI) for the understanding of sporadic nontoxic nodular goitre. *Springer Semin. Immunopathol.* **5**, 433–446.

Dons, R. F., Havlik, R., Taylor, S. I., Baird, K. L., Chernick, S. S., and Gorden, P. (1983). Clinical disorders associated with autoantibodies to the insulin receptor. *J. Clin. Invest.* **72**, 1072–1080.

Drexhage, H. A., Bottazzo, G. F., Doniach, D., Bitensky, L., and Chayen, J. (1980). Evidence for thyroid growth-stimulating immunoglobulins in some goitrous thyroid diseases. *Lancet* **2**, 287–292.

Drexhage, H. A., Bottazzo, G. F., Bitensky, L., Chayen, J., and Doniach, D. (1981). Thyroid growth-blocking antibodies in primary myxoedema. *Nature (London)* **289**, 594–596.

Dyrberg, T., Nakhooda, A. F., Baekkeskov, S., Lernmark, A., Poussier, P., and Marliss, E. B. (1982). Islet cell surface antibodies and lymphocyte antibodies in the spontaneously diabetic BB Wistar rat. *Diabetes* **31**, 278–281.

Dyrberg, T., Poussier, P., Nakhooda, A. F., Marliss, E. B., and Lernmerk, A. (1983). Humoral immunity in the spontaneously diabetic BB rat. *Metabolism* **31**, 87–91.

Dyrberg, T., Poussier, P., Nakhooda, A. F., Baekkeskov, S., Marliss, E. B., and Lernmark, A. (1984). Time course of islet cell surface antibodies in the diabetic syndrome of the "BB" Wistar rat. *Diabetologia* **26**, 159–165.

Ealey, P. A., Kohn, L. D., Ekins, R. P., and Marshall, N. J. (1984). Characterization of monoclonal antibodies derived from lymphocytes from Graves' disease patients in a cytochemical bioassay for thyroid stimulators. *J. Clin. Endocrinol. Metab.* **58**, 909–915.

Edmonds, M., Lamki, L., Killinger, D., and Volpe, R. (1973). Autoimmune thyroiditis, adrenalitis and oophoritis. *Am. J. Med.* **54**, 782–787.

Eisenbarth, G. S., and Crump, M. A. (1981). Anti-islet antibodies in patients with polyclonal beta cell activation: Mononucleosis, lupus erythematosus and rheumatoid arthritis. *Diabetes* **30** (Suppl. 1), 260A.

Eisenbarth, G. S., and Jackson, R. A. (1981). Immunogenetics of polyglandular failure and related diseases in HLA. *In* "Endocrine and Metabolic Disorders" (N. Fairid, ed.), pp. 235–264. Academic Press, New York.

Eisenbarth, G. S., Wilson, P. W., Ward, F., and Lebovitz, H. E. (1978). HLA type and occurrence of disease in familial polyglandular failure. *N. Engl. J. Med.* **298**, 92–94.

Eisenbarth, G. S., Wilson, P., Ward, F., Buckley, C., and Lebovitz, H. E. (1979). The polyglandular failure syndrome: Disease inheritance, HLA type and immune function. *Ann. Intern. Med.* **91**, 528–533.

Eisenbarth, G. S., Morris, M. A., and Scearce, R. (1981). Cytotoxic antibodies to cloned rat islet cells in serum of patients with diabetes mellitus. *J. Clin. Invest.* **67**, 403–408.

Eisenbarth, G. S., Shimizu, K., Bowring, M. A., and Wells, S. (1982). Expression of receptors for tetanus toxin and monoclonal antibody A2B5 by pancreatic islet cells. *Proc. Natl. Acad. Sci. U.S.A.* **79**, 5066–5070.

Eisenbarth, G. S., Srikanta, S., Jackson, R., and Morris, M. A. (1983a). ATGAM and prednisone immunotherapy of recent onset type I diabetes mellitus. *Clin. Res.* **31**, 500A.

Eisenbarth, G. S., Jackson, R. A., and Srikanta, S. (1983b). Type I diabetes: Autoimmunity and immunodeficiency. *In* "Monoclonal Antibodies: Probes for the Study of Autoimmunity and Immunodeficiency" (B. F. Haynes and G. S. Eisenbarth, eds.), pp. 197–218. Academic Press, New York.

Elder, M., and Maclaren, N. (1983). Identification of profound peripheral T lymphocyte immunodeficiencies in the spontaneously diabetic BB rat. *J. Immunol.* **130**, 1723–1731.

Elder, M., Maclaren, N., and Riley, W. (1981). Gonadal autoantibodies in patients with hypogonadism and/or Addison's disease. *J. Clin. Endocrinol. Metab.* **52**, 1137–1142.

Elder, M., Maclaren, N., Riley, W., and McConnell, T. (1982). Gastric parietal cell antibodies and other autoantibodies in the BB rat. *Diabetes* **31**, 313–318.

Elliott, R. B., and Martin, J. M. (1984). Dietary protein: A trigger of insulin-dependent diabetes in the BB rat. *Diabetologia* **26**, 297–299.

Elliott, R. B., Berryman, C. C., Crossley, J. R., and James, A. G. (1981). Partial preservation of pancreatic beta cell function in children with diabetes. *Lancet* **2**, 1–4.

Endo, K., Kasagi, K., Konishi, J., Ikekubo, K., Okuno, T., Takeda, Y., Mori, T., and Torizuka, K. (1978). Detection and properties of TSH-binding inhibitor immunoglobulins in patients with Graves' disease and Hashimoto's thyroiditis. *J. Clin. Endocrinol. Metab.* **46**, 734–739.

Ettienne-Deceef, J., and Winard, R. J. (1981). A sensitive technique for determination of thyroid stimulating immunoglobulin (TSI) in unfractionated serum. *Clin. Endocrinol.* **14**, 83–91.

Farid, N. R. (1981). Thyroditis. *In* "HLA in Endocrine and Metabolic Disorders" (N. R. Farid, ed.), pp. 145–176. Academic Press, New York.

Farid, N. R., Bernard, J. M., Marshall, W. H., Woolfrey, I., and O'Driscoll, R. F. (1977). Thyroid autoimmune disease in large Newfoundland family: The influence of HLA. *J. Clin. Endocrinol. Metab.* **45**, 1165–1172.

Farid, N. R., Sampson, L., Noel, E. P., Bernard, J. M., Mandevill, R., Larsen, B., and Marshall, W. H. (1979). A study of human leukocyte D locus related antigens in Graves' disease. *J. Clin. Invest.* **63**, 108–113.

Farid, N. R., Larsen, B., Payne, R., Noel, E. P., and Sampson, L. (1980). Polyglandular autoimmune disease and HLA. *Tissue Antigens* **16**, 23–29.

Farid, N. R., Sampson, L., Moens, H., and Bernard, J. M. (1981). The association of goitrous autoimmune thyroiditis is associated with HLA-DR5. *Tissue Antigens* **17**, 265–268.

Farid, N. R., Howe, B. S., and Walfish, P. G. (1983a). Increased frequency of HLA-DR3 and 5 in the syndromes of painless thyroiditis with transient thyrotoxicosis: Evidence for an autoimmune etiology. *Clin. Endocrinol.* **19**, 699–704.

Farid, N. R., Briones-Urbina, R., and Bear, J. C. (1983b). Graves' disease—The thyroid stimulating antibody and immunological networks. *Mol. Aspects Med.* **6**, 355–457.

Flier, J. S., Kahn, C. R., Roth, J., and Bar, R. S. (1975). Antibodies that impair receptor binding in an unusual diabetic syndrome with severe insulin resistance. *Science* **190**, 63–65.

Flier, J. S., Bar, R. S., Muggeo, M., Kahn, C. R., Roth, J., and Gorden, P. (1978). The evolving clinical course of patients with insulin receptor autoantibodies: Spontaneous remission or receptor proliferation with hypoglycemia. *J. Clin. Endocrinol. Metab.* **47**, 985–995.

Ganda, O. P., Srikanta, S., Brink, S. J., Morris, M. A., Gleason, R. E., Soeldner, J. S., and Eisenbarth, G. S. (1984). Differential sensitivity to beta cell secretagogues in early type I diabetes mellitus. *Diabetes* **33**, 516–521.

Gelfand, J. A. (1982). The role of complement deficiency states and SLE. *Clin. Rheum. Dis.* **8**, 29–47.

Gepts, W. (1982). Islet cell morphology in type I and type II diabetes. In "Immunology in Diabetes" (W. J. Irivine, ed.), pp. 21–35. Teviot Scientific, Edinburgh.

Gepts, W. (1984). The pathology of the pancreas in human diabetes. In "Immunology in Diabetes" (A. Andreani, U. DiMario, K. F. Federlin, and L. G. Heding, eds.), pp. 21–35. Kimpton, London.

Ginsberg, J., Segal, D., Ehrlich, R. M., and Walfish, P. G. (1978). Inappropriate triiodothyronine (T3) and thyroxine (T4) radioimmunoassay levels secondary to circulating thyroid hormone autoantibodies. *Clin. Endocrinol. (Oxford)* **8**, 133–138.

Gloor, E., and Hurlimann, J. (1984). Autoimmune oophoritis. *Am. J. Clin. Pathol.* **81**, 105–109.

Glover, R. L., and Reuber, M. D. (1967). Chronic thyroiditis in Buffalo rats with carbon tetrachloride-induced cirrhosis. *Endocrinology* **80**, 361–364.

Goldman, J., Baldwin, D., and Rubenstein, A. H. (1979). Characterization of circulating insulin and proinsulin-binding antibodies in autoimmune hypoglycemia. *J. Clin. Invest.* **63**, 1050–1059.

Gordin, A., and Lamberg, B. A. (1975). Natural course of symptomless autoimmune thyroiditis. *Lancet* **2**, 1234–1238.

Gorman, C. A. (1978). The presentation and management of endocrine opthalmopathy. *Clin. Endocrinol. Metab.* **7**, 67–96.

Gorsuch, A. N., Spencer, K. M., Lister, J., McNally, J. M., Dean, B. M., Bottazzo, G. F., and Cudworth, A. G. (1981). Evidence for a long prediabetic period in type I (insulin-dependent) diabetes mellitus. *Lancet* **2**, 1363–1365.

Gorsuch, A. N., Spencer, K. M., Lister, J., Wolf, E., Bottazzo, G. F., and Cudworth, A. G. (1982). Can future type I diabetes be predicted? A study in families of affected children. *Diabetes* **31**, 862–866.

Goudie, R. B., and Pinkerton, P. H. (1957). Anterior hypohysitis and Hashimoto's disease in a young woman. *J. Pathol. Bacteriol.* **83**, 584–585.

Gray, R. S., Borsey, D. Q., Irvine, W. J., Seth, J., and Clarke, B. F. (1983). Natural history of thyroid function in diabetics with impaired thyroid reserve: A four-year controlled study. *Clin. Endocrinol.* **19**, 445–451.

Grumet, F. C., Payne, R. O., Konishi, J., and Kriss, J. P. (1974). HLA antigens as markers for disease susceptibility and autoimmunity in Graves' disease. *J. Clin. Endocrinol. Metab.* **39**, 1115–1119.

Gupta, S., Fitrig, S. M., Khanna, S., and Orti, E. (1982). Deficiency of suppressor T cells in insulin-dependent diabetes mellitus. *Immunol. Lett.* **4**, 289–294.

Guttman, R. D., Colle, E., Michel, E., and Seemayer, T. (1983). Spontaneous diabetes mellitus syndrome in the rat. II. T lymphopenia and its association with clinical disease and pancreatic lymphocytic infiltration. *J. Immunol.* **130**, 1731–1735.

Hall, R., Soxena, K. M., and Owen, S. G. (1962). A study of the parents of patients with Hashimoto's disease. *Lancet* **2**, 1291–1292.

Hall, R., Dingle, P. R., and Roberts, D. F. (1972). Thyroid antibodies: A study of first degree relatives. *Clin. Genet.* **3**, 319–324.

Harvald, B., and Hauge, M. (1963). Selection in diabetes in modern society. *Acta Med. Scand.* **173**, 459–465.

Haspel, M. V., Onodera, T., Prabhakar, B. S., McClintock, P. R., Essani, K., Ray, U. R., Yagihaski, S., and Notkins, A. L. (1983). Multiple Organ-Reactive monoclonal autoantibodies. *Nature (London)* **304**, 73–76.

Hassan, T. H. A., Greig, W. R., Boyle, J. A., Goyle, T., and Wallace, T. J. (1966). Toxic diffuse goitre in monozygotic twins. *Lancet* **2**, 306–308.

Haywood, A. R., and Herberger, M. (1984). Culture and phenotype of activated T cells from patients with type I diabetes mellitus. *Diabetes* **30**, 319–323.

Helgason, T., and Jonasson, M. R. (1981). Evidence for a food additive as cause of ketosis-prone diabetes. *Lancet* **2**, 716–720.

Helgason, T., Ewen, S. W. B., Ross, I. S., and Stowers, J. M. (1982). Diabetes produced in mice by smoked/cured mutton. *Lancet* **2**, 1017–1022.

Herrmann, J., Rudorff, K. H., Kroner, H., and Premachandra, B. N. (1977). Antibody binding of thyroid hormone in juvenile goitrous hypothyroidism. *Horm. Metab. Res.* **9**, 394–400.

Hinds, W. E., Takai, N., Rapoport, B., Filetti, S., and Clark, O. H. (1981). Thyroid stimulating immunoglobulin bioassay using cultured human thyroid cells. *J. Clin. Endocrinol. Metab.* **52**, 1204–1210.

Hoddinott, S., Dornan, J., Bear, J. C., and Farid, N. R. (1982). Immunoglobulin levels, immunodeficiency and HLA type in type I diabetes mellitus. *Diabetologia* **23**, 326–329.

Hodge, S. E., Anderson, G. E., Nieswanger, K., Rubin, R., Sparkes, R. S., Sparkes, M. C., Crist, M., Spence, M. A., Terasaki, P. I., Rimoin, D. L., and Rotter, J. I. (1983). Accistion studies between type I (insulin-dependent) diabetes and 27 genetic markers: Lack of association between type I diabetes and the Kidd blood group. *Diabetologia* **25**, 343–347.

Horita, M., Suzuki, H., Onodera, T., Ginsberg-Fellner, F., Fauci, A. S., and Notkins, A. L. (1982). Abnormalities of immunoregulatory T cell subsets in patients with insulin-dependent diabetes mellitus. *J. Immunol.* **129**, 1246–1249.

Horowitz, D. A., and Bakke, A. C. (1984). An Fc receptor bearing, third population of human mononuclear cells with cytotoxic and regulatory function. *Immunol. Today* **5,** 148–153.

Howe, B. S., Walfish, P. G., and Farid, N. R. (1982). HLA antigens in painless thyroiditis with transient hyperthyroidism. *Tissue Antigens* **19,** 311–312.

Huang, S. W., and Maclaren, N. K. (1976). Insulin-dependent diabetes: A disease of autoaggression. *Science* **192,** 64–66.

Huen, A. H.-J., Haneda, M., Freedman, Z., Lernmark, A., and Rubenstein, A. H. (1983). Quantitative determination of islet cell surface antibodies using $^{125}$I-protein A. *Diabetes* **32,** 460–465.

Hume, R., and Roberts, G. H. (1967). Hypophysitis and hypopituitarism. A report of a case. *Br. Med. J.* **2,** 548–550.

Ichihara, K., Shima, K., Saito, Y., Nonaka, K., Tarui, S., and Nishikawa, M. (1977). Mechanism of hypoglycemia observed in a patient with insulin autoimmune syndrome. *Diabetes* **26,** 500–506.

Imahori, S. C., and Vladutiu, A. O. (1983). Autoimmune granulomatous thyroiditis in inbred mice: Resemblance to subacute (de Quevain's) thyroiditis in man. *Proc. Soc. Exp. Biol. Med.* **173,** 408–416.

Inada, M., Nishikawa, M., Naito, K., Oishi, M., Kurata, S., and Imura, H. (1980). Triiodothyronine-binding immunoglobulin in a patient with Graves' disease and its effect on metabolism and radioimmunoassay of triiodothyronine. *Am. J. Med.* **68,** 787–792.

Irvine, W. J. (1978). The immunology and genetics of autoimmune endocrine disease. *In* "Genetic Control of Autoimmune Disease" (N. R. Rose, P. E. Bigozi, and N. L. Warner, eds.), pp. 77–97. Elsevier, Amsterdam.

Irvine, W. J. (1980). Autoimmunity in endocrine disease. *Recent Prog. Horm. Res.* **36,** 509–556.

Irvine, W. J., Chan, M. M. W., Scarth, L., Kolb, F. O., Hartog, M., Bayliss, R. I. S., and Drury, M. I. (1968). Immunological aspects of premature ovarian failure associated with idiopathic Addison's disease. *Lancet* **2,** 883–887.

Irvine, W. J., Gray, R. S., Morris, P. J., and Ting, A. (1977). Correlation of HLA and thyroid antibodies with clinical course of thyrotoxicosis treated with anti-thyroid drugs. *Lancet* **2,** 898–900.

Irvine, W. J., Gray, R. S., and Steel, J. M. (1980). Islet cell antibody as a marker for early stage type I diabetes mellitus. *In* "The Immunology of Diabetes" (W. J. Irvine, ed.), pp. 117–154. Teviot, Edinburgh.

Iwatani, Y., Amino, N., Mori, H., Asari, S., Izumiguchi, Y., Kumahara, Y., and Miyai, K. (1983). T lymphocyte subsets in autoimmune thyroid diseases and subacute thyroiditis detected with monoclonal antibodies. *J. Clin. Endocrinol. Metab.* **56,** 251–254.

Jackson, R. A., and Eisenbarth, G. S. (1984). Type I diabetes mellitus of man and the BB rat: Monoclonal antibody defined T cell abnormalities. *Diagn. Immunol.* **1,** 240–244.

Jackson, R., Rassi, N., Crump, T., Haynes, B., and Eisenbarth, G. S. (1981). The BB diabetic rat. Profound T cell lymphocytopenia. *Diabetes* **30,** 887–889.

Jackson, R. A., Morris, M. A., Haynes, B. F., and Eisenbarth, G. S. (1982). Increased circulating Ia-antigen-bearing T cells in type I diabetes mellitus. *N. Engl. J. Med.* **306,** 785–788.

Jackson, R., Kadison, P., Buse, J., Rassi, N., Jegasothy, B., and Eisenbarth, G. S. (1983). Lymphocyte abnormalities in the BB rat. *Metabolism* **32** (Suppl. 1), 83–86.

Jackson, R. A., Buse, J. B., Rifai, R., Pelletier, D., Milford, E. L., Carpenter, C. B.,

Eisenbarth, G. S., and Williams, R. M. (1984a). Two genes required for diabetes in BB rats: Evidence from cyclical intercrosses and backcrosses. *J. Exp. Med.* **159,** 1629–1636.

Jackson, R. A., Buse, J., Goldstein, A. L., and Eisenbarth, G. S. (1984b). BB rat thymus: Increase of large W3/13[+], 6B2[+], OX19[−], thymocytes. *Diabetes* **33,** 60A.

Jackson, R., Haynes, B. F., Burch, W. M., Shimizu, K., Bowring, M. A., and Eisenbarth, G. S. (1984c). Ia[+] T cells in new onset Graves' disease. *J. Clin. Endocrinol. Metab.* **59,** 187–190.

Jaffe, J. P., and Mosher, D. F. (1979). Calcium binding by a myeloma protein. *Am. J. Med.* **67,** 343–346.

Jakobisiak, M., Sundick, R. S., Bacon, L. D., and Rose, N. R. (1976). Abnormal response to minor histocompatibility antigens in obese strain chickens. *Proc. Natl. Acad. Sci. U.S.A.* **73,** 2877–2880.

Jansson, R., Totterman, T. H., Sallstrom, J., and Dahlberg, P. A. (1983). The infiltrating T lymphocyte subsets in Hashimoto's thyroiditis. *J. Clin. Endocrinol. Metab.* **56,** 1164–1168.

Jansson, R., Totterman, T. H., Sallstrom, J., and Dahlberg, P. A. (1984). Intrathyroidal and circulating lymphocyte subsets in different stages of autoimmune postpartum thyroiditis. *J. Clin. Endocrinol. Metab.* **58,** 942–946.

Jaroszewski, J., Sundick, R. S., and Rose, N. R. (1978). Effects of antiserum containing thyroglobulin antibody on the chicken thyroid gland. *Clin. Immunol. Immunopathol.* **10,** 95–103.

Johnston, C., Pyke, D. A., Cudworth, A. G., and Wolf, E. (1983). HLA-DR typing in identical twins with insulin-dependent diabetes, a difference between concordant and discordant pairs. *Br. Med. J.* **286,** 253–255.

Kahn, C. R., and Harrison, L. C. (1980). Insulin receptor autoantibodies. *In* "Carbohydrate Metabolism and Its Disorders" (P. J. Randle, D. F. Steiner, and W. J. Whelan, eds.), Vol. 4, pp. 279–330. Academic Press, New York.

Kanatsuna, T., Baekkeskov, S., Lernmark, A., and Ludvigsson, J. (1982). Immunoglobulin from insulin-dependent diabetic children inhibits glucose-induced insulin release. *Diabetes* **32,** 520–523.

Karam, J. H., Lewitt, P. A., Young, C. W., Nowlain, R. E., Frankel, B. J., Fujiya, H., Freedman, Z. R., and Grodsky, G. M. (1980). Insulinopenic diabetes after rodenticide (Vacor) ingestion. A unique model of acquired diabetes in man. *Diabetes* **29,** 971–978.

Karlsson, F. A., Wibell, L., and Wide, L. (1977). Hypothyroidism due to thyroid-hormone-binding antibodies. *N. Engl. J. Med.* **296,** 1146–1148.

Kataoka, S., Satoh, J., Fujiya, H., Toyota, T., Suzuki, R., Itoh, K., and Kumagi, K. (1984). Immunologic aspects of the nonobese diabetic (NOD) mouse. Abnormalities of cellular immunity. *Diabetes* **32,** 247–253.

Khoury, E. L., Bottazzo, G. F., and Roitt, I. M. (1984). The thyroid "microsomal" antibody revisited. Its paracoxical binding to the apical surface of the follicular epithelium. *J. Exp. Med.* **159,** 577–591.

Klein, I., and Levey, G. S. (1983). Iodine excess and thyroid function. *Ann. Int. Med.* **98,** 406–407.

Koevary, S., Rossini, A., Stoller, W., Chick, W., and Williams, R. M. (1983a). Passive transfer of diabetes in the BB/W rat. *Science* **220,** 727–728.

Koevary, S., Williams, R. M., Stoller, W., and Chick W. (1983b). Passive transfer of diabetes in BB/W and Wistar-Furth rats. *Diabetes* **33** (Suppl. 1), 50A.

Kohn, L. D., Yavin, E., Yavin, A., Laccetti, P., Vitti, P., Grollman, E., and Valente, W.

(1983). Autoimmune thyroid disease studied with monoclonal antibodies to the thyrotropin receptor. *In* "Monoclonal Antibodies: Probes for the Study of Autoimmunity and Immunodeficiency" (B. F. Haynes and G. S. Eisenbarth, eds.), pp. 222–258. Academic Press, New York.

Kolb, H., Freytag, G., Kiesel, U., and Kolb-Bachofen, V. (1980). Spontaneous immune reactions against pancreatic islets in mouse strains with generalized autoimmune disease. *Diabetologia* **19**, 216–221.

Konishi, J., Iida, Y., Endo, K., Misaki, T., Nohara, Y., Matsuura, N., Mori, T., and Torizuka, K. (1983). Inhibition of thyrotropin-induced adenosine 3′,5′-monophosphate increase by immunoglobulins from patients with primary myxedema. *J. Clin. Endocrinol. Metab.* **57**, 544–549.

Kriss, J. P., and Medhi, S. Q. (1979). Cell-mediated lysis of lipid vesicles containing eye muscle protein: Implication regarding pathogenesis of Graves' ophthalmopathy. *Proc. Natl. Acad. Sci. U.S.A.* **76**, 2003–2007.

Lahita, R., Kluger, J., Drayer, D. E., Koffler, K., and Reidenberg, M. M. (1979). Antibodies to nuclear antigens in patients treated with procainamide or acetylprocainamide. *N. Engl. J. Med.* **301**, 1382–1385.

Laskin, C. A., Smathers, P. A., Reeves, J. P., and Steinberg, A. D. (1982). Studies of defective tolerance induction in NZB mice. *J. Exp. Med.* **155**, 1025–1036.

Laupacis, A., Gardell, C., Dupre, J., Stiller, C. R., Keown, P., Wallace, A. C., and Thibert, P. (1983). Cyclosporin prevents diabetes in BB Wistar rats. *Lancet* **1**, 10–13.

Laurberg, P., and Weeke, J. (1975). T3 release from thyroid slices as an assay for thyroid stimulators. *Scand. J. Clin. Lab. Invest.* **35**, 723–727.

Lazarus, J. H., Burr, M. L., McGregor, A. M., Weetman, A. P., Ludgate, M., Woodhead, J. S., and Hall R. (1984). The prevalence and progression of autoimmune thyroid disease in the elderly. *Acta Endocrinol.* **106**, 199–202.

Leer, J., Patel, B., Innes, M., and Cameron, D. P. (1980). Secondary amenorrhoea due to autoimmune ovarian failure. *Aust. N. Z. J. Obstet. Gynecol.* **20**, 177–179.

Lernmark, A., Freedman, Z. R., Hoffman, C., Rubenstein, A. H., Steiner, D. F., Jackson, R. L., Winter, R. J., and Traisman, H. S. (1978). Islet cell surface antibodies in juvenile diabetes mellitus. *N. Engl. J. Med.* **299**, 375–380.

Lervang, H., Pryds, O., Kristensen, H. P. O., Jakobsen, B. K., and Svejgaard, A. (1984). Postpartum autoimmune thyroid disorder associated with HLA-DR4? *Tissue Antigens* **23**, 250–252.

Leslie, R. D. G., and Pyke, D. A. (1980). Immunosuppression of acute insulin-dependent diabetes. *In* "Immunology of Diabetes" (W. J. Irvine, ed.), pp. 345–347. Teviot, Edinburgh.

Leslie, R. D. G., Alviggi, L., Johnston, C., Hoskins, P., and Vergani, D. (1984). Ia-positive lymphocytes and insulin-dependent diabetes. *Immunol. Diabetes Int. Symp. Rome* Abstract.

Like, A. A., and Rossini, A. A. (1984). Spontaneous autoimmune diabetes mellitus in the BioBreeding/Worcester rat. *Surv. Synth. Pathol. Res.* **31**, 131–138.

Like, A. A., Rossini, A. A., Guberski, D. L., Appel, M. C., and Williams, R. M. (1979). Spontaneous diabetes mellitus: Reversal and prevention in the BB/W rat with antiserum to rat lymphocytes. *Science* **206**, 1421–1423.

Like, A. A., Butler, A. L., Williams, R. M., Appel, M. C., Weringer, E. J., and Rossini, A. A. (1982a). Spontaneous autoimmune diabetes mellitus in the BB rat. *Diabetes* **31** (Suppl 1), 7–13.

Like, A. A., Appel, M. C., and Rossini, A. A. (1982b). Autoantibodies in the BB/W rat. *Diabetes* **31**, 816–820.

Like, A. A., Kislauskis, E., Williams, R. M., and Rossini, A. A. (1982c). Neonatal thymectomy prevents spontaneous diabetes mellitus in the BB/W rat. *Science* **216**, 644–
646.

Like, A. A., Forster, R. M., Woda, B. A., and Rossini, A. A. (1983a). T cell subsets in islets
and lymph nodes of BioBreeding/Worcester rats. *Diabetes* **32** (Suppl. 1), 51A.

Like, A. A., Weringer, E. J., Holdash, A., McGill, P., and Rossini, A. A. (1983b). Nature
of resistance to autoimmune diabetes in BioBreeding/Worcester control rats. *Diabetologia* **25**, 175.

Like, A. A., Anthony, M., Guberski, D. L., and Rossini, A. A. (1983c). Spontaneous
diabetes mellitus in the BB/W rat. Effects of glucocorticoids, cyclosporin-A and
antiserum to rat lymphocytes. *Diabetes* **32**, 326–330.

Lillehoj, H. S., and Rose, N. R. (1981). Relationship between genetic control of T-cell
mitogen response and thyroiditis susceptibility in inbred rats. *Cell Immunol.* **62**,
156–163.

Lingarde, F., and Zetterval, O. (1973). Hypercalcemia and normal ionized serum calcium
in a case of myelomatosis. *Ann. Intern. Med.* **78**, 396–399.

Livezey, M. D., Sundick, R. S., and Rose, N. R. (1981). Spontaneous autoimmune thyroiditis in chickens. II. Evidence for autoresponsive thymocytes. *J. Immunol.* **127**, 1469–
1472.

Lock, E. E. (1975). Lymphoid "hypophysitis" with end organ insufficiency. *Arch Pathol.*
**99**, 215–219.

Logothetopoulos, J., Valiquette, N., Madura, E., and Cvet, D. (1984). The onset and
progression of pancreatic insulitis in the overt, spontaneously diabetic, young adult
BB rat studied by pancreatic biopsy. *Diabetes* **33**, 33–36.

Ludwig, M., Schernthaner, G., Mayr, W. R., and Hofer, R. (1977). Lack of association
between Hashimoto's thyroiditis and SD-locus HLA antigens. *Diabetes Metab.* **3**,
127–130.

McCluskey, J., McCann, V. J., Kay, P. H., Zilko, P. J., Christiansen, F. T., O'Neill, G. J.,
and Dawkins, R. L. (1983). HLA and complement allotypes in type I (insulin-dependent) diabetes. *Diabetologia* **24**, 162–165.

McGregor, A. M., Peterson, M. M., McLachlan, S. M., Rooke, P., Rees Smith, B., and
Hall, R. (1980a). Carbimazole and the autoimmune response in Graves' disease. *N.
Engl. J. Med.* **303**, 302–307.

McGregor, A. M., Rees Smith, B., Hall, R., Petersen, M. M., Miller, M., and Dewar,
P. J. (1980b). Prediction of relapse in hyperthyroid Graves' disease. *Lancet* **1**, 1101–
1103.

McKenzie, J. M. (1958). The bioassay of thyrotropin in serum. *Endocrinology* **63**, 372–
382.

McKenzie, J. M., and Zakarija, M. (1978). LATS in Graves' disease. *Recent Prog. Horm.
Res.* **33**, 29–57.

Maclaren, N. K., and Neufeld, M. (1981). Autoimmunity and endocrine diseases. *In*
"Pediatric Endocrinology" (R. Collu, ed.), pp. 597–631. Raven, New York.

Maclaren, N. K., Elder, M. E., Robbins, V. W., and Riley, W. J. (1983). Autoimmune
diabetes and T lymphocyte immunoincompetences in BB rats. *Metabolism* **32**
(Suppl. 1), 92–96.

McNatty, K. P., Short, R. V., Barnes, I. W., and Irvine, W. J. (1975). The cytotoxic effect
of serum from patients with Addison's disease and autoimmune ovarian failure on
human granulosa cells in culture. *Clin. Exp. Immunol.* **22**, 378–384.

Makino, S., Kunimoto, K., Muraoka, Y., Mizushima, Y., Katagiri, K., and Tochino, Y.
(1980). Breeding of a non-obese, diabetic strain of mice. *Exp. Anim.* **29**, 1–13.

Marcelli-Barge, A., Poirier, J. C., Schmid, M., Deschamps, I., Lestradet, H., Prevost, P., and Hors, J. (1984). Genetic polymorphism of the fourth component of complement in type I (insulin-dependent) diabetes. *Diabetologia* **27**, 116–117.

Marliss, E. B., Sima, A. A. F., and Nakhooda, A. F. (1981). *In* "Etiology and Pathogenesis of Insulin-Dependent Mellitus" (J. M. Martin, R. M. Ehrlich, and F. J. Holland, eds.), pp. 251–274. Raven, New York.

Marner, B., Lernmark, A., Nerup, J., Molenaar, J. L., Tuk, C. W., and Bruining, G. J. (1983). Analysis of islet cell antibodies on frozen sections of human pancreas. *Diabetologia* **25**, 93–96.

Maron, R., Zerubavel, R., Friedman, A., and Cohen, I. R. (1983). T lymphocyte line specific for thyroglobulin produces or vaccinates against autoimmune thyroiditis in mice. *J. Immunol.* **137**, 2316–2322.

Marriotti, S., Russova, A., Pisani, S., and Pinchera, A. (1983). A new solid phase immunoradiometric assay for anti-thyroid microsomal antibody. *J. Clin. Endocrinol. Metab.* **56**, 467–473.

Martin, D. R., and Logothetopoulos, J. (1984). Complement-fixing islet cell antibodies in the spontaneously diabetic BB rat. *Diabetes* **33**, 93–96.

Martino, E., Safran, M., Aghini-Lombardi, F., Rajatanauin, R., Lenziardi, M., Fay, M., Pacchiarotti, A., Paronin, N., Macchia, E., Haffajee, C., Odoguardi, L., Love, J., Bigolli, A., Baschieri, L., Pinchera, A., and Braverman, L. (1984). Environmental iodine uptake and thyroid dysfunction during chronic amiodarone therapy. *Ann. Intern. Med.* **101**, 28–34.

Mascart-Lemone, F., Delespesse, G., Dorchy, H., Lemiere, B., and Servias, G. (1982). Characterization of immunoregulatory T lymphocytes in insulin-dependent diabetic children by means of monoclonal antibodies. *Clin. Exp. Immunol.* **47**, 296–300.

Mason, D. W., Arthur, R. P., Dollman, M. J., Green, J. R., Spickett, G. P., and Thomas, M. L. (1983). Function of rat T lymphocyte subsets isolated by means of monoclonal antibodies. *Immunol. Rev.* **74**, 57–82.

Matsuura, N., Yamada, Y., Nohara, Y., Konishi, J., Kasagi, K., Endo, K., Kojima, H., and Wataya, K. (1980). Familial neonatal transient hypothyroidism due to maternal TSH-binding inhibitor immunoglobulins. *N. Engl. J. Med.* **303**, 738–741.

Mizejewski, G. J., Baron, J., and Poissant, G. (1971). Immunologic investigations of naturally occurring canine thyroiditis. *J. Immunol.* **107**, 1152–1160.

Moens, H., and Farid, N. R. (1978). Hashimoto's thyroiditis is associated with HLA-DRw3. *N. Engl. J. Med.* **299**, 133–134.

Moroz, L. A., Meltzer, S. J., and Bastomsky, C. H. (1983). Thyroid disease with monoclonal (immunoglobulin G lambda) antibody to triiodothyronine and thyroxine. *J. Clin. Endocrinol. Metab.* **56**, 1009–1015.

Muktar, E. D., Smith, B. R., Pyle, G. A., Hall, R., and Vice, P. (1975). Relation of thyroid stimulating immunoglobulins to thyroid function and effect of surgery, radioiodine and antithyroid drugs. *Lancet* **1**, 713–715.

Mustonen, A., Iionen, J., Surcel, H.-M., and Akerblom, H. K. (1984). A "new" DR4-associated D specificity "JA" in type I (insulin-dependent) diabetes: A9, BW16, DJA, DR4 haplotype. *Diabetologia* **27**, 126–128.

Naji, A., Silvers, W. K., Bellgrau, D., Anderson, A. O., Plotkin, S., and Barker, C. F. (1981). Prevention of diabetes in rats by bone marrow transplantation. *Ann. Surg.* **194**, 328–338.

Naji, A., Silvers, W. K., Kimura, H., Anderson, A. O., and Barker, C. F. (1983). Influence of islets and bone marrow transplantation on the diabetes and immunodeficiency of BB rats. *Metabolism* **22**(Suppl. 1), 62–68.

Nakao, Y., Matsumoto, H., Miyazaki, T., and Farid, N. R. (1982). IgG heavy chain allotypes (Gm) in atrophic and goitrous thyroiditis. *J. Immunogenet.* **9,** 311–316.

Nakhooda, A. F., Like, A. A., Chappel, C. I., Murray, F. T., and Marliss, E. B. (1976). The spontaneously diabetic Wistar rat: Metabolic and morphologic studies. *Diabetes* **26,** 100–112.

Nakhooda, A. F., Like, A. A., Chappel, C. I., Wei, C.-N., and Marliss, E. B. (1978). The spontaneously diabetic Wistar rat (the "BB" rat). Studies prior to and during the development of the overt syndrome. *Diabetologia* **14,** 199–207.

Nakhooda, A. F., Poussier, P., and Marliss, E. B. (1983). Insulin and glucagon secretion in BB Wistar rats with impaired glucose tolerance. *Diabetologia* **24,** 58–62.

Nerup, J., and Bendixen, G. (1969). Anti-adrenal cellular hypersensitivity in Addison's disease. II. Correlation with clinical and serological findings. *Clin. Exp. Immunol.* **5,** 341–353.

Nerup, J., Andersen, O. O., Bendixen, G., Egeverg, J., and Poulsen, J. E. (1971). Anti-pancreatic cellular hypersensitivity in diabetes mellitus. *Diabetes* **20,** 424–427.

Nerup, J., Christy, M., Platz, P., Ryder, L. P., and Svejgaard, A. (1984). Aspects of the genetics of insulin-dependent diabetes mellitus. *In* "Immunology in Diabetes" (D. Andreani, U. DiMario, K. F. Federlin, and L. G. Heding, eds.), pp. 63–70. Kimpton, London.

Neufeld, M., Blizzard, R. M., and Maclaren, N. (1981). Two types of autoimmune Addison's disease associated with different polyglandular autoimmune (PGA) syndromes. *Medicine* **60,** 355–362.

Nilsson, L. A., and Rose, N. R. (1972). Restoration of autoimmune thyroiditis in bursectomized-irradiated OS chickens by bursa cells. *Immunology* **22,** 13–23.

Noble, B., Yoshida, T., Rose, N. R., and Bigazzi, P. E. (1976). Thyroid antibodies in spontaneous autoimmune thyroiditis in the Buffalo rat. *J. Immunol.* **117,** 1447–1455.

Nyulassy, S., Hnilica, P., Hirshova, B., and Buc, M. (1977). Subacute de Quervain's thyroiditis. *In* "Histocompatibility Testing" (P. I. Terasaki, ed.), p. 717. U.C.L.A. Tissue Typing Laboratory, Los Angeles.

Ochi, Y., Shiomi, K., Hachiya, T., Yoshimura, M., and Miyazaki, T. (1972). Immunological analysis of abnormal binding of thyroid hormone in the gamma globulin. *J. Clin. Endocrinol. Metab.* **35,** 743–752.

Onaya, T., Kotani, M., Yamada, T., and Ochi, Y. (1973). New *in vitro* tests to detect the thyroid stimulator in sera from hyperthyroid patients by measuring colloid droplet formation and cyclic AMP in human thyroid slices. *J. Clin. Endocrinol. Metab.* **36,** 859–866.

Orgiazzi, J., Williams, D. E., Chopra, I. J., and Solomon, D. H. (1976). Human thyroid adenyl cyclase-stimulating activity in immunoglobulin G of patients with Graves' disease. *J. Clin. Endocrinol. Metab.* **42,** 341–354.

Owerbach, D., Lernmark, A., Platz, P., Ryder, L. P., Rask, L., Peterson, P. A., and Ludgigsson, J. (1983). HLA-D region beta chain DNA endonuclease fragments differ between HLA-DR identical healthy and insulin-dependent diabetic individuals. *Nature (London)* **303,** 815–817.

Palmer, J. P., Asplin, C. M., Clemons, P., Lyen, K., Tatpaki, O., Raghu, P. K., and Paquette, T. L. (1983). Insulin antibodies in insulin-dependent diabetics before insulin treatment. *Science* **222,** 1337–1339.

Pepper, B., Noel, E. P., and Farid, N. R. (1981). The putative anti-thyrotropin receptor antibodies of Graves' disease. I. Gm allotypes. *J. Immunogenet.* **8,** 89–100.

Petz, D. (1980). Drug-induced hemolytic anemia. *Clin. Haematol.* **9,** 455–482.

Pollard, D. R., Gupta, K., Manchino, L., and Hynie, I. (1983). An immunofluorescent study of anti-pancreatic islet cell antibodies in the spontaneously diabetic BB Wistar rat. *Diabetologia* **25**, 56–59.

Polley, C. R., Bacon, L. D., and Rose, N. R. (1981). Spontaneous autoimmune thyroiditis in chickens. *J. Immunol.* **127**, 1465–1468.

Pontes de Carvalho, L. C., Wick, G., and Roitt, I. M. (1981). Requirement of T cells for the development of spontaneous autoimmune thyroiditis in obese strain (OS) chickens. *J. Immunol.* **126**, 750–753.

Pouplard, A., Bottazzo, G. F., Doniach, D., and Roitt, I. M. (1976). Binding of human immunoglobulins to pituitary ACTH cells. *Nature (London)* **261**, 142–144.

Poussier, P., Nakhooda, A. F., Falk, J. A., Lee, C., and Marliss, E. B. (1982). Lymphopenia and abnormal lymphocyte subsets in the "BB" rat: Relationship to the diabetic syndrome. *Endocrinology* **110**, 1825–1827.

Poussier, P., Sai, P., and Assan, R. (1983). BB rat immunoglobulins and lymphocytes are cytotoxic for beta cells *in vitro*. *Diabetes* **32** (Suppl. 1), 21A.

Pozzilli, P., Zuccarini, O., Iovicoli, M., Andreani, D., Sensi, M., Spencer, K. M., Bottazzo, G. F., Beverley, P. C. L., Kyner, J. L., and Cudworth, A. G. (1982). Monoclonal antibodies defined abnormalities of T lymphocytes in type I (insulin-dependent) diabetes. *Diabetes* **32**, 91–94.

Premachandra, B. N., and Blumenthal, H. T. (1967). Abnormal binding of thyroid hormone in sera from patients with Hashimoto's thyroiditis. *J. Clin. Endocrinol. Metab.* **27**, 931–936.

Prud'homme, G. J., Fuks, A., Colle, E., Seemayer, T. A., and Guttmann, R. D. (1984a). Immune dysfunction in diabetes-prone BB rats. Interleukin-2 production and other mitogen-induced responses are suppressed by activated macrophages. *J. Exp. Med.* **159**, 463–478.

Prud'homme, G. J., Fuks, A., Colle, E., and Guttmann, R. D. (1984b). Isolation of T lymphocyte lines with specificity for islet cell antigens from spontaneously diabetic (insulin-dependent) rats. *Diabetes* **33**, 801–803.

Pujol-Borrel, R., Hanafusa, T., Chiovato, L., and Bottazzo, G. F. (1983). Lectin-induced expression of DR antigen on human cultured follicular thyroid cells. *Nature (London)* **304**, 71–73.

Rabinowe, S. L., and Eisenbarth, G. S. (1984). Immunotherapy of type I (insulin-dependent) diabetes mellitus. In "Immunology in Diabetes" (D. Andreani, U. DiMario, K. Federlin, and L. G. Heding, eds.), pp. 171–175. Kimpton, London.

Rabinowe, S. L., Jackson, R. A., Dluhy, R. G., and Williams, G. H. (1984a). Ia[+] T cells in recently diagnosed idiopathic Addison's disease. *Am. J. Med.* **77**(4), 597–601.

Rabinowe, S. L., Jackson, R. A., Buse, J. B., and Eisenbarth, G. S. (1984b). A new human T cell subset defined by anti-ganglioside monoclonal antibody. *Clin. Res.* **32**, 356A.

Raum, D., Awdeh, Z., Yunis, E. J., Alper, C. A., and Gabbay, K. H. (1984). Extended major histocompatibility complex haplotypes in type I diabetes mellitus. *J. Clin. Invest.* **74**, 449–454.

Reynolds, C. W., Sharrow, S. O., Ortaldo, J. R., and Herberman, R. B. (1981). Natural killer activity in the rat. II. Analysis of surface antigens on LGL by flow cytometry. *J. Immunol.* **127**, 2204–2208.

Riley, W., and Maclaren, N. (1984). Islet cell antibodies are seldom transient. *Lancet* **1**, 1351–1352.

Rimoin, D. I., and Rotter, J. I. (1984). The genetics of diabetes. *In* "Immunology in Diabetes" (D. Andreani, U. DiMario, K. F., Federlin, and L. G. Heding, eds.), pp. 45–62. Kimpton, London.

Robbins, J., Rall, J. E., and Rawson, R. W. (1956). An unusual instance of thyroxine binding by human serum gamma globulin. *J. Clin. Endocrinol. Metab.* **16,** 573–579.

Rodriquez-Espinosa, J., Gomez-Gerique, J. A., Ordonez-Llanos, J., Soldevila-Bosch, J., and Concusteli-Bas, E. (1980). Circulant anti-triiodothyronine antibodies in a patient with Graves' disease: Effects on measurement of T3 with different RIA procedures. *Clin. Chim. Acta* **106,** 173–181.

Rose, N. R. (1982). The generation of antibody diversity. *Am. J. Hematol.* **13,** 91–99.

Rose, N. R., and Kong, Y. M. (1983). T cell regulation of experimental autoimmune thyroiditis in the mouse. *Life Sci.* **32,** 85–95.

Rose, N. R., Bacon, L. D., and Sundick, R. S. (1976). Genetic determinants of thyroiditis in the OS chicken. *Transplant. Rev.* **31,** 264–285.

Rossini, A. A., Williams, R. M., Mordes, J. P., Appel, M. C., and Like, A. A. (1979). Spontaneous diabetes in the gnotobiotic BB/W rat. *Diabetes* **20,** 1031–1032.

Rossini, A. A., Mordes, J. P., Pelletier, A. M., and Like, A. A. (1983a). Transfusions of whole blood prevent spontaneous diabetes mellitus in the BB/W rat. *Science* **219,** 975–977.

Rossini, A. A., Mordes, J. P., Gallina, D. L., and Like, A. A. (1983b). Hormonal and environmental factors in the pathogenesis of BB rat diabetes. *Metabolism* **32** (Suppl. 1), 33–36.

Rossini, A. A., Faustman, D., Woda, B. A., Like, A. A., Szymanski, I., and Mordes, J. P. (1984a). Lymphocyte transfusions prevent diabetes in the BioBreeding/Worcester rat. *J. Clin. Invest.* **74,** 39–46.

Rossini, A. A., Slavin, S., Woda, B. A., Geisberg, M., Like, A. A., and Mordes, J. P. (1984b). Total lymphoid irradiation prevents diabetes mellitus in the BioBreeding/Worcester (BB/W) rat. *Diabetes* **33,** 543–547.

Rotter, J. I. (1981). The modes of inheritance of insulin-dependent diabetes mellitus or the genetics of IDDM. No longer a nightmare, but still a headache. *Am. J. Hum. Genet.* **33,** 835–851.

Rotter, J. I., and Rimoin, D. L. (1978). Heterogeneity in diabetes mellitus—update 1978: Evidence for further genetic heterogeneity within juvenile onset insulin-dependent diabetes mellitus. *Diabetes* **27,** 599–608.

Rubenstein, P., Walker, M. E., Fendun, N., Witt, M. E., Cooper, L. Z., and Ginsberg-Fellner, F. (1982). The HLA system in congenital rubella patients with and without diabetes. *Diabetes* **32,** 1088–1091.

Ruuska, P., Ilonen, J., Mustonen, A., and Tilikainen, A. (1984). Defective erythrocyte C3b receptor function associated with low serum complement (C3, C4) in insulin-dependent diabetes mellitus. *Clin. Exp. Immunol.* **57,** 12–16.

Rynes, R. I. (1982). Inherited complement deficiency states and SLE. *Clin. Rheum. Dis.* **8,** 29–47.

Schleusener, H., Schernthaner, G., Mayr, W. R., Kotulla, P., Bogner, U., Finke, R., Meinhold, M., Koppenhagen, K., and Wenzel, K. W. (1983). HLA-DR3 and HLA-DR5 associated thyrotoxicosis—Two different types of toxic diffuse goiter. *J. Clin. Endocrinol. Metab.* **56,** 781–785.

Scott, F. W., and Trick, K. D. (1983). Dietary modification of spontaneous diabetes in the BB Wistar rat. *Can. Fed. Biol. Soc. Proc.* **26,** 222.

Seemayer, T. A., and Colle, E. (1984). Pancreatic cellular infiltrates in autoimmune prone New Zealand Black mice. *Diabetologia* **26,** 310–313.

Seemayer, T. A., Schurch, W., and Kalant, N. (1982a). B cell lymphoproliferation in spontaneously diabetic BB Wistar rats. *Diabetologia* **23,** 261–265.

Seemayer, T. A., Tannenbaum, G. S., Goldman, H., and Colle, E. (1982b). Dynamic time course studies of the spontaneously diabetic BB Wistar rat. III. Light microscopic and ultrastructural observations of pancreatic islets of Langerhans. *Am. J. Pathol.* **106,** 237–249.

Selam, J. L., Clot, J., Andary, M., and Mirouze, J. (1979). Circulating lymphocyte subpopulations in juvenile insulin-dependent diabetes. *Diabetologia* **16,** 35–40.

Silverman, D., and Rose, N. R. (1974). Neonatal thymectomy increases the incidence of spontaneous and methylcholanthrene-enhanced thyroiditis in rats. *Science* **184,** 162–163.

Silverman, D., and Rose, N. R. (1975a). Spontaneous and methylcholanthrene enhanced thyroiditis in BUF rats. *J. Immunol.* **114,** 145–147.

Silverman, D., and Rose, N. R. (1975b). Spontaneous and methylcholanthrene enchanced thyroiditis in BUF rats. II. Induction of experimental autoimmune thyroiditis without complete Freund's adjuvant. *J. Immunol.* **114,** 148–150.

Smith, B. R., and Hall, R. (1974). Thyroid-stimulating immunoglobulins in Graves' disease. *Lancet* **2,** 427–431.

Soria, J., Soria, C., Dao, C., James, J. M., Bousser, J., and Bilski-Pasquier, G. (1976). Immunoglobulin bound calcium and ultrafilterable serum calcium in myeloma. *Br. J. Haematol.* **34,** 343–344.

Sotsiou, F., Bottazzo, G. F., and Doniach, D. (1980). Immunofluorescence studies on autoantibodies to steroid-producing cells, and to germline cells in endocrine disease and infertility. *Clin. Exp. Immuinol.* **39,** 97–111.

Spira, G., Silvian, I., Tatarsky, I., and Hazani, A. (1980). A calcium binding IgG myeloma protein. *Scand. J. Hematol.* **24,** 193–198.

Sridama, V., Pacin, F., and DeGroot, L. J. (1982). Decreased suppressor T lymphocytes in autoimmune thyroid diseases detected by monoclonal antibodies. *J. Clin. Endocrinol. Metab.* **54,** 316–319.

Srikanta, S., Ganda, O. P., Eisenbarth, G. S., and Soeldner, J. S. (1983a). Islet cell antibodies and beta cell function in monozygotic triplets and twins initially discordant for type I diabetes mellitus. *N. Engl. J. Med.* **308,** 322–325.

Srikanta, S., Ganda, O. P., Jackson, R. A., Gleason, R. E., Kaldany, A., Garovoy, M. R., Milford, E. L., Carpenter, C. B., Soeldner, J. S., and Eisenbarth, G. S. (1983b). Type I diabetes mellitus in monozygotic twins: Chronic progessive beta cell dysfunction. *Ann. Intern. Med.* **99,** 320–326.

Srikanta, S., Ganda, O. P., Jackson, R. A., Brink, S. J., Fleischnick, E., Yunis, E., Alper, C., Soeldner, J. S., and Eisenbarth, G. S. (1984a). Pre-type I diabetes: Common endocrinologic course despite immunologic and immunogenetic heterogeneity. *Diabetologia* **27,** 146–149.

Srikanta, S., Ganda, O. P., Gleason, R. E., Jackson, R. A., Soeldner, J. S., and Eisenbarth, G. S. (1984b). Pre-type I diabetes: Linear loss of beta cell response to intravenous glucose. *Diabetes* **33,** 717–720.

Staeheli, V., Vallotton, M. B., and Burger, A. (1975). Detection of human anti-thyroxine and anti-triiodothyronine antibodies in different thyroid conditions. *J. Clin. Endocrinol. Metab.* **41,** 669–675.

Starzl, T. E., Porter, K. A., Iwatsuki, S., Rosenthal, J. T., Shaw, B. W., Atchison, R. W., Bahnson, H. T., Nalesnik, M. A., Ho, M., Griffith, B. P., Hakala, T. R., Hardesty, T. R., and Jaffe, R. (1984). Reversibility of lymphomas and lymphoproliferative lesions developing under cyclosporine-steroid therapy. *Lancet* **1,** 583–587.

Stastny, P., Ball, E. J., Dry, P. J., and Nunez, G. (1983). The human immune response region (HLA-D) and disease susceptibility. *Immunol. Rev.* **70,** 113–153.

Steinmetz, M., and Hood, L. (1983). Genes of the major histocompatibility complex in mouse and man. *Science* **222**, 727–733.

Sternthal, E., Like, A. A., Sarantis, K., and Braverman, L. E. (1981). Lymphocytic thyroiditis and diabetes in the BB/W rat. A new model of autoimmune endocrinopathy. *Diabetes* **30**, 1058–1061.

Stiller, C. R., Laupacis, A., Keown, P. A., Gardell, C., Dupre, J., Thibert, P., and Wall, W. (1983a). Cyclosporine: Action, pharmacokinetics, and effect in the BB rat model. *Metabolism* **32** (Suppl. 1), 69–72.

Stiller, C. R., Laupacis, A., Dupre, J., Jenner, M. R., Keown, P. A., Rodger, W., and Wolfe, B. M. J. (1983b). Cyclosporine for treatment of early type I diabetes: Preliminary results. *N. Engl. J. Med.* **308**, 1226–1227.

Stiller, C. R., Dupre, J., Gent, M., Jenner, M. R., Keown, P. A., Laupacis, A., Martell, R., Rodger, N. W., Graffenried, B. J., and Wolfe, B. M. J. (1984). Effects of cyclosporine immunosuppression in insulin-dependent diabetes mellitus of recent onset. *Science* **223**, 1362–1367.

Sundick, R. S., and Wick, G. (1976). Increased iodine uptake by obese strain thyroid glands transplanted to normal chick embryos. *J. Immunol.* **116**, 1319–1323.

Sundick, R. S., Gabchi, N., Livezey, M. D., Brown, T. R., and Mack, R. E. (1979). Abnormal thyroid regulation in chickens with autoimmune thyroiditis. *Endocrinology* **105**, 493–498.

Sutherland, D. E. R., Sibley, R., Chinn, P., Michael, A., Srikanta, S., Taub, F., Najarian, J., and Goetz, F. C. (1984). Twin-to-twin pancreas transplantation (tx): Reversal and reenactment of the pathogenesis of type I diabetes. *Clin. Res.* **32**, 561A.

Tannenbaum, G. S., Colle, E., Gurd, W., and Wannamaker, L. (1981a). Dynamic time course studies of the spontaneously diabetic BB Wistar rat. I. Longitudinal profiles of plasma growth hormone, insulin and glucose. *Endocrinology* **109**, 1872–1879.

Tannenbaum, G. S., Colle, E., Wanamaker, L., Gurd, W., Goldman, H., and Seemayer, T. A. (1981b). Dynamic time course studies of the spontaneously diabetic BB Wistar rat. II. Insulin-, glucagon-, and somatostatin-reactive cells in the pancreas. *Endocrinology* **109**, 1880–1887.

Taylor, S. I., Grunberger, G., Marcus-Samuels, B., Underhill, L. H., Dons, R. F., Ryan, J., Roddam, R. F., Rupe, C. E., and Gorden, P. (1982). Hypoglycemia associated with antibodies to the insulin receptor. *N. Engl. J. Med.* **307**, 1422–1426.

Thielemans, C., Vanhaelst, L., DeWaele, M., Jonckheer, M., and VanCamp, B. (1981). Autoimmune thyroiditis: A condition related to a decrease in T suppressor cells. *Clin. Endocrinol.* **15**, 259–263.

Tikkanen, M. J., and Lamberg, B. A. (1982). Hypothyroidism following subacute thyroiditis. *Acta Endocrinol.* **101**, 348–353.

Ting, C.-C., Yang, S. S., and Hargrove, M. E. (1984). Induction of suppressor T cells by interleukin-2. *J. Immunol.* **133**, 261–266.

Trimarchi, F., Benvenga, S., Fenzi, G., Mariotti, S., and Consolo, F. (1982). Immunoglobulin binding of thyroid hormones in a case of Waldenstrom's macroglobulinemia. *J. Clin. Endocrinol. Metab.* **54**, 1045–1050.

Truden, J. L., Sundick, R. S., Levine, S., and Rose, N. R. (1983). The decreased growth rate of obese strain chicken thyroid cells provides *in vitro* evidence for a primary target organ abnormality in chickens susceptible to autoimmune thyroiditis. *Clin. Immunol. Immunopathol.* **29**, 294–305.

Tunbridge, W. M. G., Brewis, M., French, J. M., Appelton, D., Bird, T., Clark, F., Evered, D. C., Grimley Evans, J., Hall, R., Smith, P., Stephenson, J., and Young, E. (1981). Natural history of autoimmune thyroiditis. *Br. Med J.* **282**, 258–262.

Turkington, R. W., and Lebovitz, H. (1967). Extra-adrenal endocrine deficiencies in Addison's disease. *Am. J. Med.* **43**, 499–507.

Uno, H., Sasazuki, T., Tamai, H., and Matsumoto, H. (1981). Two major genes linked to HLA and Gm control susceptibility to Graves' disease. *Nature (London)* **292**, 768–770.

Valente, W. A., Vitte, P., Yavin, Z., Yavin, E., Rotella, C. M., Grollman, E. F., Taccafondi, R. S., and Kohn, L. D. (1982). Monoclonal antibodies to the thyrotropin receptor stimulating and blocking antibodies derived from the lymphocytes of patients with Graves' disease. *Proc. Natl. Acad. Sci. U.S.A.* **79**, 6680–6684.

Verghese, M. W., Ward, F. E., and Eisenbarth, G. S. (1981). Lymphocyte suppressor activity in patients with polyglandular failure. *Hum. Immunol.* **3**, 173–179.

Vergani, D., Johnston, C., Abdullah, N. B., and Barnett, A. H. (1983). Low serum C4 concentrations: An inherited predisposition to insulin-dependent diabetes. *Br. Med. J.* **286**, 926–928.

Vladutiu, A. O. (1983). Does the amount of thyroglobulin antigen influence the severity and genetic contol of murine autoimmune thyroiditis? *Immunol. Lett.* **6**, 155–159.

Vladutiu, A. O., and Rose N. R. (1975). Cellular basis for the genetic control of immune responsive to murine thyroglobulin in mice. *Cell Immunol.* **17**, 106–113.

Volpe, R., Row, V. V., and Ezrin, C. (1967). Circulating viral and thyroid antibodies in subacute thyroiditis. *J. Clin. Endocrinol. Metab.* **27**, 1275–1284.

Wall, J. R., Henderson, J., Strakosch, C. R., and Joyner, D. M. (1981). Graves' ophthalmopathy. *Can. Med. Assoc. J.* **124**, 855–862.

Wall, J. R., Baur, R., Schleusner, H., and Dafoe-Bardy, P. (1983). Peripheral blood and intrathyroidal mononuclear cell populations in patients with autoimmune thyroid disorders enumerated using monoclonal antibodies. *J. Clin. Endocrinol. Metab.* **56**, 164–169.

Webster, A. D. (1982). Metabolic defects in immunodeficiency diseases. *Clin. Exp. Immunol.* **49**, 1–10.

Weir, G. C., Clore, E. T., Smachinski, C. J., and Bonner-Weir, S. (1981). Islet secretion in a new experimental model for non-insulin-dependent diabetes. *Diabetes* **30**, 590–595.

Weiss, M., Ingbar, S. H., Winblad, S., and Kasper, D. (1983). Demonstration of a saturable binding site for thyrotropin in *Yersinia enterocolitica. Science* **219**, 1331–1333.

Weissel, M., Hofer, R., Zasmeta, H., and Mayr, W. R. (1980). HLA-DR and Hashimoto's thyroiditis. *Tissue Antigens* **16**, 256–257.

Welch, P., Rose, N. R., and Kite, J. H. (1973). Neonatal thymectomy increases spontaneous autoimmune thyroiditis. *J. Immunol.* **110**, 575–577.

Weringer, E. J., and Like, A. A. (1984). Mechanisms of immune destruction of pancreatic beta cells in BioBreeding/Worcester (BB/W) diabetic rats. *Immunol. Diabetes Int. Symp., Rome* Abstract.

Wick, G., Kite, J. H., Cole, R. K., and Witebsky, E. (1970). Spontaneous thyroiditis in the obese strain of chickens. III. The effect of bursectomy on the development of disease. *J. Immunol.* **104**, 45–53.

Wick, G., Muller, P., and Schwarz, S. (1982). Effect of cyclosporin A on spontaneous autoimmune thyroiditis of obese strain (OS) chickens. *Eur. J. Immunol.* **12**, 877–881.

Wolf, E., Spencer, K. M., and Cudworth, A. G. (1983). The genetic susceptibility to type I (insulin-dependent) diabetes: Analysis of the HLA-DR association. *Diabetologia* **24**, 224–230.

Wright, J. R., Yates, A. J., Sharma, H. M., and Thibert, P. (1983). Pathologic lesions in the spontaneously diabetic BB Wister rat: A comprehensive autopsy study. *Metabolism* **32** (Suppl. 1), 101–105.

Wu, S.-Y., and Green, W. L. (1976). Triiodothyronine (T3)-binding immunoglobulins in a euthyroid woman: Effects on measurements of T3 (RIA) and on T3 turnover. *J. Clin. Endocrinol. Metab.* **42**, 642–652.

Yagihashi, S., Suzuki, H., Dobersen, M. J., Onodera, T., Notkins, A. L., and Ginsberg-Fellner, F. (1982). Autoantibodies to islet cells: Comparison of methods. *Lancet* **2**, 1218.

Yale, J. F., and Marliss, E. B. (1984). Altered immunity and diabetes in the BB rat. *Clin. Exp. Immunol.* **57**, 1–11.

Yanagi, Y., Hosyikai, Y., Leggett, K., Clark, S. P., Alksander, I., and Mak, T. W. (1984). A human T cell-specific cDNA clone encodes a protein having extensive homology to immunoglobulin chains. *Nature (London)* **308**, 145–149.

Yoon, J. W., Austin, M., Onodera, T., and Notkins, A. L. (1979). Virus-induced diabetes mellitus: Isolation of a virus from the pancreas of a child with diabetic ketoacidosis. *N. Engl. J. Med.* **300**, 1173–1179.

Zakarija, M., and McKenzie, J. M. (1983). Pregnancy associated changes in the thyroid-stimulating antibody of Graves' disease and the relationship to neonatal hyperthyroidism. *J. Clin. Endocrinol. Metab.* **57**, 1036–1040.

Zier, K. S., Leo, M. M., Spielman, R. S., and Baker, L. (1984). Decreased synthesis of interleukin 2 (IL-2) in insulin-dependent diabetes mellitus. *Diabetes* **33**, 552–555.

Zinkernagel, R. M., and Doherty, P. C. (1980). MHC-restricted cytotoxic T-cells: Studies on the biologic role of polymorphic major transplantation antigens determining T-cell restriction, specificity, function, and responses. *Adv. Immunol.* **27**, 51–177.

# Role of Cytochromes *P*-450 in the Biosynthesis of Steroid Hormones

## PETER F. HALL

*Worcester Foundation for Experimental Biology*
*Shrewsbury, Massachusetts*

## I. WHAT IS *P*-450?

Is it an enzyme? Why is it called *P*-450? These questions, which are still asked today, illustrate the confusion caused by this inappropriate name and the inadequacy of the treatment accorded the subject in standard textbooks. This is disappointing because *P*-450 is the most widely studied of all enzymes—in 1982, more than 650 papers appeared on this subject in the Enlgish language alone. The cytochromes *P*-450 consitute a family of oxygenases that use atmospheric or molecular oxygen to oxidize diverse substrates that are, for the most part,

315

lipophilic. They belong to that group of oxygenases that insert one of the two atoms of oxygen into the substrate—the so-called monooxygenases (three Os), and as the name cytochrome implies, they are heme proteins. As it happens, the term "cytochrome" is applied to electron carriers which are not strictly enzymes in that they do not permanently alter a substrate. This should not, of course, mean that some members of the cytochome family cannot serve as enzymes—the properties of the protein moiety of $P$-450 justify the term "cytochrome." Moreover, there is much to be said for emphasizing the similarities between enzymes and carriers of oxygen and electrons. After all, the allosteric properties of hemoglobin have long served as a model for the study of this property of enzymes. In spite of all this, it is not unlikely that cytochrome $P$-450 will eventually appear under an unexceptional, but uninteresting name. In the meantime, we should notice that all cytochromes $P$-450 show important similarities that justify their consideration as a family, and yet they also display sufficient differences to distinguish one from another.

## II. Discovery of Cytochrome $P$-450

Although articles in this publication do not usually discuss the history of the subject at hand, the discovery of $P$-450 serves to illustrate the major functions of these enzymes. In 1958, Garfinkel and Klingenberg separately discovered the presence of an absorbance maximum at 450 nm when liver microsomes were treated with carbon monoxide (Garfinkel, 1958; Klingenberg, 1958). This discovery was made possible by spectrophometers developed by Chance (1957) which permitted examination of turbid samples by difference, i.e., absorbance by untreated sample is subtracted from that of sample treated with carbon monoxide. The unknown compound responsible for the peak at 450 nm was called pigment 450, or "$P$-450" for short. It was subsequently discovered that steroid 21-hydroxylation by adrenal microsomes is inhibited by carbon monoxide (Ryan and Engel, 1957). Six years later, it was reported that this inhibition can be reversed by light with maximal reversal at a wavelength of 450 nm (Estabrook et al., 1963). This photochemical action spectrum demonstrated the involvement of $P$-450 in a steroid hydroxylation reaction essential for the synthesis of corticosteroids. Two years later, it was found that $P$-450 is involved in the hydroxylation of drugs by hepatic microsomes (Cooper et al., 1965). These observations established $P$-450 as a component in enzyme systems responsible for hydroxylation of lipophilic substrates—both in synthetic reactions (steroid synthesis) and in reactions involved in metabolic disposal systems in which the new hydroxyl group renders the substrate more hydrophilic, which facilitates filtration in the kidney and discourages nonspecific entry into cells. The most intensely studied cytochromes $P$-450 are those of hepatic microsomes, the $P$-450 of *Pseudomonas putida,* and more recently, those of the steroid-forming organs—adrenal, testis, ovary, and placenta.

## III. Structure of Cytochromes $P$-450

Cytochromes $P$-450 consist of an apoprotein of 30,000–60,000 Da together with a prosthetic group—protoheme. So far, only one protein species has been found with each $P$-450, although the number of protein subunits in the active form of the enzyme is, in most cases, unknown. The heme is bound to the protein rather loosely by a combination of noncovalent forces so that it can be readily removed by solvent extraction. The nature of the association between the heme and the protein is of considerable importance, since it is responsible for many of the distinctive properties of $P$-450, and it is believed to be the same in all cytochromes $P$-450 so far studied. In addition to hydrophobic and Coulombic forces which bind the heme to the protein, the heme iron is attached to the protein. The heme iron can exist in either of two valence states—pentacoordinate or hexacoordinate. Four of the valencies are associated with the four pyrrole nitrogens of the heme. As the result of many spectroscopic studies of $P$-450 using a variety of methods and the synthesis of so-called model compounds (Jefcoate and Gaylor, 1969; Koch *et al.,* 1975; Collman and Sorrell, 1975; Ullrich *et al.,* 1977), there is now general agreement that the fifth bond involves a sulfur atom in the protein, taking the form of a thiolate bond with cystein (Ullrich, 1979; White and Coon, 1980). Using extended X-ray absorption, Cramer *et al.* (1978) concluded that in one form of hepatic $P$-450, the iron–sulfur bond length is 2.3 Å. Data from these various sources have eliminated the alternative candidate for the fifth ligand, namely, oxygen. These five bonds account for the pentacoordinate form of the heme iron. The nature of the sixth ligand in the hexacoordinate form of the iron is less clear. Although nitrogen from histidine has received some support (Chevion *et al.,* 1977), oxygen appears more likely, and it may be present as the OH group of water or an amino acid (Ullrich *et al.,* 1979). A recent publication approaching this question by specific modification of tyrosine suggests that this amino acid may serve as the sixth ligand in at least one $P$-450 (Janig *et al.,* 1983). In view of these doubts, the sixth ligand must remain uncertain for the present. In what follows, OH⁻ from water will be accepted as the sixth ligand for the purpose of discussion. No comments or conclusions made here will require modification if another ligand turns out to occupy the sixth coordinate.

The protein components of different cytochromes P-450 show important differences in size and amino acid composition. However, cytochromes P-450 from bacteria, liver, and steroid-forming organs show conserved amino acid sequences (Yuan *et al.*, 1983; Nakajin *et al.*, 1984). As mentioned above, a fundamental dogma in the field is that the attachment of heme to protein is the same in all cytochromes P-450. This attachment is responsible for those properties which set P-450 apart from all other heme proteins.

Not only are most of the substrates for P-450 hydrophobic, but the enzymes themselves are often very hydrophobic—in some cases they are insoluble in water (Nakajin *et al.*, 1981). It is suggested that the active sites of these enzymes, which must include the heme group to which the substrate oxygen binds, take the form of hydrophobic crevices (White and Coon, 1980). It may be useful, as a framework for discussion, to illustrate these ideas with a diagram.

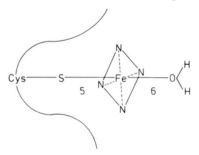

The four bonds to pyrrole nitrogen are called planar because they lie in the plane of the heme ring. The fifth and sixth bonds and the atoms involved are called axial bonds and ligands, respectively.

IV. Spectral Properties of Cytochromes P-450

Heme compounds, including heme proteins, are conjugated throughout the heme moiety and are therefore highly colored. Absorption spectroscopy of heme compounds reveals a conspicuous band at ~420 nm called the Soret band after the French chemist who first discovered it. In addition, $\alpha$, $\beta$, and $\delta$ bands are seen at various wavelengths between

400 and 600 nm. The exact locations and intensities of these absorbance maxima are influenced by details of the chemistry of the heme, the nature of its attachment to the protein by the protein itself, and the solvent used. The Soret band is described as "strong," i.e., of high extinction, so that details of this band are important in the study of heme proteins. Moreover, the conjugated bond system of heme is strongly influenced by changes in the nearby protein which may affect the distribution of electrons in the heme and hence the position and intensity of the Soret peak. The heme is said to serve as a reporter group. Two important examples of such influences on the Soret peak are seen when *P*-450 combines with carbon monoxide and when substrates are added to the enzyme.

## A. CO SPECTRA

Carbon monoxide can combine with reduced heme, i.e., with ferroprotoporphyrins. In doing so, CO competes with oxygen for binding to iron. If CO is bubbled through a solution of reduced *P*-450, the Soret peak shifts to 450 nm.

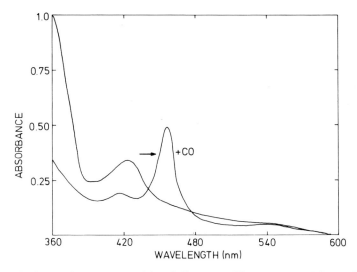

This shift can be measured by difference. If we start with a solution of oxidized *P*-450 saturated with CO in both sample and reference cuvette and set the instrument to subtract absorbance in the reference cuvette from that in the sample, it will produce a straight line (no difference). If the contents of the sample cuvette are now reduced (e.g., by adding sodium dithionite), CO will bind to the iron and the Soret peak will shift to 450 nm. The instrument now reveals this peak at 450 nm.

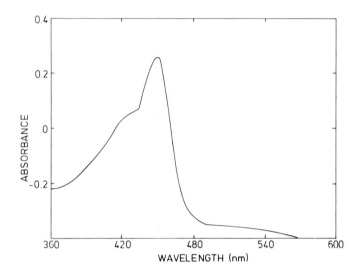

This peak, which shows a molar extinction coefficient of 91,000 (Omura and Sato, 1964), represents what is perhaps the most important single property of $P$-450. In addition to giving the protein its name, the CO spectrum provides the most common method of identifying and measuring all forms of cytochrome $P$-450. The importance of this approach is further emphasized by the use of difference spectroscopy which, with modern spectrophotometers, makes it easy to obtain accurate measurements of the amount of $P$-450 in such crude samples as suspensions of microsomes and mitochondria. To ensure rapid and complete reduction of $P$-450, dithionite is routinely used in such measurements rather than enzymatic reduction with NADPH and electron carriers.

### B. Substrate-Induced Difference Spectra

When a substrate for $P$-450 is added to a solution of the enzyme, the Soret peak shifts from ~420 nm to ~390 nm (Narasimhula *et al.*, 1965; Remmer *et al.*, 1966; Schenkman *et al.*, 1982). The basis of this shift is considered below. At this point, it should be noticed that the shift in the Soret peak provides a useful means of measuring the amount of bound substrate (ES) in a sample of $P$-450 (E) and substrate (S). The

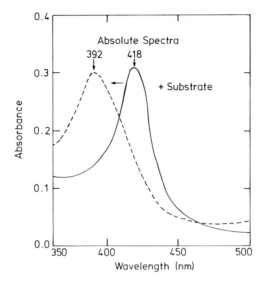

measurement can be made by difference, i.e., *P*-450 + substrate (Soret peak at 390nm) minus *P*-450 + solvent (Soret peak at 420 nm).

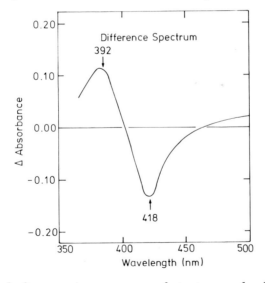

This method of measuring enzyme–substrate complex has three important advantages: first, the signal for a given number of bound molecules is increased by measuring peak-to-trough; second, difference spectroscopy reduces background by subtraction so that accurate values can be obtained with turbid samples, and third, the spectral shift is all or nothing, i.e., for each molecule of $P$-450, the Soret peak is either at 420 or at 390 nm. Therefore, $A_{392-418}$ is directly proportional to the number of molecules of ES.

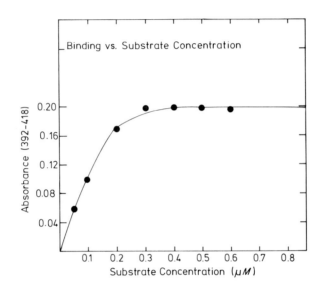

This method provides a simple and direct procedure for determining the affinity of the enzyme for its substrate—one that does not involve the complexities of catalysis and one that does not destroy the enzyme (Schenkman *et al.*, 1982; Nakajin and Hall, 1981b).

## C. *P*-420

This term is a general name for those forms of $P$-450 in which the attachment of the heme iron to the protein via a thiolate bond has been disrupted (Jung *et al.*, 1979). The protein loses enzymatic activity and the reduced CO spectrum shows a peak at 420 nm—hence the name. Presumably, many possible changes in the protein can cause formation of $P$-420—sometimes the changes can be reversed, but in some cases, it appears to involve irreversible denaturation (Yu and Gunsalus, 1974a,b). Since various forms of harsh treatment produce $P$-420, it is necessary to examine the absolute CO spectrum of any sample of $P$-450 with some care. The spectrum always shows a shoulder at 420 nm due to a vibrational mode of the iron. Notice, however, that the pen goes down and never up. An upward deflection means that some $P$-420 is

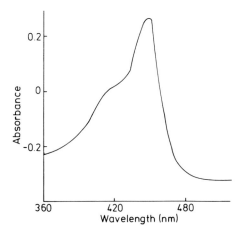

present. A useful rule of thumb is that if $A_{450}/A_{420}$ exceeds 2.4, *P*-420 is not present in the sample. The spectral properties of *P*-450 have been reviewed by a number of authors (Griffen *et al.*, 1979; Sligar, 1976).

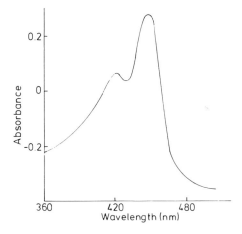

## V. CATALYTIC CYCLE OF *P*-450

Like all enzymes, *P*-450 displays a cycle of events that begins with binding of substrate and ends with the release of product to make way for another molecule of substrate. In oxidzing the substrate, *P*-450 must be reduced; reduction involves the iron to which substrate oxygen is bound. The reduced enzyme must be restored to the ferric state to repeat the cycle, and the substrate must be converted to product. These cyclic events are collectively referred to as the catalytic cycle. Details of the cycle provide insights into the mechanism of action of *P*-450 and reveal problems which are not currently understood. It is generally believed that all cytochromes *P*-450 make use of the same catalytic cycle. The cycle requires the regulated output of a single electron per molecule of *P*-450 at each of two steps. We will consider the source of the electrons later. The cycle can be seen as several consecutive steps, although such a division represents a descriptive artifact—the steps are smoothly coordinated into a continuous cycle:

STEP 1. Formation of the enzyme–substrate complex

$$Fe^{3+} + RH \rightarrow Fe^{3+}\!\!-\!\!RH$$

where the oxidized enzyme is represented as $Fe^{3+}$ and RH is the substrate which will eventually be converted to the product R—OH. This step is driven by the hydrophobic attraction of the lipophilic substrate for the heme pocket of the enzyme. We will see that with steroidogenic cytochromes *P*-450, this attraction shows the usual specificity expected of an enzyme, but apparently much less specificity is seen between xenobiotic enzymes and their substrates.

It will be recalled that this step leads to a striking shift of the Soret band (420 → 390 nm). This change results from a reorganization of the *d* orbital electrons of iron. Before the substrate binds, the iron is ferric and hexacoordinate. Ferric iron contains five electrons in the *d* orbitals which are paired as follows:

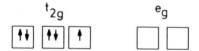

This distribution of electrons is referred to by the shorthand nomenclature of 1/2 (one unpaired electron), and the iron is said to be low spin. The nomenclature of group theory uses the terms $t_{2g}$ and $e_g$ to designate the symmetry of the orbitals of the *d* electrons. In the low-spin form of iron, all five *d* orbitals are of the same symmetry ($t_{2g}$), which is lower than the energy of the $e_g$ orbital. Such a change in the coordination of the metal atom is common during the catalytic activity of metalloenzymes. In the case of *P*-450, this change results from the loss of a weak sixth bond, so that the iron is attached to the protein only through the thiolate bond. The electrons of the *d* orbitals rearrange to the following orbitals:

$$t_{2g} \qquad e_g$$
$$\uparrow\uparrow\uparrow \qquad \uparrow\uparrow$$

This arrangement is referred to as 5/2: five unpaired electrons with two electrons in the higher energy ($e_g$) orbital, and the iron is said to be high spin. We can therefore associate the Soret band at 420 nm with hexacoordinate iron and substrate-free *P*-450, while the 390 peak is commonly associated with pentacoordinate iron and bound substrate (Rein and Ristau, 1978; Ullrich, 1969).

| Coordination Valance | Ferric Iron Spin State | d Electrons | Soret Band nm | Substrate |
|---|---|---|---|---|
| 6 | Low | ⬆⬇⬆⬇⬆ | 420 | Absent |
| 5 | High | ⬆⬆⬆⬆⬆ | 390 | Bound |

It should, however, be pointed out that factors other than binding of substrate affect the spin state of the iron in *P*-450. It should also be added that the conversion of low-spin iron to the pentacoordinate high-spin form is associated with displacement of the iron from the plane of the ring toward the thiolate sulfur.

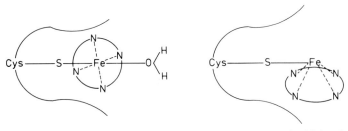

Hexacoordinate; low spin                Pentacoordinate; high spin

This step, in addition to producing the enzyme–substrate complex, promotes the flow of the first electron to the iron from an electron carrier (see below). The mechanism of this effect is not entirely clear (Gunsalus *et al.*, 1974). It should be noted, however, that the position vacated by the sixth ligand will subsequently be occupied by oxygen. The substrate binds to the active site on the same side of the heme as the oxygen.

STEP 2: The first electron:

$$Fe^{3+}-RH + e^- \rightarrow Fe^{2+}-RH$$

The enzyme–substrate complex accepts an electron from an electron carrier. This exchange is accomplished by the formation of a complex between the electron carrier and *P*-450 (White and Coon, 1980). The iron is now reduced.

STEP 3: Binding of oxygen:

$$Fe^{2+}\text{---}RH + O_2 \rightarrow Fe^{2+}\underset{\overset{|}{O_2}}{\text{---}}RH$$

In the catalytic cycle under consideration, one step facilitates the next. In this case, loss of the sixth coordinate bond when the substrate binds promotes binding of oxygen to the sixth position. It is characteristic of ferrous heme proteins with a vacant sixth ligand position that they readily bind molecular oxygen (Gunsalus *et al.*, 1974; Ishimura *et al.*, 1971; Estabrook *et al.*, 1971).

STEP 4: The second electron:

$$Fe^{2+}\underset{\overset{|}{O_2}}{\text{---}}RH + e^- \rightarrow Fe^{3+}\underset{\overset{|}{O_2^{2-}}}{\text{---}}RH$$

The enzyme–substrate–oxygen complex now accepts a second electron from an electron carrier. This electron activates oxygen to a form capable of completing the reaction cycle. The iron now reverts to the ferric form as the result of an internal rearrangement of electrons.

STEP 5: Oxygen cleavage:

$$Fe^{3+}\underset{\overset{|}{O_2^{2-}}}{\text{---}}RH + 2H^+ \rightarrow (Fe\text{---}O)^{3+}\underset{\overset{|}{RH}}{} + H_2O$$

The two oxygen atoms separate and water is formed from one atom (Ullrich *et al.*, 1979; Hoa *et al.*, 1978).

STEP 6: Oxygen insertion:

$$(Fe\text{---}O)^{3+}\underset{\overset{|}{RH}}{} \rightarrow Fe^{3+}OH^-\underset{\overset{|}{R}}{} \rightarrow Fe^{3+}(ROH)$$

The exact mechanism of this step is not clear, but a reasonable formulation is shown above. Hydrogen is removed from the substrate to leave a carbon radical. The hydrogen forms a hydroxyl radical with the oxygen, and this radical recombines with the carbon radical to form a hydroxylated substrate—so-called rebound. The hydroxylated substrate represents the major product of the reaction; the second product is water. This mechanism is sometimes called oxygen rebound (Hori *et al.*, 1977; Groves and van der Puy, 1974, 1976; Groves and McCluskey, 1976).

STEP 7: Dissociation of the product:

The product of the reaction is relatively polar (ROH), so that it is easily discharged from the active site to leave a hexacoordinate low-spin ferric iron ready to start the cycle again by binding another molecule of substrate:

$$Fe^{3+}(ROH) \rightarrow Fe^{3+} + ROH$$

These seven steps can be represented as a cycle:

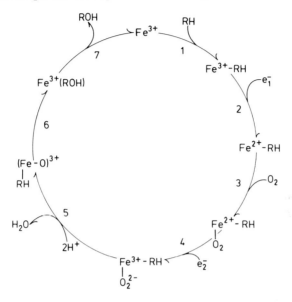

VI. Electron Donors

The electrons for the catalytic cycle come from reduced pyridine nucleotide via protein carriers. In mitochondrial and bacterial cytochromes $P$-450, the transfer of electrons requires two proteins—a flavoprotein and an iron–sulfur protein (Omura $et\ al.$, 1966). By contrast, the microsomal cytochromes $P$-450 require a single flavoprotein (Yasukochi and Masters, 1976). The two systems are specific for the source of $P$-450, i.e., the mitochondrial electron carriers cannot support the activity of microsomal $P$-450, and vice versa. The mitochondrial system involves reduction of the flavoprotein, which contains FAD, and this in turn passes electrons to the iron–sulfur protein, and finally to $P$-450.

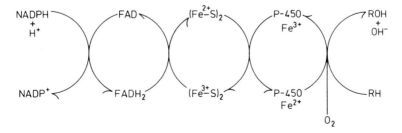

The exact redox state of the flavoprotein that is responsible for transferring electrons to the iron–sulfur protein is not clear at this time. The iron–sulfur protein contains a region of two iron–two acid-labile sulfurs which accepts and donates a single electron (Kimura, 1968; Dunham *et al.*, 1971).

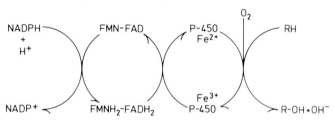

The microsomal system consists of a single flavoprotein containing FMN and FAD. The protein can be fully reduced to $FMNH_2$, $FADH_2$, although the form of the protein that denotes an electron to $P$-450 is not known (Iyanagi and Mason, 1973; Vermilion and Coon, 1978). This protein is called cytochrome $P$-450 reductase and is not specific for a particular $P$-450, e.g., the enzyme from hepatic microsomes is capable of reducing testicular microsomal $P$-450 (Nakajin and Hall, 1981b). However, details in the molecular differences between various microsomal cytochrome $P$-450 reductase enzymes have not yet been determined.

The nomenclature for the iron–sulfur proteins is not entirely settled. They can be referred to as the ferridoxins, since they resemble plant ferridoxins rather closely. In general, they are known by the suffix "-doxin," with a prefix to designate the tissue in question, e.g., adrenodoxin for the protein from adrenal mitochondria, and testodoxin for the testis. The reductase enzymes follow this nomenclature, e.g., adrenodoxin reductase. These two groups of proteins were formerly called nonheme iron and diaphorase, respectively. These names should no longer be used.

The major uncertainty concerning electron transport in the microsomal system lies in the possible involvement of the cytochrome $b_5$. Addition of cytochrome $b_5$ to a variety of reconstituted microsomal systems causes increase or inhibition of enzyme activity or no effect, depending on the conditions used. It has been pointed out that details of the ratios of protein to lipid used are critical to determining the effects of $b_5$ on reconstituted systems (Bosterling *et al.*, 1982). Hildebrandt and Estabrook (1971) suggested that cytochrome $b_5$ may supply the second electron which, as discussed above, is responsible for activation of oxygen and hence for the catalytic activity of $P$-450. It appears safe to conclude that $b_5$ is not an obligatory component of the $P$-450 system, since some reconstituted systems prepared without $b_5$ show turnover numbers as great as or greater than those observed for the analogous reactions measured in microsomes (Lu and West, 1978; Haugen *et al.*, 1975). Miki *et al.* (1980) have isolated a hepatic cytochrome $b_5$ with high affinity for $P$-450. A system containing $b_5$, NADH-$b_5$ reductase and detergent, was reconstituted from purified components. The authors showed that $b_5$ can influence the reduction of $P$-450. Recent studies with microsomes suggest that $b_5$ may be important for reduction of ferrous oxy-$P$-450 in the microsomal membrane (Werringloer and Kawano, 1980). These investigators measured the rates and extent of reduction of $P$-450 and $b_5$ under a variety of conditions. Their results suggest that the environment provided by the membrane is important in the regulation of electron transport (Werringloer and Kawano, 1980).

The role of cytochrome $b_5$ must therefore be considered uncertain at this time. However, in steroidogenic microsomes from the testis, some interesting observations have been made (Ohba *et al.*, 1981; Onoda and Hall, 1982). Leydig cell microsomes contain $b_5$ and $b_5$ reductase (Ohba *et al.*, 1981; Onoda and Hall, 1982). NADH supports weak $P$-450 activity in the $C_{21}$ side-chain cleavage system. Activity is too low to determine whether NADH acts via $b_5$ reductase or via $P$-450 reductase as a weak reductant (Onoda and Hall, 1982). In a system reconstituted from highly purified $P$-450 and $P$-450 reductase, addition of $b_5$ greatly increases enzyme activity and alters the ratio of lyase to hydroxylase activities (Onoda and Hall, 1982). Clearly the $b_5$ is not acting via $b_5$ reductase, so that it must be concluded that $b_5$ is capable of influencing the activity of $P$-450 presumably by direct interaction between the two cytochromes, as suggested by the observations of Miki *et al.* for hepatic $P$-450 (Miki *et al.*, 1982).

In some microsomal systems phospholipid or detergent is necessary for the reconstitution of an active $P$-450 system from purified components (Lu *et al.*, 1973). The function of the phospholipid is not known.

## VII. BIOSYNTHESIS OF STEROID HORMONES

By comparing the structure of cholesterol, from which steroid hormones are synthesized, with that of the major classes of steroid hormones, we can see that all four steroid hormones differ from cholesterol in the A and B rings; these changes do not involve $P$-450 in the first three groups of hormones. In addition, the glucocorticoids cortisol has

(1) lost part of the side chain of cholesterol ($C_{22}$–$C_{27}$), and (2) has acquired three hydroxyl groups (II$\beta$, 17$\alpha$, and 21-). These four changes require four separate cytochromes $P$-450 (Shikita and Hall, 1973; Omura et al., 1966; Nakajin et al., 1984; Estabrook et al., 1963). The mineralocorticoid shows an aldehyde at $C_{18}$ in place of the methyl group in cholesterol; this change involves another $P$-450. The androgens have lost the side chain of $C_{21}$ steroids (i.e., $C_{20}$ and $C_{21}$), which requires yet another $P$-450. Finally, the aromatic A ring of the major estrogens requires the activity of a special $P$-450 called aromatase (Ryan, 1959).

Steroid hormones are synthesized in the adrenal cortex, testis, ovary, and placenta. Each organ produces a characteristic mix of steroid hormones using enzymes which are fundamentally similar in each case. Differences in the hormones secreted by these organs result from differences in the amounts of the various enzymes present. For example, the testis produces large amounts of $C_{19}$ androgens because it possesses a very active $C_{21}$ steroid side-chain cleavage system. The ovary secretes high levels of estrogens because it is rich in aromatase. Such differences reflect specific regulation of the expression of the corresponding genes. In addition, it is also clear, as we will see, that the activities of the various enzymes are subject to local regulation within the mitochondrial and microsomal membranes of the steroidogenic organs.

Not only are the enzymes themselves similar from organ to organ, but the arrangement of the enzymes within the various steroidogenic cells is similar (Samuels, 1960; Hall, 1970a,b):

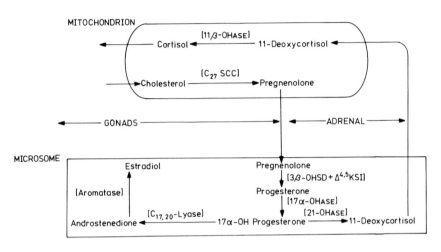

OHASE : Hydroxylase
OHSD  : Hydroxysteroid Dehydrogenase
KSI   : Ketosteroid Isomerase
SCC   : Side-chain Cleavage

It will be seen that steroid synthesis requires contributions from mitochondria and microsomes. The placenta produces steroids of all the major functional groups (corticosteroids, androgens, progesterone, and estrogens). Steroid synthesis begins in all cases with the conversion of cholesterol to pregnenolone:

CHOLESTEROL    PREGNENOLONE

This reaction, which takes place in the inner mitochondrial membrane (Yago *et al.*, 1970), is referred to as $C_{27}$ side-chain cleavage to distinguish it from the later step of $C_{21}$ side-chain cleavage. Pregnenolone then moves to the microsomal compartment in which it is converted to the $\Delta^4$-3-ketone progesterone.

PREGNENOLONE            PROGESTERONE

In the gonads, progesterone is subjected to $C_{21}$ side-chain cleavage by two enzymatic activities, namely, $17\alpha$-hydroxylase and $C_{17,20}$-lyase.

Progesterone                    Androstenedione

In the testis, the 17-ketone is reduced to the $17\beta$-alcohol by $17\beta$-hydroxysteroid dehydrogenase to give testosterone, the principal androgen.

In the ovary, testosterone is converted to estradiol by the $P$-450 enzyme system called aromatase.

Testosterone                    Estradiol

In the adrenal cortex, on the other hand, $17\alpha$-hydroxylation results in the production of a $17\alpha$-hydroxy-$C_{21}$ steroid, $17\alpha$-hydroxyprogesterone, which is not cleaved to a $C_{19}$ steroid, but subjected to 21-hydroxylation to give 11-deoxycortisol.

$17\alpha$-Hydroxyprogesterone       11-Deoxycortisol

This intermediate returns to the mitochondrion for the final step in the pathway, namely, 11β-hydroxylation (Samuels, 1960), which takes place in the inner membrane of the organelle (Yago *et al.*, 1970). The product of 11β-hydroxylation is cortisol:

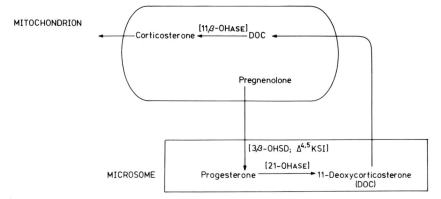

At this point, an important species difference must be noted, namely, in the adrenal cortex of some species, including the rat, 17α-hydroxylation does not take place, so that progesterone is subjected to 21-hydroxylation to give 11-deoxycorticosterone (DOC):

DOC is taken to the inner mitochondrial membrane to be converted to corticosterone by 11β-hydroxylation. These schemes must be modified for the synthesis of aldosterone which is formed from DOC by 11β-hydroxylation followed by 18-hydroxylation (Sharma *et al.*, 1967):

18-Hydroxycorticosterone is converted to aldosterone by an oxidase. This scheme reveals an important feature of the pathway in those

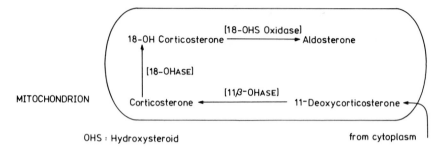

OHS : Hydroxysteroid

species that synthesize cortisol as opposed to corticosterone. In such species, including man, both 11-deoxycortisol and DOC must return to mitochondria to serve as substrates for the synthesis of cortisol and aldosterone, respectively. We must later consider the problem of whether these two pathways can proceed side by side in the same cells and in the same mitochondria or whether they are situated in different regions of the adrenal cortex.

SEQUENCE OF ENZYME ACTIVITIES

A glance at the pathways just outlined will show that the reactions catalyzed by the various enzymes need not proceed in the order given above but could, at least in theory, proceed in different sequences. If, for example, we begin by considering the synthesis of androgens, it can be seen that the conversion of pregnenolone to androstenedione could proceed by two alternative routes:

There are, however, certain limitations to these possibilities; for example, the $3\beta$-hydroxysteroid dehydrogenase and the isomerase appear as an enzyme pair in the sense that the intermediate $\Delta^5$-$3\beta$-one never appears in detectable quantities, and although $17\alpha$-hydroxyprogesterone and $17\alpha$-hydroxypregnenolone can be readily isolated from the gonads and from the adrenal cortex, we will see that $17\alpha$-hydroxylation and $C_{17,20}$-lyase activity result from the action of a single enzyme—indeed, from a single active site. It does not therefore seem possible for such sequences as

$$17\alpha\text{-OHase} \rightarrow 3\beta\text{-OHSD} \rightarrow C_{17,20}\text{-lyase} \rightarrow \Delta^{4,5}\text{KSI}$$

to occur *in vivo*.

In the adrenal, a second limitation may arise from the transport of intermediates to and from the mitochondrion. There is, for example, no evidence for the pathway

$$17\alpha\text{-OHase} \rightarrow 11\beta\text{-OHase} \rightarrow 21\text{-OHase}$$

Evidently, $11\beta$-hydroxylation is always the last step in the pathway.

For the synthesis of androgens then, there are two possible pathways conveniently referred to as the progesterone or $\Delta^4$ pathway and the dehydroepiandrosterone or $\Delta^5$ pathway. It appears that both pathways occur *in vivo* (Samuels, 1960). Moreover, the relative proportion of the two pathways is species specific and highly reproducible. For example, the rat uses largely the $\Delta^4$ pathway (Samuels, 1960); the dog (Eik-Nes and Hall, 1962), rabbit (Hall *et al.*, 1964), and pig (Ruokonen and Vihko, 1974) make extensive use of the $\Delta^5$ pathway. The mechanism(s) by which the microsomal membrane regulates the extent to which synthesis proceeds by one or other pathway will be discussed below.

In the adrenal, the choices are more complex. On p. 336 we see three possible pathways between pregnenolone and 11-deoxycortisol. The two alternatives shown in the diamond at the left resemble the situation in the pathway to androgens, except that there is no lyase activity, so that the product of this part of the pathway is $17\alpha$-hydroxyprogesterone rather than androstenedione. The third alternative in the upper right is peculiar to the synthesis of $C_{21}$ steroids:

$$17\alpha\text{-OHase} \rightarrow 21\text{-OHase} \rightarrow \begin{cases} 3\beta\text{-OHSD} \\ \Delta^{4,5}\text{KSI} \end{cases}$$

These pathways occur in the microsomal membrane so that there would seem to be two possible mechanisms by which the choice of pathway could be determined—either by the relative affinities of the

$\boxed{1}$ $\boxed{2}$ and $\boxed{3}$ : Alternative pathways
17α,21-DiOHP: 17α,21-Dihydroxypregnenolone

various enzymes for the possible substrates or by the organization of the enzymes and substrates within the microsomal membrane (or perhaps by some combination of these mechanisms).

The first possibility could be considered in the context of the three possibilities for the adrenal cortex (see above). Pathway 3 appears to be of minor importance in most species, if indeed it occurs at all *in vivo*. Little or no use of this pathway could come about as the result of the relative affinities of 3β-hydroxysteroid dehydrogenase for the two alternative substrates, namely, 17α-hydroxypregnenolone (high) and 17,21-dihydroxypregnenolone (low), and/or as the result of a preference of 21-hydroxylase for 17α-hydroxyprogesterone as opposed to 17α-hydroxypregnenolone or a combination of both these relative affinities. Other possibilities can be developed by examining this scheme in greater detail (above). It should be added that such affinities of an enzyme for competing substrates can be accurately measured with the pure enzyme, although the possible influence of the lipid membrane on the relative affinities of the enzymes for their putative substrates should be considered in measuring kinetic constants with lipophilic substrates.

The second possibility could be envisaged by considering the microsomal membrane not as a three-dimensional solution, but as a two-dimensional liquid. The loss of one degree of freedom may allow the microsome to regulate the flow of steroid intermediates in a linear or near-linear fashion resembling a factor belt. In this event, the intermediates must pass from enzyme to enzyme in a sequence determined by the linear sequence of enzymes within the lipid bilayer:

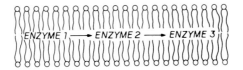

Now it is well known that biological membranes are best considered as two-dimensional liquids (Singer and Nicolson, 1972). However, to maintain a fixed linear organization would require either low mobility of enzymes within the plane of the bilayer or some anchoring device. One might, for example, propose that there is a pregnenolone-binding protein in the microsomal membrane that is specifically associated with one of the steroidogenic enzymes. Pregnenolone would then enter the membrane through what might be called entry ports and may pass inevitably from the binding protein to the associated enzyme which would then ipso facto become the first enzyme in the pathway. At this time, we have little information upon which to decide between various possibilities. It should be noticed that either of the two main possibilities could explain any mixture of alternative pathways from all one pathway to all the other pathways. Finally, the second possibility cannot, by definition, be examined with the pure enzymes. It is here that reconstitution studies with liposomes prepared in the laboratory may prove invaluable.

## VIII. Steroidogenic Enzymes

The conversion of cholesterol to corticosteroids, androgens, and estrogens requires the following changes in the structure of the initial substrate:

| Activity | C atoms or steroid ring |
| --- | --- |
| Hydroxylation | 22, 20, 17$\alpha$, 21, 11$\beta$ 18 |
| Dehydrogenation | 3$\beta$ |
| Oxidase activity | 18 |
| C—C cleavage | 20, 22 and 17, 20 |
| Aromatization | A ring |
| Isomerization | $\Delta^{4,5}$ |

Hydroxylation, C—C cleavage, and aromatization require specific cytochromes $P$-450 (mitochondrial and microsomal). Dehydrogenation requires a typical pyridine nucleotide dehydrogenase. Oxidation at $C_{18}$ requires an enzyme that has not so far been studied in detail, and isomerization of the $\Delta^5$ to the $\Delta^4$ structure requires an isomerase.

## A.  $C_{27}$ SIDE-CHAIN CLEAVAGE

The conversion of cholesterol to pregnenolone occurs in the inner mitochondrial membrane (Yago *et al.*, 1970). The classical hydroxylase activity of $P$-450 is used at two adjacent C atoms in the side chain of cholesterol, and the intervening bond is then cleaved to release isocapraldehyde and pregnenolone from which the various steroid hormones are synthesized *in vivo* (Lynn *et al.*, 1954; Solomon *et al.*, 1956; Shimizu *et al.*, 1960; Constantopoulos and Tchen, 1961; Hall and Koritz, 1964a):

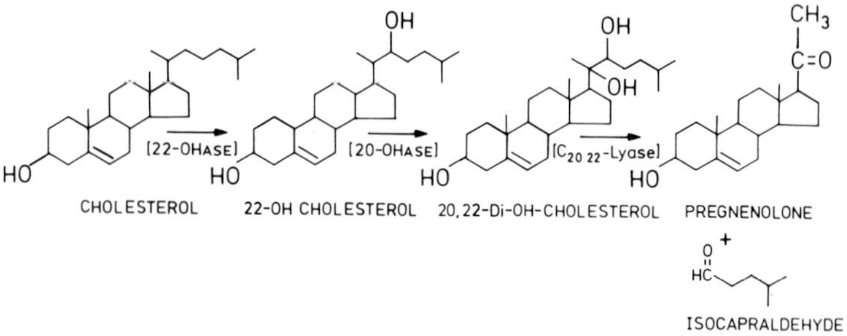

The correct nomenclature for the two intermediates is as follows: (22R)-22-hydroxycholesterol and (2OR,22R)-20,22-dihydroxycholesterol. Throughout this discussion, the names given below the above structures will be used for the sake of brevity.

An important feature of the pathway is that neither of the intermediates can be detected in significant amounts when the pure enzyme is reconstituted *in vitro* (Hall and Koritz, 1964a,b; Koritz and Hall, 1964a,b). This stands in marked contrast to $C_{21}$ side-chain cleavage enzyme with which the intermediate 17$\alpha$-hydroxyprogesterone accumulates during the reaction (Slaun *et al.*, 1956).

The $C_{27}$ side-chain cleavage enzyme was first purified by use of conventional chromatographic methods applied to cholate extracts of mitochondria (Shikita and Hall, 1973, 1974). The use of cholate introduced by Horie (Mitani and Horie, 1969) has remained standard procedure for all cytochromes $P$-450. The purified enzyme was shown to be homogenous by rigorous criteria and to be essentially devoid of substrate (cholesterol). The enzyme was found to appear in various states of aggregation—4, 8, and 16 subunit forms were isolated in aqueous buffers and characterized by analytical ultracentrifugation (Shikita and Hall, 1974). The monomeric form was only observed in the presence of denaturing agents such as guanadinium chloride and SDS. Three different criteria—electrophoresis on acrylamide gels, chromatography on Sephadex with SDS, and analytical ultracentrifugation—the molecular weight of the monomer was found to be 52,000 and the 4, 8, and 16 oligomeric forms gave appropriate values for molecular weights determined in the analytical ultracentrifuge (Shikita and Hall, 1973, 1974). The yield of enzyme was greatly increased by means of affinity chromatography with pregnenolone as the ligand (Tilley *et al.*, 1977). Numerous modifications of the original methods of preparation have appeared and lower molecular weights have been reported for the monomer (e.g., Ramseyer and Harding, 1973; Takimori *et al.*, 1975).

Obviously, this enzyme catalyzes a complex reaction in which two hydroxylation reactions are followed by cleavage of a carbon–carbon bond. Since the enzyme can be prepared in homogenous form, the three reactions are catalyzed by a single protein. The first step in clarifying the underlying mechanism was the determination of stoichimetry of the reaction. It was shown that each of these three steps requires 1 mol of NADPH and 1 mol of oxygen, so that the overall stoichiometry is as follows (Shikita and Hall, 1974):

$$C_{27}H_{46}O + 3O_2 + 3NADPH + 3H^+ \rightarrow C_{21}H_{32}O_2 + C_6H_{12}O + 3NADP^+ + 4H_2O$$

This also means that the cleavage of the 20,22 bond shows the stoichiometry of a typical monooxygenase. It therefore became important to determine whether the heme moiety of the $P$-450 is involved in this third step of the reaction. The photochemical action spectrum for the conversion of 20,22-dihydroxycholesterol to pregnenolone unequivocally demonstrated the involvement of heme in this conversion (Takagi *et al.*, 1975). Reversal of inhibition for the enzyme by light was maximal at 450 nm.

Meanwhile, the apparent failure of the two hydroxylated intermediates to appear during the reaction was difficult to understand. The two intermediates are rapidly converted to pregnenolone by the enzyme (Shikita and Hall, 1973; Constantopoulos and Tchen, 1962; Hall and Koritz, 1964a). Eventually Burstein and Gut (1976), using vast quantities of a crude mitochondrial extract, isolated small amounts of the two intermediates under conditions that strongly supported the three-step scheme presented above. Earlier claims that hydroxylation at $C_{20}$ preceded that at $C_{22}$ have evidently been eliminated.

The next question is whether the enzyme has three active sites or one. Kinetic and binding studies point to a single active site (Duque *et al.*, 1978). This conclusion immediately presents another problem which takes us back to the catalytic cycle. It was pointed out that the hydroxylated reaction product should readily leave the hydrophobic active site and that the stimulus for initiation of a new cycle is the binding of a new molecule of hydrophobic (unhydroxylated) substrate which triggers reduction of iron by the first electron (Ullrich, 1979; White and Coon, 1980).

A detailed study of the binding of substrate, intermediates, and product to the pure enzyme using electron spin resonance, absorbance spectroscopy, and equilibrium dialysis revealed one binding site for each of these steroids (Orme-Johnson *et al.*, 1979). Moreover, the dissociation constants for these steroids are as follows:

| Steroid | $K_D$ (n$M$) |
|---------|--------------|
| 22$R$-cholesterol | 4.9 |
| 20$R$,22$R$-diOH cholesterol | 81 |
| Pregnenolone | 2900 |

It is at once obvious that the two intermediates are tightly bound. Moreover, 22$R$-OH cholesterol shows a dissociation frequency of less than 5 per second. It is equally clear that the product of the reaction dissociates relatively easily from the enzyme. This provides an explanation for the difficulty of isolating the intermediates. Evidently the catalytic cycle is modified in such a way as to permit a second cycle to occur with the product of the previous cycle still bound to the enzyme. When pregnenolone is formed, the product dissociates and the next cycle of three reactions is initiated by binding of cholesterol.

An interesting approach to this problem has been initiated by Skeets and Vickery (1982), who have synthesized a series of steroids bearing an amine on side chains of various lengths at $C_{17}$. It is assumed that these molecules bind in the same way as cholesterol, at least as far as the steroid ring system is concerned. The amine gives a spectral shift in the Soret band if it is close enough to interact with the heme iron. One such steroid, 22-amino-23,24-bisnor-5-cholen-3$\beta$-ol, is capable of such interaction. Kendrew skeletal molecular models show that $C_{17}$ must be less than 5.5 Å from the iron. This should permit direct attack of Fe-bound oxygen on $C_{22}$. If we consider the oxygen-rebound mechanism discussed above, we can envisage hydrogen extraction by the Fe-O from $C_{22}$ to form a carbon radical which could then react with the iron-bound OH causing this group to rebound to or react with the $C_{22}$ radical to form 22-hydroxycholesterol. Unfortunately, apart from some uncertainty about this mechanism, the important question is left open regarding the next step in the reaction. $C_{20}$ would be an additional 1.54 Å from the iron if enzyme and substrate maintain the same relative positions. Can the hydroxylation of this carbon atom take place over this greater distance, or must the substrate (intermediate) move relative to the enzyme to take up position closer to the iron? It is conceivable that such movement might result from a change in the conformation of the enzyme so that not only does $C_{20}$ become closer to the iron, but the flow of the first electron for the next catalytic cycle is triggered.

The third step in the reaction, cleavage of the $C_{20,22}$ bond, is an unusual reaction for $P$-450, although we will encounter a second example of C—C cleavage in steroidogenesis (see below). The photochemical action spectrum and the stoichiometry of the cleavage step are those of typical monooxygenation (Shikita and Hall, 1974; Takagi *et al.*, 1975). Evidently heme is required for this step. It is possible to propose several plausible chemical mechanisms for carbon–carbon cleavage by $P$-450, but so far there is no experimental evidence to support any of them.

When pregnenolone is added to purified $C_{27}$ side-chain cleavage $P$-450, a spectral shift occurs that is the inverse of the typical type I shift discussed above (peak at 420, trough at 390 nm) (Orme-Johnson *et al.*, 1979). It has been suggested that such a shift results from binding to a site other than the site which produces the typical type I shift (Schenkman *et al.*, 1967). It therefore follows that the second site to which pregnenolone binds is different from the active site. Such a second site may be responsible for the inhibition of side-chain cleavage produced by pregnenolone (Koritz and Hall, 1964a). It is interesting to notice that the inhibition of side-chain cleavage by pregnenolone shows some characteristics of an allosteric mechanism (Koritz and Hall, 1964b).

## B. $C_{21}$ Side-Chain Cleavage

Cytochrome $P$-450 is full of surprises. Since the adrenal cortex is capable of forming $17\alpha$-hydroxy-$C_{21}$ steroids while the gonads produce

$C_{18}$ and $C_{19}$ steroids, it was reasonable to expect that the two steps in $C_{21}$ side-chain cleavage (hydroxylase and lyase) would be catalyzed by two different enzymes:

PROGESTERONE          17α-OH PROGESTERONE          ANDROSTENEDIONE

The hydroxylase would be found in both adrenal and gonads and lyase would be largely confined to the gonads. Differential inhibition of the two reactions by carbon monoxide with a microsomal system seemed to confirm this idea (Betz *et al.*, 1976). It came as a complete surprise to find that the two activities copurify to homogeneity from testicular microsomes (Nakajin and Hall, 1981a). The evidence for homogeneity is based upon gel electrophoresis and immunochemistry. More important, the amino acid sequence has been determined for ~50% of the protein, and no evidence of more than one protein has been found (Nakajin *et al.*, 1981a,b). Surprise no longer seems necessary when it is realized that this enzyme shows much in common with the $C_{27}$ system—two steps instead of three because one oxygen function is already present in the substrate. Because of this similarity, the term $C_{21}$ steroid side-chain cleavage and the abbreviation $P$-450 $C_{21scc}$ have been used to refer to the enzyme and the reaction.

Substrate-induced difference spectra and equilibrium dialysis showed that this enzyme possesses a single active site for which the substrate per mole of heme and progesterone can displace 17α-hydroxyprogesterone from the enzyme, and vice versa (Nakajin *et al.*, 1981). Similar competition was seen with the $\Delta^5$ substrates pregnenolone and 17α-hydroxypregnenolone. Although this enzyme shows much in common with the $C_{27}$ side-chain cleavage enzyme, there is at least one important difference, namely, that whereas with the $C_{27}$ system the intermediate hydroxysteroids do not accumulate and can only be detected by special methods, 17α-hydroxyprogesterone accumulates freely in the surrounding medium. Clearly, this intermediate leaves the enzyme quite readily and yet it also binds to the enzyme with a $K_m$ similar to that of progesterone (Nakajin and Hall, 1981c) (see tabulation below).

| Substrate | $K_m$ ($\mu M$) | $V_{max}$ ($n$ moles product/min/$n$ mole $P$-450) |
|---|---|---|
| Pregnenolone | 0.8 | 3.9 |
| 17α-OH pregnenolone | 0.9 | 2.5 |
| Progesterone | 1.8 | 10.0 |
| 17α-Hydroxypregnenolone | 2.5 | 6.1 |

Similar values are observed with substrate-induced difference spectra (Nakajin and Hall, 1981c). Once again, the photochemical action spectrum shows that heme is required for the lyase reaction (Nakajin and Hall, 1983). Moreover, since there is one heme per protein subunit, the substrates for the two reactions must bind close to the heme. These considerations make the active site a subject of great interest.

To examine the active site in greater detail, the substrate analog 17α-bromo[$^3H$]acetoxyprogesterone was used as an affinity probe. This

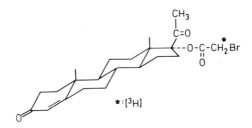

substance inactivates both hydroxylase and lyase activities with a single linear relationship as a function of time, with $t_{1/2}$ of ~3 hours for each activity (Onoda *et al.*, 1984). The fact that the analog inactivates both activities over the same time course strongly suggests inactivation of a single active site. Again the enzyme is protected from inactivation by the analog if either substrate is present. Each substrate protects both activities from inactivation by the analog (Onoda *et al.*, 1984). These observations provide further support for the conclusion that the enzyme possesses a single active site.

The bromoacetoxysteroid forms a covalent bond with the enzyme at room temperature, releasing HBr.

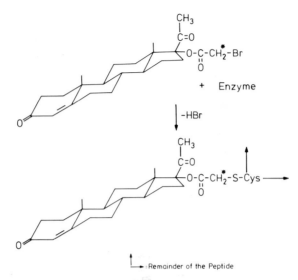

The scheme shows cysteine as the residue attacked by the bromine for diagrammatic purposes. However, other amino acids such as lysine and tryptophan can react with the analog which can be used to detect any one of nine amino acids at the active site. When the enzyme has formed the appropriate steroid derivative, the sample is divided into two parts. One part is subjected to acid hydrolysis and amino acid analysis to give the component amino acids, one of which will be found as a derivative. Acid hydrolysis removes the steroid moiety by cleaving the ester bond, leaving a carboxymethyl derivative of the amino acid attacked at the active site by the bromine:

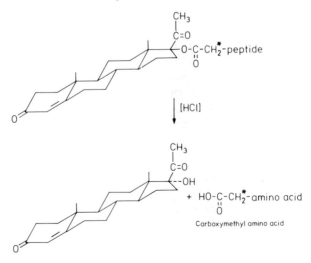

The carboxymethyl group is radioactive (*) and the relevant derivatives of the various reactive amino acids can be readily identified on the amino acid analyzer.

The second part of the sample is subjected to enzymatic digestion to produce a peptide map in which the radioactive amino acid derivative can be detected. This identifies the particular peptide containing the amino acid attacked by the steroid analog; this allows identification of a unique residue within the primary structure of the enzyme. When such a study with the $C_{21}$ steroid side-chain cleavage enzyme system from pig testicular microsomes using $17\alpha$-bromo[$^3H$]acetoxyprogesterone was conducted, the following peptide was isolated (Onoda *et al.*, 1984):

Ser-Asp-Leu-Glu-Leu-Pro-Asp-Asp-Gly-Gln-Leu-Leu-Gly-Cys

$$S-CH_2^*-\underset{\underset{O}{\|}}{C}-OH$$

This peptide is evidently highly conserved, since very similar peptides have been found in $P$-450 from rat liver and that from *Pseudomonas putida* (Nakajin *et al.*, 1981). Presumably this peptide is concerned with some aspect of the cytochrome that is not specific for steroid synthesis, but is rather of a more general character. Since $C_{17}$ is involved in $C_{21}$ side-chain cleavage, this peptide is presumed to contribute to the catalytic center of the active site. It should be pointed out that similar bromoacetoxy derivates at other parts of the progesterone molecule can be expected to form covalent bonds with other amino acids situated elsewhere within the active site.

The mechanism of carbon–carbon bond cleavage by this enzyme is likely to be similar to that of the $C_{27}$ side-chain cleavage enzyme, although the ease with which the intermediate $17\alpha$-hydroxyprogesterone leaves the active site and accumulates in the medium stands in marked contrast to the almost complete absence of intermediates in the side-chain cleavage of cholesterol. On the other hand, photochemical action spectra show that heme is involved in both hydroxylase and lyase activities (Nakajin and Hall, 1983). Presumably the cleavage step follows the same mechanism with both enzymes.

## C. 17$\alpha$-HYDROXYLASE

More surprises have come with purification of the $17\alpha$-hydroxylase from pig adrenal microsomes. It was pointed out above that $17\alpha$-hydroxylation represents a branch point in steroidogenesis—one that distinguishes the synthesis of $17\alpha$-hydroxy-$C_{21}$ steroids in the adrenal from the $C_{21}$ side-chain cleavage system in the gonads. In the rat adrenal, steroids are produced without a $17\alpha$-hydroxy group. It was therefore believed that in animals such as man and pig that produce $17\alpha$-hydroxy-$C_{21}$ adrenal steroids, the adrenal cortex must possess an enzyme different from that in the testis, one capable of $17\alpha$-hydroxylation without lyase activity; interesting contrasts between the enzymes were anticipated. The relatively small amount of androgen made by the adrenal has been attributed to the activity of different cells—possibly those of the *zona reticularis* which would presumably contain a hydroxylase/lyase like the testis. Pig adrenal microsomes convert progesterone to $17\alpha$-hydroxy-$C_{21}$ steroids. Androgenic $C_{19}$ steroids are not detected:

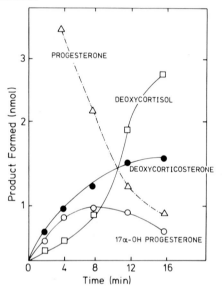

However, the purified $17\alpha$-hydroxylase from pig adrenal shows both hydroxylase and lyase activities (Nakajin *et al.*, 1983):

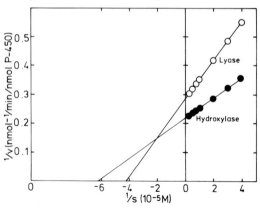

Clearly, the enzyme shows strong lyase activity like the testicular enzyme. Further examination of the two enzymes showed that kinetic constants with substrates for hydroxylase and lyase were very similar for the two enzymes. Again, antibody cross-reactivity on double diffusion does not distinguish the two enzymes using antibodies to the adrenal enzyme and antibodies to the testicular enzyme (Nakajin *et al.*, 1984). Finally, the amino acid sequences at the $NH_2$ termini of the two enzymes are extremely similar (Nakajin *et al.*, 1984). We must conclude that a very similar enzyme exists in both testicular and adrenal microsomes. In testicular microsomes, the enzyme acts as a hydroxylase/lyase, i.e., $C_{21}$ side-chain cleavage system. In the adrenal microsomes, a similar enzyme acts chiefly as a hydroxylase, whereas it acts like the testicular enzyme when released from the microsomal membrane. Clearly, some regulatory mechanism within the microsomal compartment must influence the activity of this interesting enzyme. Incidentally, such local regulation would explain the changes in hydroxylase relative to lyase seen in response to numerous regulatory changes (Fevold, 1983).

## D. 21-Hydroxylase

This microsomal $P$-450 was first purified from beef adrenal by Kominami *et al.* (1980). The enzyme has also been purified from pig adrenal (Yuan *et al.*, 1983). The cystein-containing peptides of this enzyme show significant homology with liver and bacterial cytochromes $P$-450 (Yuan *et al.*, 1983). Two interesting features of the porcine enzyme are worth noting, namely, it shows lower $K_m$ with $17\alpha$-hydroxyprogesterone than with progesterone and the corresponding $\Delta^5$ steroids are poor substrates for this enzyme. The first point is interesting in view of the earlier suggestion of Hechter and co-workers who observed that 17-hydroxylation precedes 21-hydroxylation in beef adrenal and proposed that 21-hydroxylase does not bind $17\alpha$-hydroxyprogesterone (Eichorn and Hechter, 1957; Hechter and Pincus, 1954). The pure enzyme shows that on the basis of values for $K_m$, this steroid is actually preferred to progesterone. Clearly other microsomal factors must regulate the sequence in which these reactions occur. The second observation suggests that 21-hydroxylation of $\Delta^5$ substrates is not important, at least in pig.

## E. 11$\beta$-18-Hydroxylase

This enzyme catalyzes the last reaction in the pathway to glucocorticoids and an essential step in the pathway to aldosterone. The 11$\beta$-/18-

hydroxylase is found in the inner mitochondrial membrane and is clearly distinct from the $C_{27}$ side-chain cleavage system (Yago *et al.,* 1970). The 11$\beta$-hydroxylase is a typical *P*-450, and like the other mitochondrial *P*-450 of the adrenal, it requires both a flavoprotein and an iron–sulfur protein as electron carriers. The enzyme is very unstable under all conditions examined so far (Watanuki *et al.,* 1978). Studies with adrenal cells suggest that this instability may result from lipid peroxidation (Hornsby, 1980). It is interesting that the $C_{27}$ side-chain cleavage enzyme is relatively stable compared to the 11$\beta$-hydroxylase.

The enzyme was purified from beef adrenal cortex. In view of the studies by Bjorkham and Kalmar showing that under a variety of physiological and pathological conditions the two activities of 11$\beta$- and 18-hydroxylation changed in unison (Bjorkham and Kalmar, 1977; Bjorkham and Kalmar, 1977b), these workers suggested that a single enzyme might be responsible for catalyzing both reactions. Indeed, the pure enzyme does catalyze both 11$\beta$- and 18-hydroxylation of DOC. However, the enzyme does not catalyze 18-hydroxylation of corticosterone (Watanuki *et al.,* 1978). The evidence for a single enzyme includes a single $NH_2$-terminal amino acid, cross-reactivity to antibodies, and inhibition of both reactions by a variety of inhibitors, including antibodies to the enzyme. The purified enzyme contains one heme group per peptide molecule so that it is likely that both reactions are catalyzed by a single active site, although this has not been demonstrated by direct approaches.

The functional significance of the 18-hydroxylation of DOC is not clear. At least two possibilities must be considered: Either this enzyme comes from the *zona fasiculata* and is therefore not concerned with the synthesis of aldosterone or the enzyme has changed during isolation.

The first possibility would mean that a second enzyme would be expected to catalyze 18-hydroxylation of corticosterone. It was pointed out above that the synthesis of aldosterone is believed to proceed via corticosterone and not via 18-hydroxy DOC (see scheme on p. 348) (Ayers *et al.*, 1960; Sheppard *et al.*, 1963).

It is no doubt significant that the *zona fasciculata* of the rat contains much 18-hydroxy DOC, some of which is secreted (Fraser and Lantos, 1978). The physiological significance of the secretion of 18-hydroxy DOC is not known, nor has this steroid been isolated from beef adrenal. It is conceivable that the enzyme isolated by Watanuki *et al.* (1977) may catalyze the 11$\beta$- and 18-hydroxylation of DOC in the *zona fasciculata*. On the other hand, it seems equally possible that some form of regulation exists within the mitochondrion so that once the enzyme is released from the inner membrane it changes specificity. The situation would then be reminiscent of the microsomal 17$\alpha$-hydroxylase discussed above, that is, the enzyme shows different specificity when released from the membrane (in that case the microsomal membrane).

The situation is made more intriguing by recent observations showing that beef adrenal 11$\beta$-hydroxylase can also catalyze hydroxylation of $C_{19}$ (Momoi *et al.*, 1983):

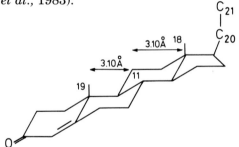

So far, 19-hydroxysteroids do not appear to have been isolated from the adrenal cortex. This situation may again represent an activity displayed by the pure enzyme, but suppressed in the membrane of the mitochondrion. Measurements in molecular models show that $C_{18}$ and $C_{19}$ are equidistant from $C_{11}$. It is interesting to notice that the distance between $C_{18}$ and $C_{11}$ is approximately twice that of a C—C bond, as in the side chain of cholesterol:

CHOLESTEROL

PARTIAL STRUCTURE OF
ALDOSTERONE

These intriguing observations must be explained when the mechanisms of reactions catalyzed by $P$-450 are finally elucidated. It was pointed out above that the work of Skeets and Vickery suggests that for side-chain cleavage of cholesterol, $C_{22}$ must approach to within 5.5 Å of the heme iron. This leaves open the question of whether the hydroxylation of $C_{20}$ can occur over this distance plus 1.54 Å (i.e., the additional distance of a C—C bond). The alternative would be a readjustment of the substrate within the active site between the two hydroxylation reactions. The $11\beta$-/18-hydroxylase provides an even greater distance (5.5 + 3.1 Å) over which the second hydroxylation must occur. Clearly, the possibility of movement by the substrate relative to the enzyme must be considered.

### F. 18-Oxidase

The enzyme responsible for the conversion of 18-hydroxycorticosterone to aldosterone is presumed to reside in the inner mitochondrial membrane, although there is no direct proof of this assumption. The enzyme has not been purified, so that elucidation of this reaction must await further investigation.

### G. Zones of the Adrenal Cortex

The adrenal cortex consists of three distinct zones, namely (from within out): *reticularis, fasciculata,* and *glomerulosa.* The *reticularis* appears to be a remnant of the fetal adrenal and may be responsible for the production of androgens after birth. It is generally agreed that the *fasciculata* synthesizes glucocorticoids, while the *zona glomerulosa* is responsible for the production of aldosterone. It has been proposed that all adrenal cells that secrete steroids arise from the periphery (capsule and/or *glomerulosa*) and that cells migrate toward the *reticularis,* undergoing morphological and functional transformation as they progress through the three zones. This view is not generally accepted, and for the purposes of this discussion, it will be assumed that after birth, the adrenal cortex consists of three largely independent zones which secrete the three classes of steroids as described above. It may be that the functional significance of the zones differs in different species. The subject is complex, but need not concern us here. It has been well reviewed by Long (1975). Incidentally, it should be pointed out that qualification of the independence of the three zones, implied above by the word "largely," is occasioned by consideration of the remarkable blood supply to the adrenal cortex which flows from the periphery toward the medulla. The products of peripheral cells are thereby taken past more centrally located cells so that the possibility for complex but indirect interactions between the three zones must be considered. Again, this subject has been well reviewed by Coupland (1975).

With this background, two aspects of steroidogenesis need to be considered briefly.

1. If androgens are synthesized by the adrenal cortex, is there a 17$\alpha$-hydroxylase/$C_{17,20}$-lyase different from the 17$\alpha$-hydroxylase of the *fasciculata*? It was pointed out above that Nakajin and Hall (1981b) discovered that the enzyme from pig adrenal serves as a 17$\alpha$-hydroxylase in the microsome, but as a hydroxylase/lyase when purified. Moverover, these authors could find no evidence of a second enzyme, that is, a pure 17$\alpha$-hydroxylase (no lyase), in spite of a careful search in extracts of pig adrenal (Nakajin and Hall, 1981b). One possibility is that the enzyme may be regulated by other microsomal factors (protein or lipid). This regulation could be fixed in the sense that the *reticularis* always expresses some lyase activity which results in the synthesis of androgens and the *fasciculata* does not express lyase activity. On the other hand, the expression of lyase activity may be variable and subject to regulation. Alternatively, both *reticularis* or *fasciculata* might be capable of producing androgens under regulated conditions. In this connection, the synthesis of some androstenedione by microsomes incubated with high levels of 17$\alpha$-hydroxyprogesterone may be significant (Nakajin *et al.*, 1983). Could it be that the regulation of androgen synthesis lies in the levels of available 17$\alpha$-hydroxyprogesterone? The matter is important for the understanding of those congenital abnormalities that involve high levels of 17$\alpha$-hydroxyprogesterone and androgens (Miller *et al.*, 1983). The purification of the relevant enzymes should resolve this problem by revealing the distribution of each of these enzymes. In this connection, the rat may be important. Rat adrenal secretes androgens *in vivo,* and yet it does not hydroxylate $C_{21}$ steroids at the 17$\alpha$- position. Is this because the hydroxylase/lyase occurs only in the *reticularis*? The alternative would be a hydroxylase/lyase in the *fasciculata* that is permanently inactive, at least under normal conditions.

2. How does the synthesis of aldosterone proceed without 17$\alpha$-hydroxylation? We must presume that in those species that produce cortisol, the smooth endoplasmic reticulum of the *glomerulosa* lacks this enzyme, while that of the *fasciculata* possesses 17$\alpha$-hydroxylase. Presumably, the cytoplasm of the *glomerulosa* cells contains a transport protein for DOC, and that of *fasciculata* cells contains the same or a

different protein for 11-deoxycortisol; these binding proteins would be responsible for transporting the intermediates to the mitochondrion. When these two intermediates reach their respective mitochondria, it must be supposed that DOC in the *glomerulosa* will be subjected to 11$\beta$- and 18-hydroxylation, while 11-deoxycortisol in the *fasciculata* will become a substrate for 11$\beta$-hydroxylation, but not 18-hydroxylation. It is interesting to observe that 18-hydroxycortisol has been isolated from adrenal and urine of patients suffering from primary aldosteronism (Chu and Ulick, 1982), and 18-ketocortisol has been isolated from adrenal tissue (Ulick *et al.*, 1983).

## H. AROMATASE

The conversion of a $\Delta^4$-3-ketosteroid to a steroid with an aromatic A ring is likely to be a complex multistep reaction.

Androstenedione        Estrone

The angular methyl group ($C_{19}$) must be removed and the A ring must be converted to the phenol. At first glance, cytochrome *P*-450 would not seem to be a likely candidate for such a reaction. However, it was reported by Ryan (1959) that microsomes from human placenta convert androstenedione to estrone and that NADPH and oxygen are required for this conversion. This suggested that monooxygenation may be involved in removing $C_{19}$. It was logical to determine whether a 19-nor-$\Delta^4$-3-ketosteroid steroid could be converted to the corresponding phenol. It was indeed shown that 19-nortestosterone is converted to estradiol by the same microsomal system and that oxygen and NADPH are also required (Ryan, 1959; Morato *et al.*, 1961). It seems likely that removal of $C_{19}$ and subsequent formation of the phenolic A ring both involve monooxygenation. Meyer (1955) isolated 19-hydroxyandrostenedione from placental microsomes, and several workers showed that both 19-hydroxy- and 19-ketoandrostenedione are rapidly converted to estrone in the presence of NADPH and oxygen (Morato *et al.*, 1961; Akhtar and Skinner, 1968; Skinner and Akhtar, 1969). More recently, it has been shown that 19-ketoandrostenedione may serve as a precursor of estrone (Braselton *et al.*, 1972). Further examination of the rates of formation and disappearance of 19-hydroxyandrostenedione suggested that this substance behaves like a true biosynthetic intermediate in the aromatization of androstenedione (Wilcox and

Engel, 1965). In addition, it has been shown that the second product of the aromatization of androstenedione is formic acid (Skinner and Akhtar, 1969).

These are the available facts; intepretation must remain uncertain. It would be reasonable to propose that hydroxylation at $C_{19}$ is followed by oxidation to the ketone which could, in turn, be followed by oxidative elimination of formic acid. Formic acid has in fact been isolated from a placental system during the conversion of androstenedione to estrone (Skinner and Akhtar, 1969).

ANDROSTENEDIONE     19-OH ANDRO-STENEDIONE     19-KETOANDRO-STENEDIONE     ESTRONE

The mechanism of step II is not clear. One possibility would be a second hydroxylation by monooxygenation. The gem diol 19,19-dihydroxyandrostenedione could collapse to the ketone. Alternatively, dehydrogenation of the single hydroxyl group in 19-hydroxyandrostenedione could also be responsible for the formation of 19-ketoandrostenedione from 19-hydroxyandrostenedione. It would seem unlikely that a single dehydrogenation would occur in the midst of a series of monooxygenase reactions, so that a common formulation for step II is as follows:

19-HYDROXYANDROSTENEDIONE     19,19-DIHYDROXYANDROSTENEDIONE     19-KETOANDROSTENEDIONE

The gem diol would be highly unstable and conversion to the ketone would be spontaneous. The stoichiometry for the conversion of androstenedione to estrone was measured with placental microsomes and high concentrations of cyanide (Thompson and Siiteri, 1974a). The stoichiometry $NADPH:O_2:product$ (estrone) was as follows: $3:3:1$. Oxygen and NADPH were required for the conversion of 19-hydroxyandrostenedione to 19-ketoandrostenedione. Measurement of stoichiometry raises a number of significant technical problems so that caution is necessary in interpreting the results. However, these findings are compatible with the sequence

Adione → 19-OHAdione → 19,19-dihydroxvAdione → estrone

the last step proceeding via the ketone. A third hydroxylation is excluded by the formation of formate—a trihydroxy intermediate would produce $CO_2$.

The aromatization of 19-ketoandrostenedione is even more obscure than the steps leading to this intermediate. Stereospecific loss of hydrogen from the $1\beta$ and $2\beta$ positions of androstenedione during aromatization suggests that hydroxylation at one or both of these positions may be involved in aromatization (Fishman et al., 1969; Townsley and Brodie, 1968; Brodie et al., 1969). However, $1\beta$- and $2\beta$-Hydroxyandrostenedione, are poor precursors of estrone, i.e., aromatization of these steroids in vitro is slow (Brodie et al., 1969; Townsley and Brodie, 1966). Again, 19-norsteroids are poor precursors of estrogens (Thompson and Siiteri, 1974a). These observations do not provide the basis for any mechanism, and indeed, it should be pointed out that the fact that a substance is a poor intermediate, in the sense that conversion to the product is slow, does not necessarily exclude this substance as an intermediate in the reaction. We shall have occasion to consider instances in which the access of exogenous steroids to the active sites of enzymes is limited, and the intermediate generated at the active site from a precursor may be greatly favored when compared to the same compounds presented exogenously by the experimenter. It is a serious mistake to consider that because steroids are lipophilic they have unrestricted access to the active sites of membrane-bound enzymes.

Even if we agree to accept hydroxylated steroids as intermediates in aromatization and even if these hydroxylation reactions require NADPH and oxygen, these facts do not establish that the aromatase is a cytochrome $P$-450. The picture is once again unclear. The two convincing ways of establishing the involvement of $P$-450 in any reaction are enzymological and photochemical. Purification of an enzyme to homogeneity demonstrates that the pure enzyme is a $P$-450, and reconstitution of the enzyme activity with the obligatory addition of the pure $P$-450 provides strong evidence for the involvement of this enzyme in the reaction. A typical photochemical action spectrum with inhibition of enzyme activity by CO and reversal of inhibition by light, specifically that of wavelength 450 nm, is also compelling evidence for involvement of $P$-450. Neither of these criteria has been met with aromatase. However, Thompson and Siiteri (1974b) provided some indirect evidence for the involvement of $P$-450 in aromatization of androstenedione by human placental microsomes. It is, however, something of a problem that the conversion of androstenedione to estrone is not inhibited by carbon monoxide (Thompson and Siiteri, 1974b).

Perhaps these problems will be resolved when the enzyme is finally purified. Certainly it is axiomatic that studies on crude microsmal fractions can be misleading; a pure enzyme will leave no doubt as to the involvement of *P*-450 in aromatization. Problems of stoichiometry, details of the intermediates, and the number of active sites may provide difficulties for some time after the pure enzyme becomes available. Indirect approaches suggest a single active site (Kelly *et al.*, 1977; Kautsky and Hagerman, 1980). Some success has been reported with solubilization of aromatase (Thompson and Siiteri, 1976; Pasanen and Pelkonen, 1981). However, it is clear that present preparations are far from pure.

## IX. STEROIDOGENIC INNER MITOCHONDRIAL MEMBRANE

This interesting membrane must be fully explored before we can understand the regulation of the three important biosynthetic reactions involving *P*-450 that take place within the membrane, namely, $C_{27}$ side-chain cleavage, 11$\beta$-hydroxylation, and 18-hydroxylation. The available approaches are those of classical biochemistry, namely, investigation of the native membrane, fractionation of the membrane to release pure components, and reconstitution of enzyme activity in the hope of restoring the native membrane from the pure components. These ambitious goals are still far from completion. Moreover, there is the added problem of the membrane itself which provides an environment quite unlike that of the usual aqueous buffer. An intervening step in the cycle from native membrane to reconstituted membrane is therefore based upon incorporation of pure components into lipid vesicles prepared from pure phospholipids. The native membrane has not been intensively studied, although methods are available for preparing this membrane from adrenal cells (Yago *et al.*, 1970). Important approaches must be based on freeze fracture and a variety of biophysical methods capable of recording rapid interactions between proteins and lipids within the membrane.

In aqueous buffers, the $C_{27scc}$ system appears as a high-molecular-weight form (MW 850,000), but it can also be isolated in forms showing molecular weights of 425,000 and 212,000 (Shikita and Hall, 1973a,b). The monomeric form (MW 52,000) can only be isolated under denaturing conditions (Shikita and Hall, 1973b). Moreover, if either the hexadecamer (850,000), the octomer, or tetramer is sedimented through a sucrose density gradient containing NADPH, adrenodoxin, and adrenodoxin reductase, enzymatic activity is found only in that part of the gradient corresponding to the 16 subunit form (Takagi *et al.*, 1975).

Clearly, the hexadecamer is the active species in an aqueous system. The enzyme preparation used in these studies contained 80 nmol of phospholipid per nanomole of $P$-450, which may well influence the ability of the enzyme to aggregate.

The importance of the lipid environment in regulating the side-chain cleavage system has been studied by incorporating the pure enzyme in vesicles prepared from purified phospholipids. In vesicles composed of an equal mixture of phosphatidylethanolamine and phosphatidylcholine, the enzyme is converted to the low-spin form and shows a greatly reduced $K_m$ for the substrate cholesterol (Hall $et$ $al.$, 1979). Moreover, the two electron carriers adrenodoxin and adrenodoxin reductase can be incorporated into liposomes with $P$-450 and cholesterol so that side-chain cleavage occurs upon addition of NADPH. The details of incorporation of the side-chain cleavage system were examined by Seybert and colleagues (1978), who showed that the active site of the enzyme is closely associated with the hydrophobic region of the bilayer, while a site on the $P$-450 that binds adrenodoxin is found on the surface of the vesicle facing the external water phase. As these observations would suggest, $P$-450 in one vesicle cannot bind cholesterol in another vesicle (Seybert $et$ $al.$, 1978).

The same group of investigators showed that one molecule of adrenodoxin reductase can reduce more than one molecule of adrenodoxin as the result of dissociation of the reduced adrenodoxin from the reductase followed by association with another molecule of oxidized adrenodoxin (Seybert $et$ $al.$, 1978). It appears that the affinity of adrenodoxin for the reductase is influenced by the state of oxidation of adrenodoxin, so that the oxidized iron–sulfur protein shows a higher affinity for the reductase than the reduced form. Therefore, oxidized adrenodoxin binds to reductase and becomes reduced. Reduced adrenodoxin does not bind well to reductase, but binds to $P$-450 and thereby becomes oxidized once more. In this manner, adrenodoxin is said to shuttle between the reductase and $P$-450 as it transfers electrons from the flavoprotein to the heme protein (Lambeth $et$ $al.$, 1979). Moreover, the shuttle is promoted by cholesterol bound to $P$-450 because the enzyme–substrate complex binds adrenodoxin more readily than enzyme without substrate (Lambeth $et$ $al.$, 1980a).

Clearly, the lipid is important in regulating the functions of the side-chain cleavage system. Little was learned, however, from careful analysis of mitochondrial lipid. No difference was seen in the composition of phospholipid associated with the pure enzyme and the bulk phospholipid of mitochondrial membrane (Hall $et$ $al.$, 1979). Moreover, there was nothing unusual about the mitochondrial phospholipids when compared with phospholipids of other mitochondria except for the high concentration of arachidonate in the adrenal mitochondria (Hall *et al.*, 1979). However, when the composition of synthetic vesicles was varied it was found that cardiolipin stimulates binding of cholesterol by the enzyme. Addition of cardiolipin and polyphosphoinositides to adrenal mitochondria has been reported to lead to increased conversion of cholesterol to pregnenolone (Lambeth *et al.*, 1980b). The significance of these observations remains in doubt, since there is little cardiolipin in bovine adrenocortical mitochondria, and ACTH does not apparently alter the amount of cardiolipin in rat adrenal, although it increases the amounts of polyphosphoinositides present (Farese, 1983).

## X. STEROIDOGENIC ENDOPLASMIC RETICULUM

By contrast to the inner mitochondrial membrane, the microsomal system possesses only a single electron carrier, although this flavoprotein contains both FAD and FMN. Again, the possible sequences of reactions in the mitochondrion are invariant, but the microsomal steps can proceed in several possible sequences and the proportion of the various alternative pathways is regulated. In addition, we must consider the important question of cytochrome $b_5$ which may play a significant role in electron transport to microsomal *P*-450.

### A. ORGANIZATION OF PROTEINS IN THE MEMBRANE

Samuels and co-workers were the first investigators to consider the organization of the steroidogenic microsome. Beginning with two assumptions, namely, that the usual methods of cell fractionation produce right-side-out vesicles and that proteolytic enzymes and phopholipase enzymes cannot penetrate the bilayer, these workers made two important observations by exposing testicular microsomes to such enzymes (Samuels *et al.*, 1975): (I) Phospholipases A and C cause decrease in 3$\beta$-hydroxysteroid dehydrogenase and loss of the ability to bind pregnenolone; and (II) mild treatment with trypsin causes loss of 3$\beta$-hydroxysteroid dehydrogenase activity, loss of hydroxylase/lyase activity, and loss of pregnenolone binding.

Earlier studies of the distribution of labeled steroids in aqueous suspensions of microsomes showed a third important finding (Samuels and Matsumoto, 1974): (III) Hydroxylase/lyase acts on intramembranous substrate, whereas the dehydrogenase acts on substrate from the surrounding water phase.

Studies performed with liver $P$-450 showed that this enzyme is situated on the inner side of the microsomal membrane and hence on the side remote from the bulk (external) aqueous phase in right-side-out vesicles (Welton and Aust, 1974).

These findings suggest that pregnenolone binding involves a protein (observation II) that is readily released from the membrane (observation I) and, as expected, this protein is accessible from the external water phase (observation II) because this corresponds to the cytoplasmic surface in the cell, from which pregnenolone must presumably reach the endoplasmic reticulum. On the other hand, $3\beta$-hydroxysteroid dehydrogenase requires some organized membrane structure (observation I) and is also on the external surface of the membrane (observations II and III). The hydroxylase/lyase $P$-450 does not require an organized membrane (observation I). Presumably trypsin inhibits this enzyme (observation II) because the reductase is on the external surface of the membrane so that inhibition results from interference with reduction of $P$-450 and not from proteolytic digestion of the enzyme itself. Finally, the substrate must enter the lipid bilayer to reach the active site of $P$-450 (observation III). This last observation is in agreement with findings from the inner mitochondrial membrane (see above). These facts can be illustrated diagrammatically as follows:

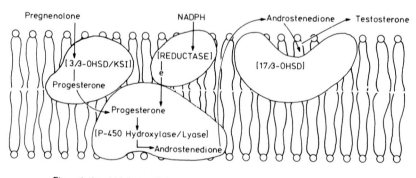

⟶ Flow of steroid intermediates
—e→ Flow of electrons

The diagram may serve to suggest new experimental approaches to the problem of microsomal organization. Obviously the available data are not sufficiently complete to permit a hard and fast description of microsomal organization. The figure has in fact been through several earlier versions and will no doubt be modified in the future.

## B. ORGANIZATION OF ALTERNATE PATHWAYS

It was pointed out above that two pathways are possible in microsomes for the conversion of pregnenolone to androstenedione. Too little is known about the organization of the microsome to comment on the important possibility that the arrangement of enzymes within the lipid bilayer may regulate the preferred pathway. However, the experiments of Samuels and colleagues (1975), have revealed a pregnenolone binding activity that is susceptible to proteolytic digestion of the microsome. Presumably the steroidogenic microsome contains a pregnenolone binding protein, and if this protein is closely associated with the dehydrogenase-isomerase, the $\Delta^4$ pathway would be favored, whereas association with hydroxylase-lyase would facilitate the $\Delta^5$ pathway. Methods are now available for cross-linking proteins in membranes so that such organizational factors can be approached experimentally when more is known about the pregnenolone binding protein.

The organization of *P*-450 and reductase in hepatic microsomes has been studied by a number of indirect approaches to determine the relative distributions of these two proteins. The results are of interest, since similar questions have not been approached in the steroidogenic microsome. There are many more molecules of *P*-450 than molecules of reductase in such microsomes—the ratio depending on a variety of factors. It might be asked whether one molecule of reductase is fixed within a cluster of molecules of *P*-450 to all of which this reductase provides electrons. The idea is not attractive because current views on biological membranes present the membrane as a dynamic two-dimensional solution of proteins in the bilayer. Certainly the diffusion coefficients for proteins in membranes are high even in the plasma membrane where cytoskeletal attachment may limit freedom of movement by proteins to a considerable degree (Wu *et al.*, 1982; Tank *et al.*, 1982a,b). Less is known about movement of proteins in internal membranes, although the available evidence points to rapid movement of proteins in internal membranes as well (Hochli and Hackenbrock, 1979). There is therefore no need to postulate the existence of clusters, and diffusion appears capable of explaining monooxygenase activity of hepatic microsomes (Dean and Gray, 1982). It will be interesting to study the less complex steroidogenic microsome from this point of view. So far, the numbers of molecules of *P*-450 and reductase are not known. It should be pointed out that the protein content of the microsome is higher relative to lipid than that of the plasma membrane, so that it may be unwise to assume that the mobility of proteins in this membrane is as high as that of plasma membranes.

ACKNOWLEDGMENTS

This work was supported by grants from the National Institutes of Health (AM28113, HD16525, CA29497, AM32236).

The author is grateful to Allyn McIntyre for excellent editorial assistance and for the execution of all the artwork in this manuscript.

## REFERENCES

Akhtar, M., and Skinner, S. J. (1968). The intermediary role of a 19-oxoandrogen in the biosynthesis of oestrogen. *Biochem. J.* **109**, 318–21.

Ayers, J., Eichhorn, J., Hechter, O., Saba, N., and Tait, S. A. S. (1960). Some studies on the biosynthesis of aldosterone and other adrenal steroids. *Acta Endocrinol.* **33**, 27–58.

Betz, G., Tsai, P., and Weakley, R. (1976). Heterogeneity of cytochrome $P$-450 in rat testis microsomes. *J. Biol. Chem.* **251**, 2839–2841.

Bjorkhem, I., and Karlmar, K. E. (1968). A novel technique for assay of side-chain cleavage of exogenous and endogenous cholesterol in adrenal mitochondrial and submitochondrial preparations. *Anal. Biochem.* **68**, 404–414.

Bjorkhem, I., and Karlmar, K. E. (1977a). Common characteristics of the cytochrome $P$-450 system involved in 18- and 11-$\beta$-hydroxylation of deoxycorticosterone in rat adrenals. *J. Lipid Res.* **18**, 592–603.

Bjorkhem, I., and Kalmar, K. E. (1977b). 18-Hydroxylation of DOC by reconstituted systems from rat and bovine adrenals. *Eur. J. Biochem.* **51**, 145–154.

Bosterling, B., Trudell, J. R., Trevor, A. J., and Bendix, M. (1982). Lipid–protein interactions as determinants of activation or inhibition by cytochrome $b_5$ of cytochrome $P$-450-mediated oxidations. *J. Biol. Chem.* **257**, 4375–4380.

Braselton, W. E., Orr, J. D., and Engel, L. L. (1972). Proc. Int. Congr. Endocrinol., 4th, Washington, D.C. p. 123.

Brodie, H. J., Kripalani, K. J., and Possanza, G. (1969). Studies on the mechanism of estrogen biosynthesis. VI. The stereochemistry of hydrogen elimination at C-2 during aromatization. *J. Am. Chem. Soc.* **91**, 1241–1242.

Burstein, S., and Gut, M. (1976). Intermediates in the conversion of cholesterol to pregnenolone: Kinetics and mechanism. Steroids **28**, 115–131.

Chance, B. (1957). Techniques for assay of the respiratory enzymes. *In* "Methods in Enzymology" (S. P. Colowick and N. O. Kaplan, eds.), Vol. 4, p. 273. Academic Press, New York.

Chevion, M., Peisach, J., Blumberg, W. E. (1977). Imidazole, the ligand trans to mercaptide in ferric cytochrome $P$-450. An EPR study of proteins and model compounds. *J. Biol. Chem.* **252**, 3637–3645.

Chu, M. D., and Ulick, S. (1982). Isolation and identification of 18-hydroxycortisol from the urine of patients with primary aldosteronism. *J. Biol. Chem.* **257**, 2218–2224.

Collman, J. P., and Sorrell, T. N. (1975). A model for the carbamyl adduct of ferrous cytochrome $P$-450. *J. Amer. Chem. Soc.* **97**, 4133–4134.

Constantopoulos, G., and Tchen, T. T. (1961). Cleavage of cholesterol side chain by adrenal cortex. I. Cofactor requirement and product of cleavage. *J. Biol. Chem.* **236**, 65–67.

Cooper, D. Y., Levin, S. S., Narasimhulu, S., Rosenthal, O., and Estabrook, R. W. (1965). Photochemical action spectrum of the terminal oxidase of mixed function oxidase systems. *Science* **147**, 400–402.

Coupland, R. E. (1975). *Handb. Physiol. Sec.* **6**, 2.

Cramer, S. P., Dawson, J. H., Hodgson, J. O., and Hager, L. P. (1978). Studies on the ferric forms of cytochrome *P*-450 and chloroperoxidase by extended X-ray absorption fine structure. Characterization of the FE-S distances. *J. Amer. Chem. Soc.* **100,** 7282–7290.

Dean, W. L., and Gray, R. D. (1982). Relationship between state of aggregation and catalytic activity for cytochrome *P*-450LM2 and NADPH-cytochrome *P*-450 reductase. *J. Biol. Chem.* **25,** 14679–14685.

Debrunner, P. G., Gunsalus, I. C., Sligar, S. G., and Wagner, G. C. (1978). *In* "Metal Ions in Biological Systems" (H. Siegel, ed.), Vol. 7, pp. 241–247. Dekker, New York.

Dunham, W. R., Palmer, G., Sands, R. H., and Bearden, A. J. (1971). On the structure of the iron–sulfur complex in the two-iron ferredoxins. *Biochem. Biophys. Acta* 253, 373–384.

Duque C., Morisaki, M., Ikekawa, N., and Shikita, M. (1978). The enzyme activity of bovine adrenocortical cytochrome *P*-450 producing pregnenolone from cholesterol: Kinetic and electrophoretic studies on the reactivity of hydroxycholesterol intermediates. *Biochem. Biophys. Res. Commun.* **82,** 179–187.

Eichorn, J., and Hechter, O. (1957). Status of deoxycorticosterone as intermediary in the biosynthesis of cortisol. *Proc. Soc. Exp. Biol. Med.* **95,** 311–315.

Eik-Nes, K. B., and Hall, P. F. (1962). Isolation of dehydroepiandrosterone-[14]C from dogs infused with cholesterol-4-[14]C by the spermatic artery. *Proc. Soc. Exp. Biol. Med.* **111,** 280–282.

Estabrook, R. W., Cooper, D. Y., and Rosenthal, O. (1963). The light reversible carbon monoxide inhibition of the steroid $C_{21}$-hydroxylase system of the adrenal cortex. *Biochem. Z.* **338,** 741–755.

Estabrook, R. W., Hildebrandt, A. G., Baron, J., Netter, K., and Leibman, K. (1971). A new spectral intermediate associated with cytochrome *P*-450 function in liver microsomes. *Biochem. Biophys. Res. Commun.* **42,** 132–139.

Farese, R. V. (1983). The role of the phosphatidate–inositide cycle in the action of steroidogenic agents. *J. Steroid. Biochem.* **19,** 1029–1032.

Fevold, H. R. (1983). Regulation of the adrenal and gonadal microsomal mixed function oxygenases of steroid hormone biosynthesis. *Annu. Rev. Physiol.* **45,** 19–36.

Fishman, J., Guzik, H., and Dixon, D. (1969). Stereochemistry of estrogen biosynthesis. *Biochemistry* **8,** 4304–309.

Fraser, R., and Lantos, C. P. (1978). 18-Hydroxycorticosterone: A review. *J. Steroid Biochem.* **9,** 273–296.

Garfinkel, D. (1958). Preparation and properties of microsomal DPNH-cytochrome *c* reductase. *Arch. Biochem. Biophys.* **71,** 111–121.

Griffin, B. W., Peterson, J. A., and Estabrook, R. W. (1979). *In* "The Porphyrins" (D. Dolphin, ed.), Vol. VII, pp. 333–368. Academic Press, New York.

Groves, J. T., and McClusky, G. (1976). Aliphatic hydroxylation via oxygen rebound. Oxygen transfer catalyzed by iron. *J. Am. Chem. Soc.* **98,** 859–860.

Groves, J. T., and van Der Puy, M. (1974). Stereospecific aliphatic hydroxylation by an iron-based oxidant. *J. Am. Chem. Soc.* **96,** 5274–5275.

Groves, J. T., and van der Puy, M. (1976). Stereospecific aliphatic hydroxylation by iron-hydrogen peroxide. Evidence for a stepwise process. *J. Am. Chem. Soc.* **98,** 5290–5297.

Gunsalus, I. C., Meeks, J. R., Lipscomb, J. D., DeBrunner, P., and Miinck, E. (1974). *In* "Molecular Mechanisms of Oxygen Activation" (O. Hayiashi, ed.), p. 559. Academic Press, New York, London.

Hall, P. F. (1970a). Gonadotropic regulation of testicular function. *In* "Androgens of the Testis" (K. B. Eik-Nes, ed.), Ch. 3, pp. 73–115. Dekker, New York.

Hall, P. F. (1970b). Endocrinology of the testis. *In* "Testicular Physiology and Biochemistry" (A. D. Johnson, W. R. Gomes, and V. L. Van Denmark, eds.), Vol. II, pp. 1–71. Academic Press, New York.

Hall, P. F., and Koritz, S. B. (1964a). The conversion of cholesterol and 20$\alpha$-hydroxycholesterol to steroids by acetone powder of particles from bovine corpus luteum. *Biochemistry* **3**, 129–134.

Hall, P. F., and Koritz, S. B. (1964b). Inhibition of the biosynthesis of pregnenolone by 20$\alpha$-hydroxycholesterol. *Biochim. Biophys. Acta* **93**, 441–444.

Hall, P. F., Sozer, C. C., and Eik-Nes., K. B. (1964). Formation of dehydroepiandrosterone during *in vivo* and *in vitro* biosynthesis of testosterone by testicular tissue. *Endocrinology* **74**, 35–43.

Hall, P. F., Watanuki, M., DeGroot, J., and Rouser, G. (1979a). Composition of lipids bound to pure cytochrome $P$-450 of cholesterol side-chain cleavage enzyme from bovine adrenocortical mitochondria. *Lipids* **14**, 148–151.

Hall, P. F., Watanuki, M., and Hamkalo, B. A. (1979b). Adrenocortical cytochrome $P$-450 side-chain cleavage: Preparation of membrane-bound side-chain cleavage system from purified components. *J. Biol. Chem.* **254**, 547–552.

Haugen, D. A., van der Hoeven, T. A., and Coon, M. J. (1975). Purified liver microsomal cytochrome $P$-450. Separation and characterization of multiple forms., *J. Biol. Chem.* **250**, 3567–3570.

Hechter, O., and Pincus, G. (1954). Genesis of the adrenocortical secretion. *Physiol. Rev.* **34**, 459–496.

Hildebrandt, A., and Estabrook, R. W. (1971). Evidence for the participation of cytochrome $b_5$ in hepatic microsomal mixed-function oxidation reactions. *Arch. Biochem. Biophys.* **143**, 66–79.

Hoa, G. H., Begard, E., Debey, P., and Gunsalus, I. C. (1978). Two univalent electron transfers from putidaredoxin to bacterial cytochrome $P$-450 at subzero temperature. *Biochemistry* **17**, 2835–2839.

Hochli, M., and Hackenbrock, C. R. (1979). Lateral translational diffusion of cytochrome $c$ oxidase in the mitochondrial energy-transducing membrane. *Proc. Natl. Acad. Sci. U.S.A.* **76**, 1236–1240.

Hori, A., Takamuku, S., and Sakurai, J. (1977). Reaction of atomic oxygen with alkanes. Regioselective alcohol formation on $\gamma$-radiolysis of liquid carbon dioxide solutions of alkanes *J. Org. Chem.* **42**, 2318.

Hornsby, P. J. (1980). Regulation of cytochrome $P$-450-supported 11$\beta$-hydroxylation of deoxycortisol by steroids, oxygen, and antioxidants in adrenocortical cell cultures. *J. Biol. Chem.* **255**, 4020–4027.

Ishimura, Y., Ullrich, V., and Peterson, J. A. (1971). Oxygenated cytochrome $P$-450 and its possible role in hydroxylation. *Biochem. biophys. Res. Commun.* **42**, 140–144.

Ishimura, Y., Ullrich, V., Pedersen, T. C., Austin, R. H., and Gunsalus, I. C. (1977). *In* "Microsomes and Drug Oxidations" (V. Ullrich, ed.), p. 275. Pergamon, Oxford.

Iyanagi, T., and Mason, H. S. (1973). Some properties of hepatic reduced nicotinamide adenine dinucleotide phosphate—Cytochrome $c$ reductase. *Biochemistry* **12**, 2297–2308.

Janig, G. R., Dettmer, R., Usanov, S. A., Ruckpaul, K. (1983). Identification of the ligand trans to thiolate in cytochrome $P$-450 LM2 by chemical modification. *Febs Lett.* **159**, 58–62.

Jefcoate, C. R., and Gaylor, J. L. (1969). Ligand interactions with hemoprotein $P$-450. II.

Influence of phenobarbital and methylcholanthrene induction processes on *P*-450 spectra. *Biochemistry* **8**, 3464–3472.

Jung, C., Friedrich, J., and Ristau, O. (1979). Quantum chemical interpretation of the spectral properties of the CO and $O_2$ complexes of hemoglobin and cytochrome *P*-450. *Acta Biol. Med. Ger.* **38**, 363–377.

Kautsky, M. P., and Hagerman, D. D. (1980). Kinetic properties of steroid 19-hydroxy-lase and estrogen synthetase from porcine ovary microsomes. *J. Steroid Biochem.* **13**, 1283–1290.

Kelly, W. G., Judd, D., and Stolee, A. (1977). Aromatization of $\Delta^4$-androstene-3,17-dione, 19-hydroxy-$\Delta^4$-androstene-3,17-dione, and 19-oxo-$\Delta^4$-androstene-3,17-dione at a common catalytic site in human placental microsomes. *Biochemistry* **16**, 140–145.

Kimura, T. (1968). Biochemical aspects of iron–sulfur linkage in non-heme iron protein with special reference to adrenodoxin. *Struct. Bond.* **5**, 1–35.

Klingenberg, M. (1958). Pigments of rat liver microsomes. *Arch. Biochem. Biophys.* **75**, 376–386.

Koch, S., Tang, S. C., Holm, R. H., Fraenkel, R. B., and Ibers, J. A. (1975). Ferric porphyrin thiolates. Possible relationships to cytochrome *P*-450 enzymes and the structure of (*p*-nitrobenzene thiolate) iron (III). Protoprophyrin IX dimethyl ester. *J. Am. Chem. Soc.* **97**, 916–918.

Kominami, S., Ochi, H., Kobayashi, Y., and Takemori, S. (1980). Studies on the steroid hydroxylation system in adrenal cortex microsomes. Purification and characteriza-tion of cytochrome *P*-450 specific for steroid $C_{21}$ hydroxylation. *J. Biol. Chem.* **255**, 3386–3394.

Koritz, S. B., and Hall, P. F. (1964a). End-product inhibition of the conversion of choles-terol to pregnenolone in an adrenal extract. *Biochemistry* **3**, 1298–1304.

Koritz, S. B., and Hall, P. F. (1964b). Feedback inhibition by pregnenolone: A possible mechanism. *Biochim. Biophys. Acta* **93**, 215–217.

Lambeth, J. D., Seybert, D. W., and Kamin, H. (1979). Ionic effects on adrenal steroido-genic electron transport. The role of adrenodoxin as an electron shuttle. *J. Biol. Chem.* **254**, 7255–7264.

Lambeth, J. D., Kamin, H., and Seybert, D. W. (1980a). Phosphatidylcholine vesicle reconstituted cytochrome *P*-450scc. Role of the membrane in control of activity and spin state of the cytochrome. *J. Biol. Chem.* **255**, 8282–288.

Lambeth, J. D., Seybert, D. W., and Kamin, H. (1980b). Adrenodoxin reductase. Adreno-doxin complex. Rapid formation and breakdown of the complex and a slow conforma-tional change in the flavoprotein. *J. Biol. Chem.* **255**, 4667–4672.

Lambeth, J. D., Seybert, D. W., and Kamin, H. (1980c). Phospholipid vesicle-reconsti-tuted cytochrome *P*-450scc. Mutually facilitated binding of cholesterol and adreno-doxin. *J. Biol. Chem.* **255**, 138–143.

Lambeth, J. D., Lancaster, J. R., Jr., and Kamin, H. (1981). Steroidogenic electron transport by adrenodoxin reductase and adrenodoxin. Use of acetylated cytochrome *c* as a mechanistic probe of electron transfer. *J. Biol. Chem.* **256**, 3674–3678.

Long, J. A. (1975). *Handb. Physiol. Sect.* 7 **VI**, 13–24.

Lu, A. Y. H., and West, S. B. (1978). Pharmac. Ther. A. 2 337–358. Reconstituted mammalian mixed-function oxidases: Requirements, specifications, and other prop-erties.

Lu, A. Y., Levin, W., West, S. B., Jacobson, M., Ryan, D., Kuntzman, R., and Conney, A. H. (1973). Reconstituted liver microsomal enzyme system that hydroxylates drugs, other foreign compounds, and endogenous substrates. VI. Different substrate specificities of the cytochrome P-450 fractions from control and phenobarbital-treated rats. *J. Biol. Chem.* **248,** 456–460.

Lynn, W. S., Jr., Staple, E., and Gurin, S. (1954). The degradation of cholesterol by mammalian tissue extracts. *J. Am. Chem. Soc.* **76,** 4048.

Meyer, A. D. (1955). The substrate specificity of liver glucose-6-phosphatase. *Biochim. Biophys. Acta* **17,** 441–442.

Miki, N., Sugiyama, T., and Yamano, T. (1980). Purification and characterization of cytochrome P-450 with high affinity for cytochrome $b_5$. *J. Biochem. (Tokyo)* **88,** 307–310.

Miller, W. L., Rosenthal, R. L., and Miller, W. L. (1983). Congenital adrenal hyperplasia. *In* "Hirsutism and Virilism" (V. B. Mahesh, R. B. Greenblatt, and John Wright, eds.), pp. 87–120. PSG, Boston.

Mitani, F., and Horie, S. (1969). Studies on P-450. V. On the substrate-induced spectral change of P-450 solubilized from bovine adrenocortical mitochondria. *J. Biochem. (Tokyo)* **65,** 269–280.

Momoi, K., Okamoto, M., Fujii, S., Kim, C. Y., Miyake, Y., and Yamano, T. (1983). 19-Hydroxylation of 18-hydroxy-11-deoxycorticosterone catalyzed by cytochrome P-450 (11$\beta$) of bovine adrenocortex. *J. Biol. Chem.* **258,** 8855–8860.

Morato, T., Hayano, M., Dofman, R. I., and Axelrod, L. R. (1961). The intermediate steps in the biosynthesis of estrogens from androgens. *Biochem. Biophys. Res. Commun.* **6,** 334–338.

Nakajin, S., and Hall, P. F. (1981a). Microsomal cytochrome P-450 from neonatal pig testis: Two enzymatic activities (17$\alpha$-hydroxylase and $C_{17,20}$-lyase) associated with one protein. *Biochemistry* **20,** 4037–4042.

Nakajin, S., and Hall, P. F. (1981b). Microsomal cytochrome P-450 from neonatal pig testis: Purification and properties of a $C_{21}$ steroid side-chain cleavage system (17$\alpha$-hydroxylase and $C_{17,20}$-lyase). *J. Biol. Chem.* **256,** 3871–3876.

Nakajin, S., and Hall, P. F. (1981c). Side-chain cleavage of $C_{21}$ steroids to $C_{19}$ steroids by testicular microsomal cytochrome P-450: 17$\alpha$-Hydroxy $C_{21}$ steroids as obligatory intermediates. *J. Steroid. Biochem.* **14,** 1249–1252.

Nakajin, S., and Hall, P. F. (1983). Side-chain cleavage of $C_{21}$ steroids by testicular microsomal cytochrome P-450 (17$\alpha$-hydroxylase/lyase): Involvement of heme. *J. Steroid Biochem.* **1,** 1345–1348.

Nakajin, S., Hall, P. F., and Onada, M. (1981). Testicular microsomal cytochrome P-450 for $C_{21}$ steroid side-chain cleavage: Spectral and binding studies. *J. Biol. Chem.* **256,** 6134–6139.

Nakajin, S., Shinoda, M., and Hall, P. F. (1983). Purification and properties of 17$\alpha$-hydroxylase from microsomes of pig adrenal: A second $C_{21}$ side-chain cleavage system. *Biochem. Biophys. Res. Commun.* **111,** 512–517.

Nakajin, S., Shinoda, M., Hanniu, M., Shively, J. E., and Hall, P. F. (1984). The $C_{21}$ steroid side-chain cleavage enzyme from porcine adrenal microsome: Purification and characterization of the 17$\alpha$-hydroxylase/$C_{17,20}$-lyase cytochrome P-450 *J. Biol. Chem.* **256,** 3971–3976.

Narasimhulu, S., Cooper, D. Y., and Rosenthal, O. (1965). Spectrophotometric properties of a Triton-clarified steroid 21-hydroxylase system of adrenocortical microsomes. *Life Sci.* **4,** 2101–2107.

Ohba, H., Inano, H., and Tamaoki, B. (1981). Contribution of microsomal cytochrome $b_5$ electron transport system coupled with $\Delta^5$-3$\beta$-hydroxysteroid dehydrogenase to androgen synthesis from progesterone. *Biochem. Biophys. Res. Commun.* **103,** 1273–280.

Omura, T., and Sato, R. (1964). The carbon monoxide-binding pigment of liver microsomes. II. Solubilization, purification, and properties. *J. Biol. Chem.* **239**, 2379–2385.

Omura, T., Sanders, E., Estabrook, R. W., Cooper, D. Y., and Rosenthal, O. (1966). Isolation from adrenal cortex of a nonheme iron protein and a flavoprotein functional as a reduced triphosphapyridine nucleotide-cytochrome $P$-450 reductase. *Arch. Biochem. Biophys.* **117**, 660–673.

Onoda, M., and Hall, P. F. (1982). Cytochrome $b_5$ stimulates purified testicular microsomal cytochrome $P$-450 ($C_{21}$ side-chain cleavage). *Biochem. Biophys. Res. Commun.* **108**, 454–460.

Onoda, M., Sweet, F., Shively, J. E., and Hall, P. F. (1984). Affinity alkylation of the active site of $C_{21}$ steroid side-chain cleavage cytochrome $P$-450: A unique cysteine residue alkylated by 17α-bromoacetoxyprogesterone. *Biochemistry* (submitted).

Orme-Johnson, N. R., Light, D. R., White-Stevens, R. W., and Orme-Johnson, W. H. (1979). Steroid binding properties of beef adrenal cortical cytochrome $P$-450 which catalyzes the conversion of cholesterol into pregnenolone. *J. Biol. Chem.* **254**, 2103–2111.

Pasanen, M., and Pelkonen, O. (1981). Solubilization and partial purification of human placental cytochromes $P$-450. *Biochem. Biophys. Res. Commun.* **103**, 1310–1317.

Peterson, J. A. (1971). Oxygenated cytochrome $P$-450 and its possible role in enzyme hydroxylation. *Biochem. Biophys. Res. Commun.* **42**, 140–146.

Ramseyer, J., and Harding, B. W. (1973). Solubilization and properties of bovine adrenal cortical cytochrome $P$-450 which cleaves the cholesterol side-chain. *Biochim. Biophys. Acta* **315**, 306–316.

Rein, H., and Ristau, O. (1978). The importance of the high-spin/low-spin equilibrium existing in cytochrome $P$-450 for the enzymatic mechanism. *Pharmazie* **33**, 325–8.

Remmer, H., Schenkman, J., Estabrook, R. W., Sasame, H., Gillette, J., Narashimhulu, S., Cooper, D. Y., and Rosenthal, O. (1966). *Mol. Pharmacol.* **2**, 187.

Rosenfield, R. L., and Miller, W. L. (1983). Congenital adrenal hyperplasia. *In* "Hirsutism and Virilism" (V. Mahesh and R. B. Greenlat, eds.), pp. 87–121. PSG, Boston.

Ruokonen, A., and Vihko, R. (1974). Steroid metabolism in testis tissue: Concentration of unconjugated and sulfated neutral steroids in boar testis. *J. Steroid Biochem.* **5**, 33–38.

Ryan, K. J. (1959). Biological aromatization of steroids. *J. Biol. Chem.* **234**, 268–272.

Ryan, K. J., and Engel, L. L. (1957). Hydroxylation of steroids at carbon 21. *J. Biol. Chem.* **225**, 103–114.

Samuels, L. T. (1960). *In* "Metabolic Pathways" (D. M. Greenberg, ed.), Vol. I, 2nd Ed. Ch. 11, p. 431. Academic Press, New York.

Samuels, L. T., and Matsumoto, J. (1974). Localization of enzymes involved in testosterone biosynthesis by the mouse testis. *Endocrinology* **94**, 55–60.

Samuels, L. T., Bussman, L., Matsumoto, K., and Huseby, R. A. (1975). Organization of androgen biosynthesis in the testis. *J. Steroid. Biochem.* **6**, 291.

Schenkman, J. B., Remmer, H., and Estabrook, R. W. (1967). Spectral studies of drug interaction with hepatic microsomal cytochrome. *Mol. Pharmacol.* **3**, 113–23.

Schenkman, J. B., Sligar, S. G., and Cinti, D. L. (1982). *In* "Hepatic Cytochrome $P$-450 Monoxygenase Systems" (J. B. Schenkman and D. Kupfer, eds.), p. 587. Pergamon, Oxford.

Schneider, H., Hochli, M., and Hackenbrock, C. R. (1982). Relationship between the density distribution of intramembrane particles and electron transfer in the mitochondrial inner membrane as revealed by cholesterol incorporation. *J. Cell Biol.* **94**, 387–393.

Sedzik, J., Blaurock, A. E., and Hochli, M. (1984). Lipid/myelin basic protein multilayers. A model for the cytoplasmic space in central nervous system myelin. *J. Mol. Biol.* **174**, 385–409.

Seybert, D. W., Lambeth, J. D., and Kamin, H. (1978). The participation of a second molecule of adrenodoxin in cytochrome *P*-450-catalyzed 11β-hydroxylation. *J. Biol. Chem.* **253**, 8355–8358.

Seybert, D. W., Lancaster, J. R., Jr., Lambeth, J. D., and Kamin, H. (1979). Participation of the membrane in the side chain cleavage of cholesterol. Reconstitution of cytochrome *P*-450scc into phospholipid vesicles. *J. Biol. Chem.* **254**, 12088–12098.

Sharma, D. C., Nerenberg, C. A., and Dorfman, R. I. (1967). Studies on aldosterone biosynthesis *in vitro*. II. *Biochemistry* **67**, 3472–3479.

Sheppard, H., Swanson, R., and Mowles, F. (1963). Purification of cytochrome *P*-450 from bovine adrenocortical mitochondria. *Biophys. Res. Commun.* **50**, 289–293.

Shikita, M., and Hall, P. F. (1973). Cytochrome *P*-450 from bovine adrenocortical mitochondria: An enzyme for the side-chain cleavage of cholesterol. II. Subunit structure. *J. Biol. Chem.* **248**, 5605–5609.

Shikita, M., and Hall, P. F. (1974). The stoichiometry of the conversion of cholesterol and hydroxycholesterols to pregnenolone (3β-hydroxypregn-5-en-20-one) catalyzed by adrenal cytochrome *P*-450. *Proc. Natl. Acad. Sci. U.S.A.* **71**, 1441–1445.

Shimizu, J., Dorfman, R. I., and Gut, M. (1960). Isocaproic acid, a metabolite of 20α-hydroxycholesterol. *J. Biol. Chem.* **235**, PC25.

Singer, S. J., and Nicolson, G. L. (1972). The fluid mosaic model of the structure of cell membranes. *Science* **175**, 720–731.

Skeets, J. J., and Vickery, L. E. (1982). Proximity of the substrate binding site and the heme-iron catalytic site in cytochrome *P*-450scc. *Proc. Natl. Acad. Sci. U.S.A.* **79**, 5773–5777.

Skinner, S. J., and Akhtar, M. (1969). The stereospecific removal of a C-19 hydrogen atom in oestrogen biosynthesis. *Biochem. J.* **114**, 75–81.

Slaun White, W. R., Jr., and Samuels, L. T. (1956). Progesterone as a precursor of testicular androgens. *J. Biol. Chem.* **220**, 341–352.

Sligar, S. G. (1976). Coupling of spin, substrate, and redox equilibria in cytochrome *P*-450. *Biochemistry* **15**, 5399–5406.

Solomon, S., Levitan, P., and Lieberman, S. (1956). Possible intermediator between cholesterol and pregnenelone in corticosteroidogenesis. *Rev. Can. Biol.* **15**, 282.

Takagi, Y., Shikita, M., and Hall, P. F. (1975). The active form of cytochrome *P*-450 from bovine adrenocortical mitochondria. *J. Biol. Chem.* **250**, 8445–8448.

Takimori, S., Sato, H., Gomi, T., Suhara, K., and Katagiri, M. (1975). Purification and properties of cytochrome *P*-450 (11β) from adrenocortical mitochondria. *Biochem. Biophys. Res. Commun.* **67**, 1151–1157.

Tank, D. W., Miller, C., and Webb, W. W. (1982a). Isolated-patch recording from liposomes containing functionally reconstituted chloride channels from *Torpedo* electroplax. *Proc. Natl. Acad. Sci. U.S.A.* **79**, 7749–7753.

Tank, D. W., Wu, E. S., and Webb, W. W. (1982b). Enhanced molecular diffusibility in muscle membrane blebs: Release of lateral constraints. *J. Cell Biol.* **92**, 207–212.

Thompson, E. A., and Siiteri, P. K. (1974a). Utilization of oxygen and reduced nicotinamide adenine dinucleotide phosphate by human placental microsomes during aromatization of androstenedione. *J. Biol. Chem.* **249**, 5364–5372.

Thompson, E. A., and Siiteri, P. K. (1974b). The involvement of human placental microsomal cytochrome *P*-450 in aromatization. *J. Biol. Chem.* **249**, 5373–5378.

Thompson, E. A., and Siiteri, P. K. (1976). Partial resolution of the placental microsomal aromatase complex. *J. Steroid Biochem.* **7**, 635–663.

Tilley, B. E., Watanuki, M., and Hall, P. F. (1977). Preparation and properties of side-chain cleavage cytochrome *P*-450 from bovine adrenal cortex by affinity chromatography with pregnenolone as ligand. *Biochim. Biophys. Acta* **493**, 260–271.

Townsley, J.D., and Brodie, H.J. (1966). A new placental metabolite of oestr-4-ene-3,17-dione: A possible source of error in oestrogen estimation. *Biochem. J.* **101**, 25C–27C.

Townsley, J. D., and Brodie, H. J. (1968). Studies on the mechanism of estrogen biosynthesis. III. The stereochemistry of aromatization of $C_{19}$ and $C_{18}$ steroids. *Biochemistry* **7**, 33–40.

Ulick, S., Chu, M. D., and Land, M. (1983). Bosynthesis of 18-oxocortisol by aldosterone-producing adrenal tissue. *J. Biol. Chem.* **258**, 5498–502.

Ullrich, V. (1969). On the hydroxylation of cyclohexane in rat liver microsomes. *Hoppe Seylers Z. Physiol. Chem.* **350**, 357–365.

Ullrich, V. (1979). Cytochrome *P*-450 and biological hydroxylation reactions. *Curr. Top. Chem.* **83**, 67–104.

Ullrich, V., Ruf, H. H., and Wende, P. (1977). Models for ferric cytochrome *P*-450 characterization of hemin mercaptide complexes by electronic and ESR spectra. *Croat. Chem. Acta* **49**, 213 (From *Chem. Abstracts*).

Ullrich, V., Sakurai, H., and Ruf, H. H. (1979). Model systems for the coordination chemistry of cytochromes *P*-450. *Acta Biol. Med.* **38**, 287–297.

Vermilion, J. L., and Coon, M. J. (1978). Purified liver microsomal NADPH-cytochrome *P*-450 reductase. Spectral characterization of oxidation–reduction states. *J. Biol. Chem.* **253**, 2694–2704.

Watanuki, M., Tilley, B. E., and Hall, P. F. (1977). Purification and properties of cytochrome *P*-450 (11$\beta$- and 18-hydroxylase) from bovine adrenocortical mitochondria. *Biochim. Biophys. Acta* **483**, 236–247.

Watanuki, M., Tilley, B. E., and Hall, P. F. (1978). Cytochrome *P*-450 for 11$\beta$- and 18-hydroxylase activities of bovine adrenocortical mitochondria: One enzyme or two. *Biochemistry* **17**, 127–130.

Welton, A. F., and Aust, S. D. (1974). The effects of 3-methylcholanthrene and phenobarbital induction on the structure of the rat liver endoplasmic reticulum. *Biochim. Biophys. Acta* **373**, 197–210.

Werringloer, J., and Kawano, S. (1980). Spin state transitions of liver microsomal cytochrome *P*-450. *Acta Biol. Med.* **38**, 163–175.

White, R. E., and Coon, M. J. (1980). Oxygen activation by cytochrome *P*-450. *Ann. Rev. Biochem.* **49**, 315–356.

Wilcox, B. R., and Engel, L. L. (1965). 19-Hydroxyandrostonedione in estrogen biosynthesis. *Steroids Suppl.* **1**, 49–57.

Wu, E. S., Tank, D. W., and Webb, W. W. (1982). Unconstrained lateral diffusion of concanavalin A receptors on bulbous lymphocytes. *Proc. Natl. Acad. Sci. U.S.A.* **79**, 4962–4966.

Yago, N., Kobayashi, S., Sekiyama, S., Kurokawa, H., and Iwai, Y. (1970). Further studies on the submitochondrial localization of cholesterol side chain-cleaving enzyme system in hog adrenal cortex by sonic treatment. *J. Biochem.* (*Tokyo*) **68**, 775–783.

Yasukochi, Y., and Masters, B. S. S. (1976). Some properties of a detergent-solubilized NADPH–cytochrome *c* (cytochrome *P*-450) reductase purified by biospecific affinity chromatography. *J. Biol. Chem.* **251**, 5337–5344.

Yu, C. A., and Gunsalus, I. G. (1974a). Cytochrome *P*-450 III. Removal and replacement of ferriprotoporphyrin IX. *J. Biol. Chem.* **249**, 107–110.

Yu, C. A., and Gunsalus, I. G. (1974b). Cytochrome *P*-450. II. Interconversion with *P*-420. *J. Biol. Chem.* **249,** 102–106.

Yuan, P. M., Nakajin, S., Hanniu, M., Hall, P. F., and Shively, J. E. (1983). Steroid 21-hydroxylase (cytochrome *P*-450) from porcine adrenocortical microsomes: Microsequence analysis of cysteine-containing peptides. *Biochemistry* **22,** 143–149.

# Index

## A

ACTH, *see* Adrenocorticotropic hormone
Actin, exocytosis and, 139–141
Addison's disease, 284–286
Adrenal cortex
  ascorbic acid in, 41–48
    compartmentalization, 42
    content and transport, 41–42
    dynamic behavior, 42–48
    function, 42–48
    subcellular localization, 42
  zones of, 350–352
Adrenal gland, ascorbic acid concentration in, 3
Adrenal medulla, *see also* Chromaffin cell
  ascorbic acid in, 21–41
    compartmentalization, 26–30
    content and transport, 21–26
    dynamic behavior, 38–41
    function, 30–38
    subcellular localization, 26–30
Adrenocorticotropic hormone, 43–47
Aldosterone, synthesis, 329–337
Androgens, synthesis, 329–337
Androstenedione, synthesis, 329–337
Antibodies, *see* Autoimmune endocrine disease
Antisera, site-specific 240–242
Aromatase, 352–355
Ascorbic acid
  assays, 9–14
  biosynthesis, 14
  biosynthetic rates in mammals, 4, 16–20
  chemistry, 5–9
  distribution, 14–15
  history, 5
  minimum daily requirements, 15, 20–21

recommended daily allowance, 15–20
  tissue concentrations, 3
Autoimmune endocrine disease, 253–295
  defined, 253–256
  in humans, 267–277, 281–292
Autoimmune polyglandular syndromes, 284–286

## B

BB rat, diabetes in, 256–266
  active autoimmunity, 261–265
  genetics, 256–257
  immunodeficiency, 258–261
  immunotherapy, 265–266
  prediabetic physiology, 261–262
  triggering events, 261
$\beta$-cell, *see* Diabetes mellitus
BGP, *see* Bone Gla protein
Bone
  mineralization, 89–93
  plasma BGP and, 82–89
  warfarin and, 93–102
Bone Gla protein, 65–108
  biosynthesis, 74–77
  chemical modification, 71–72
  chemotactic activity, 101–102
  interaction with $Ca^{2+}$ and hydroxyapatite, 72–74
  isolation, 67–68
  message, structure of, 70
  in metabolic bone disease, 86–89
  in mineralizing tissue, 89–93
  occurrence, 66–67
  in plasma, 82–89
  primary structure, 68–69
  properties, 70–74
  regulation by 1,25-$(OH)_2D_3$, 77–82
  regulation of hydroxyapatite formation, 74
  warfarin and, 93–102
Bromine, in ascorbic acid assay, 10, 11

369

## Date Due